More Praise for *Elderhood*

Winner of the Wayne State University Academy of Scholars
Thomas N. Bonner Award

"A serious, useful, and important book." —*The Wall Street Journal*

"Exquisitely written . . . [Aronson] advocates a new paradigm: a rebalancing act in which technology has a role but the focus returns to care. Unlike the high-tech, algorithmic march of modern medicine, her idea of truly 'personalized medicine' incorporates the patient's past experiences and current expectations. This integrative, humanistic model of geriatrics is rare. One can only hope its practices are adopted swiftly." —*Nature*

"A passionate, deeply informed critique of how our health care system fails in its treatment of the elderly . . . Vitally important . . . Though the subject of this provocative book is the elderly, its message touches the entire span of human life." —*BookPage*

"Eloquent and impressive . . . A landmark work . . . In a world of increasing numbers of older adults, Aronson's highly readable, absorbing, and thought-provoking book should serve as a guide for how our culture must change in order to provide a future in which all of us can age well throughout the span of our lives." —ChangingAging

"[A] penetrating meditation on geriatrics . . . Aronson's deep empathy, hard-won knowledge, and vivid reportage makes for one of the best accounts around of the medical mistreatment of the old." —*Publishers Weekly* (starred review)

"An examination of aging and the human condition encompassing poignant stories and the viewpoints of medical experts, writers, historians, and scientists . . . Empathetic, probing, and often emotionally moving narratives on appreciating the power and the pain of aging." —*Kirkus Reviews* (starred review)

"A bold critique of our antiaging society and of the medical care seniors receive . . . This book, part memoir, part critique, and part prescription, encourages readers to help put an end to the antiaging industry and its profiteers, to engage in better self-care, and to collectively ask the medical community to look at elderhood not as a disease." —*The Missourian*

"One of the most significant books on aging and ageism in America . . . *Elderhood* should be required reading, alongside Dr. Atul Gawande's best-selling *Being Mortal*." —*GBO News*

"I loved reading this book and recommend it to all health professionals, policy makers, service providers, and researchers involved in the aging enterprise; anyone who has an aging relative; and all of us who are growing older every day. The book is beautifully written and inspirational." —*Health Affairs*

"[A] vast and penetrating analysis . . . With strong empathy that comes from both a professional understanding of and personal experience with the challenges of aging, Aronson provides an essential guide to how society in general and the health care industry in particular must recalibrate their approach to providing concerned and competent elder care. Thought provoking and wise, Aronson's memoir-cum-treatise should be required reading for medical professionals and will be of great use for seniors and those who support them." —*Booklist* (starred review)

"*Elderhood*, like the life station it studies, is dynamic, multifaceted, and full of wonder. Aronson's writing, too, flexes with vibrant energy as she discusses in lucid, candid detail the ways she has seen the health care system neglect the overall well-being of her patients, her colleagues, and herself . . . Monumental . . . Intimidating as it may seem, elderhood becomes welcoming and generous in Aronson's deft care." —*Shelf Awareness* (starred review)

"An in-depth, unusually frank exploration of biases that distort society's view of old age and that shape dysfunctional health policies and medical practices." —Kaiser Health News

"Louise Aronson pushes us to think differently . . . I found this book provocative in the best sense of the word. It has stayed with me and pulled me back into multiple readings . . . There's not much more I could ask of a book." —*The Christian Century*

"Aronson's *Elderhood* is dazzling, rich with knowledge gleaned from her professional work as a geriatrician, her personal experience as a daughter, her common sense, and her thorough analysis of our social supports and cultural messaging. Her arguments are powerful, and her conclusions are revolutionary. I hope everyone who has a stake in older people, which is ultimately all of us, will read this book." —Mary Pipher, author of *Women Rowing North*

"In the latter years there are possibilities for joy, transcendence, and meaning, but also for just the opposite. Aronson writes like a memoirist while giving us scientific insight, philosophical wisdom, and wise counsel for a journey and destination we all share. *Elderhood* is a lovely and thoughtful exploration of this voyage." —Abraham Verghese, author of *Cutting for Stone*

"In *Elderhood*, the physician-writer Louise Aronson provides an honest and humane analysis of what it means to grow old in America. Her book—part memoir, history, and social critique—is deeply sympathetic to elders and sharply critical of the "anti-aging industry" that has tried to turn being elderly into some sort of disease. I highly recommend this wonderful book to anyone who plans on growing old in this country." —Sandeep Jauhar, author of *Heart: A History*

"As Louise Aronson says, 'Life offers just two possibilities: die young or grow old.' This searing, luminous book is for everyone who hopes to accomplish the latter and remain fully human as they do. It will challenge your assumptions and open your mind—and it just might change your life." —Lucy Kalanithi, MD, editor of *When Breath Becomes Air*

"In *Elderhood*, Louise Aronson draws on the experiences of her own life and the many lives she has touched as a geriatrician to think about age and aging, combining the insights of science and medicine with the wisdom of literature and human history, all narrated with the practical realism of the caring clinician. It's a wise and beautiful book, to be cherished by anyone who hopes to keep on growing, aging, and learning." —Perri Klass, MD, author of *The Mercy Rule* and *Treatment Kind and Fair*

"The book that every one of us has been or will be looking for—a passionate, illuminating, brilliant, and beautifully written meditation on aging and caring for elders, *Elderhood* is a godsend." —Pauline Chen, MD, author of *Final Exam*

"A book that needs to be consulted by every caregiver and health professional for the wisdom it contains." —*Sun News Tucson*

*A History of the Present Illness: Stories*

# ELDERHOOD

## REDEFINING AGING, TRANSFORMING
## MEDICINE, REIMAGINING LIFE

### LOUISE ARONSON

BLOOMSBURY PUBLISHING

NEW YORK · LONDON · OXFORD · NEW DELHI · SYDNEY

For my mother
and
for Jane

BLOOMSBURY PUBLISHING
Bloomsbury Publishing Inc.
1385 Broadway, New York, NY 10018, USA

BLOOMSBURY, BLOOMSBURY PUBLISHING, and the Diana logo are trademarks of
Bloomsbury Publishing Plc

First published in the United States 2019

This edition published 2021

ISBN: HB: 978-1-62040-546-8; PB: 978-1-6-2040-5-475; eBook: 978-1-62040-548-2

Library of Congress Cataloging-in-Publication Data

Names: Aronson, Louise, author.
Title: Elderhood : redefining aging, transforming medicine, reimagining life / Louise Aronson.
Description: New York : Bloomsbury Publishing, 2019. | Includes bibliographical references.
Identifiers: LCCN 2018040491 | ISBN 9781620405468 (hardback) | ISBN 9781620405482 (e-book)
Subjects: LCSH: Older people—Health and hygiene—United States. | Aging—United States. |
Older people—Medical care—United States.
Classification: LCC RA564.8 .A76 2019 | DDC 362.60973—dc23 LC record available at
https://lccn.loc.gov/2018040491

2 4 6 8 10 9 7 5 3 1

Typeset by Westchester Publishing Services
Printed and bound in the U.S.A. by Berryville Graphics Inc., Berryville, Virginia

To find out more about our authors and books visit www.bloomsbury.com and
sign up for our newsletters.

Bloomsbury books may be purchased for business or promotional use. For information
on bulk purchases please contact Macmillan Corporate and Premium Sales Department at
specialmarkets@macmillan.com.

*Old age will only be respected if it fights for itself, maintains its rights . . . and asserts control over its own to its last breath.*

—CICERO

# CONTENTS

**Conception**
Author's note    xiii

**Birth**
1. Life    3

**Childhood**
2. Infant    13
   MEMORIES · LESSONS
3. Toddler    24
   HISTORY · SICK · ASSUMPTIONS
4. Child    41
   HOUSES · RESURRECTION · CONFUSION · STANDARDS · OTHER
5. Tween    63
   NORMAL · DIFFERENT
6. Teen    75
   EVOLUTION · PERVERSIONS · REJUVENATION · GAPS · CHOICES

**Adulthood**
7. Young Adult    105
   TRAUMA · MODERN · INDOCTRINATION · MISTAKES · COMPETENCE ·
   SHAME · BIAS
8. Adult    137
   OBLIVIOUS · LANGUAGE · VOCATION · DISTANCE · VALUES · TRUTH ·
   BIOLOGY · ADVOCACY · OUTSOURCED · ZEALOT

9. Middle-aged  192
STAGES · HELP · PRESTIGE · COMPLEXITY · COMBUSTION · SEXY ·
DISILLUSIONMENT · PRIORITIES · SYMPATHY

10. Senior  241
AGES · PATHOLOGY · COMMUNICATION · FREEDOM · BACKSTORY ·
LONGEVITY · CHILDPROOF · RECLAMATION

**Elderhood**
11. Old  273
EXCEPTIONAL · FUTURE · DISTRESS · WORTH · BELOVED · PLACES ·
COMFORT · TECH · MEANING · IMAGINATION · BODIES ·
CLASSIFICATION

12. Elderly  324
INVISIBILITY · DUALITY · CARE · EDUCATION · RESILIENCE ·
ATTITUDE · DESIGN · HEALTH · PERSPECTIVE

13. Aged  363
TIME · NATURE · HUMAN · CONSEQUENCES · ACCEPTANCE

**Death**
14. Stories  397

**Coda**
Opportunity  403

Acknowledgments  405
Notes  407
Bibliography  433
Index  436

# CONCEPTION

*The aging body is never just a body subjected to the imperatives of cellular and organic decline, for as it moves through life it is continuously being inscribed and reinscribed with cultural meanings.*
—Mike Featherstone and Andrew Wernick

# AUTHOR'S NOTE

This began as an old age book, and then became more than that, including a book about medicine and what it means to be a human being. Its evolution surprised me, as a doctor and as an aging person. It turned into something at once conventional and countercultural, fact- and story-based, affectionate and opinionated, part battle cry and part lament, a verbal potpourri of joy, wonder, frustration, outrage, and hope about old age, medicine, and American life.

The stories in this book are true to the best of my recollection. Hearing about the same crisis from a doctor's perspective or a patient's, and from a nurse's or administrator's or family member's, the same events can sound unrelated. Memory is flawed, malleable, and significant. Perspective depends on where you're standing and who you are, on context, role, attitude, and values.

Given how much variation in story occurs in the immediate aftermath of an event, it can only be more so after time passes. I have done my best to be both accurate and true to my own thoughts and feelings. I have changed patient names throughout the book and often avoided mention of colleagues' or friends' names. Where I lacked a patient's or family's permission to tell their story, I have changed select telling details. Those measures were taken not only in keeping with core tenets of medicine and the stipulations of federal health privacy laws but also out of profound gratitude for the many people who entrusted me with their well-being and in so doing taught me about what old age is, what it should be, and what it could be.

This book also owes a substantial debt to many scientists, scholars, and writers, past and present. These powerful thinkers have created an enormous body of work on old age that should have far more influence on our aging lives and policies. One of my great hopes for this book is that it leads readers to the work of historians like Thomas Cole and Pat Thane; anthropologists, psychologists, and sociologists like Sharon Kaufman, Becca Levy, and Carroll Estes; physicians like Robert Butler, Bill Thomas, and Muriel Gillick; and more scientists and writers than I can list but whose work appears in these pages or in the notes and bibliography at the end of the book.

There's just one more thing you need to know before turning the page or swiping to the next screen: this book doesn't always walk a straight line from here to there. It dances—or so I hope.

# BIRTH

*Our humanity is our burden, our life; we need not battle for it; we need
only to do what is infinitely more difficult—that is, accept it.*
—James Baldwin

# 1. LIFE

Like many doctors, I went into medicine because I wanted to help people. And like many medical students, I quickly discovered that medical education is more about chemical structures and biology, diseases and organs, than about humanity and healing.

Midway through my first year, I knew every dean and had a collection of catalogs to other graduate programs: public health and medical anthropology, English, policy, and psychology. This wasn't entirely surprising; as a history major who'd chosen my undergraduate college for its lack of math or science requirements, I was an unlikely medical student. But I believed medicine would allow me to make a difference in people's lives in ways those other fields might not. Still, for two years I kept the glossy booklets hidden in my dorm room, and late at night I pored over their disparate course offerings with the zeal of a kid set free in a candy shop. My secret catalogs provided glimpses of a worldview absent from my medical textbooks and the lectures I attended. Here were courses and professions that acknowledged the particularity, complexity, and ambiguity of human lives without reducing them to disembodied cells, parts, and processes.

In our third year, my class entered the hospital: a gauntlet of challenges and humiliations. It sometimes seemed as if the frequent changes in place, people, and specialty had been designed to keep us anxious and off-balance. We learned to work without sleeping, eating, or urinating, without fresh air or clean clothes or feelings of horror or disgust, without tears or time off. It was brutal, and yet, for me, so much better than the two years before. At last my days included learning about actual people with stories no less seductive or meaningful than those in my favorite novels. My hospital work gave me some of the deep human understanding that great literature provides and combined it with opportunities to be useful to people in need. Once I began taking care of patients, medicine became exactly what I'd hoped for when I chose it over all those other fields that more inherently interested me and for which I seemed more naturally suited. I returned home each night feeling not only that my time had been well spent but also that my life mattered in a larger way, even if my contribution to the larger world was itself small. It was a wonderful feeling.

Nearly thirty years later, I still get that pleasure from being a doctor. I also now know that medicine routinely undermines its mission by dismissing the sorts of knowledge I looked for in those course catalogs. So many parts of our complicated human lives don't easily lend themselves to measurement or experimentation. Although science provides invaluable information, and technology can be transformative, both are beholden to the interests and beliefs of the relatively few humans who wield them, and neither is well suited to addressing critical aspects of human life, from individuality to suffering to wellness. This is especially true in the years after a person turns sixty, the ages of the patients I care for as a geriatrician. That may be why, though I thought I was working for them, my patients ended up teaching me what questions really matter as we age and how people can increase their chances of living well and meaningfully throughout their lives.

On a foggy morning in 2015, I arrived at the University of California, Berkeley, for an appointment with Professor Guy Micco. I had heard about an exercise he did every fall with his new medical students, and I wanted to see it for myself.

Standing at the front of a cramped classroom, Micco asked a group of sixteen medical students to put down the first words that came to mind when he used the word *old* in reference to a person.

"Don't filter," he said. "Just write."

With his thick white mustache and ring of flyaway hair, Micco bore a vague resemblance to Albert Einstein, an effect compounded over the next two hours by his wide-ranging curiosity and distractibility.

The young men and women around the single large table were first-year students in a joint medicine–public health graduate program that describes its matriculates as "passionately dedicated to improving the world's health."

They ranged in age from early to middle twenties, and their résumés attested to extraordinarily idealistic good intentions.

The students began scribbling on the scratch paper Micco provided so he could collect responses and assess trends over time. When a minute elapsed, he told them to stop, then repeated his instructions, but this time with the word *elder*.

A few students shook their heads—they knew they were being manipulated.

Micco had been doing this exercise with his students for years. The faces in the room changed, but their responses to the two prompts did not. There were no trends reflecting shifts in how his students thought and felt about old age. Not yet anyway.

He wasn't surprised when the most common associations with the word *old* included *wrinkled, bent over, slow moving, bald*, and *white hair*. ("Sorry, Guy," a student once said to him without irony.) Many also wrote *weak, fragile, feeble, frail*, or *sick*. A sizable minority put down a variation of *grandparent*, and several listed their mothers, though generally the parents of medical students range in age from late forties to early sixties, years most people consider part of middle age. Some used words like *wisdom*, but more chose *sad, pejorative, stubborn*, and *lonely*. One wrote, "smelling of mothballs and stale smoke."

For *elder*, the list looked different. By far the most common word was *wise*. Other responses were *respect, leader, experience, power, money*, and *knowledge*.

Micco's students were in their first months of a process that would take years. Over their four years in medical school and three to ten years of residency and fellowship training, doctors in training are taught that human beings come in two age categories that matter: children and adults. After required classes and rotations elucidating differences in physiology, social behaviors, and health needs between those two age groups, they choose whether to work in children's hospitals or adult hospitals, and as pediatric specialists or adult specialists. If they happen to notice that older adults make up 16 percent of the population but over 40 percent of hospitalized adults, or that patients over sixty-five are the group most likely to be harmed by medical care, that knowledge will be tempered not only by medicine's predilections for saves and cures but also by comments from their teachers and mentors such as "Unless you really like changing adult diapers, don't waste your time" learning geriatrics.

Micco doesn't do this exercise to convince his students that old people are worthy of their time and attention as doctors. He knows he can't win that battle. The problem, he told me one sunny winter morning a few months later when I met him for coffee, isn't the students' youth or inexperience. He has given hospital colleagues and friends with jobs that have nothing to do with medicine the same prompts and has been told the same words, even when those doctors and nurses and friends themselves qualify as old. His feeling is that the word *old* "is lost. Gone. Too loaded with negativity to be used for people anymore."

Micco pulled a pen from his pocket and slid a paper napkin into the space between us on the table. He drew a basic graph. "Here's how most people see old age."

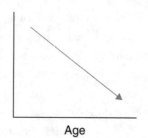

Age

"What's the other axis?" I asked. In other words, what did people think dropped so relentlessly from youth through old age?

Micco stared at me. "Anything," he said. "Everything."

I knew he was right. Although this view of aging is no more than very partially accurate, everyone believes it, including old people. Micco's idealistic students and caring friends and colleagues define *old* with negatives because that is our culture's prevailing view. At this point in history, it's also the prevailing view on the planet. But of course this singular negative vision of old age doesn't tell the whole story. They write positives in response to *old*'s synonym *elder*, because those affirmative attributes are also true. This disconnect suggests they—and the rest of us—are missing something when we think about old age. At the very least, we are losing an opportunity to look at the final third of life with the same concern, curiosity, creativity, and rigor as we view the first two-thirds.

In the months leading up to my meeting with Micco, like many doctors these days, I'd sometimes found myself feeling furious, hurt, and helpless. I obsessed about the forces and people working to undermine patients, doctors, and our health care system generally. In the twentieth century, American medicine became more interested in cosmetics and catastrophes than in promoting and preserving human health and well-being. In the twenty-first century, it worships machines, genes, neurons, hearts, and tumors, but cares little about sanity, walking, eating, frailty, or suffering. It values adults over the young and old, and hospitals and intensive care units over homes and clinics. It prioritizes treatment over prevention, parts over wholes, fixing over caring, averages over individuals, and the new over the proven.

Working as a geriatrician in such a system, I have had to wage daily, often fruitless battles against these structural forces to get my patients what they needed. In such a system, what was most helpful to the people I cared for (as a doctor) and about (as a human being) was neither billable (which mattered to my bosses and institution) nor part of my recognized workday (which mattered to me). My patients, whether old or ancient, healthy or sick, hale or frail, could easily get dialysis, surgeries that fixed a damaged part but destroyed their lives, months of fruitless chemotherapy, long stays in intensive care units, the latest high-tech scans, and all sorts of wildly expensive drugs of no proven benefit in their age group or state of health.

What most of them could *not* get were the sorts of things that would have made them more comfortable, more functional, healthier, and happier— things like hearing aids, enough time with their doctor, or exercise classes that would help treat many of their chronic diseases while increasing their chances of remaining independent. Nor could they get two of medical care's most essential elements: scientific data about the pros and cons of the care they received, or being treated as a human being worthy of resources and concern.

Questioning the system's priorities, tools, and structures is verboten in medicine. Someone who questions is seen as being a complainer or bad team player. For years I'd either squelched my concerns or been reprimanded for raising questions I felt were essential to good patient care and a more compassionate and effective health system. But in 2015 I'd begun having health problems myself, including vision loss, anxiety, and arthritis, that were worrisome in both practical and existential ways. These changes brought me face-to-face with the likelihood of ongoing discomfort and disability at a far earlier age than I'd expected. As I adjusted to my new reality, my ability to understand how medicine fit into our larger social, cultural, economic, and political worlds became more acute. Suddenly, still mostly healthy but with chronic challenges as well, I found myself positioned between youth and old age in a way that gave me a panoramic view of life.

It was then that I saw what had been right in front of me my entire career: that the experiences of older people in our health care system are indicative of how current medical care is broken for all of us. We have created a society where we do everything possible to stay alive yet dread being old, a culture that discards people who don't fit the latest human "product specifications," and a health care system in which the work of medicine is often incompatible with both care and health.

Over two thousand years ago, Aristotle defined a whole as "that which has a beginning, a middle, and an end." He showed that in three-act dramas each part contains multiple scenes and serves a unique purpose. Most human lives follow a similar progression, from setup through complications to conclusion. Until recently in human history, people's individual dramas often ended early in the first act and certainly before the curtain fell on what we now consider Act II. The average life span was thirty to forty years, with childbirth, accidents, and infections routinely cutting lives short. These days, average longevity has doubled. With so much more time, each act contains more scenes, and most of us make it to Act III. Now, alongside childhood and adulthood, the vast majority of us can also expect a third act, or elderhood, that begins at sixty or seventy and lasts for decades. This third act is not a repeat of the first or second. More often, it is in life what it is in drama: the site of our story's climax, denouement, and resolution.

Those last two scare us. We desperately want our elderhood to be long, meaningful, and satisfying, yet most of us refuse to approach it with the same shameless ambition we reflexively accord childhood and adulthood. For the first years of my career, I thought I understood old age and how to create a comfortable, meaningful Act III for my patients. But once my parents entered their eighties and I turned fifty, I realized I had been mistaken. I found myself making all the same sorts of cracks and feeling all the same feelings about aging as everyone else.

Up until that point, I had believed that geriatrics, with its specialized tools and knowledge, had all the answers about old age. But if geriatrics adequately addressed old age, wouldn't the rest of medicine and everyone else have adopted our philosophy and strategies? Clearly, geriatrics was to elderhood what we doctors call "necessary but not sufficient," and I began to wonder what I was missing.

This book is my attempt to fill in those gaps by looking at old age in new ways. It draws from science and medicine, history, anthropology, literature, and popular culture. Who we are and what we value and believe is revealed in how we care for the sick. But although many of the stories in this book involve people who are old and sick, this is a book about life. If we want old age to be something other than a loathsome expanse of years or decades, we need to begin examining the hows and whys of our current approach.

For most of us, Act III is long and varied. If we see it differently, our feelings about it might also change. And if we see and feel differently about old age, we can make different choices, ones that change our experience of elderhood for the better.

# CHILDHOOD

*We're all old people in training.*
—Joanne Lynn, MD

# 2. INFANT

MEMORIES

Among my earliest memories of old age are breasts. The sighting took place on the eighth floor of the hilltop building where Kim Novak's character lived in Hitchcock's *Vertigo*. Twelve years after that movie made audiences scream, my great-grandmother casually removed her robe and I willed my six-year-old self not to gasp. Granny sat on an overstuffed stool in her dressing room, a narrow space with mirrored closet doors and small windows whose lowered shades glowed with yellow light. The air smelled sweet and stale, like used books in a space too long without fresh air. She must have been just out of the bath or shower. My little sister and I held hands but didn't dare look at each other as Granny eased one gigantic breast and then the other into her bra and pulled the straps up over her shoulders, chatting as she moved through her tasks. It's hard to say, even now, what made me most uncomfortable, the shock of her nudity, the heft of her bosom, or the strangeness of her aged body.

Granny would have been in her eighties then, and since I considered my grandparents old, my great-grandmother clearly qualified as ancient. In some ways, my grandparents and great-grandparents were members of that large category known as adults, people who knew a lot and could tell a kid what to do. But they were also clearly an altogether different class of person than my parents and their friends, and only part of what distinguished them came from their wrinkled skin and gray, white, or absent hair. The older generations of my family also had more formal clothes, behavior, and belongings. If they joined our regular Sunday picnics in Golden Gate Park, the women wore dresses or skirts and sat on folding chairs instead of with the rest of us on blankets spread on the grass. With the exceptions of pajamas at sleepovers and bathing suits on the beach, we never saw the men in anything but collared sport tops or button-down shirts. Their apartments were similarly distinct, with furnishings that made family dinners feel more like visits to an old hotel or historic site than a meal in someone's home.

During this same phase of my life, I would sometimes find myself with my sister and cousins just a block away from Granny's at the top of a steep hill with an incline so acute, most locals drove around it, sparing their engines, brakes, and nerves. Not my grandfather, especially not if he had one or more of his five granddaughters in the car. After a Chinatown dinner and before the ice-cream cones, he would drive us to the top of that crazy hill and let the car teeter on its precipice. Then he'd release the hand brake, let go of the steering wheel, and put his hands up in the air. Each time, we grabbed each other and squealed, gasping and laughing. And each time his foot was still on the brake pedal and the pace, though it felt like speed to us, would have elicited honks and frustration on most other blocks. Each time we spent a night out with Gramps, it was hard to imagine having more fun.

Those two memories show why I should have known better about old age. But, like many people, I never gave it much thought, even when it was right in front of me. I thought more about Granny's exposed breasts than about how her softened skin, odor, and the look and feel of her apartment affected my experience of them. And I thought about all the fantastic nights out with my grandfather but not about how much fun he was having being a grandparent, a role that not a few people describe as the best of their lives. Nor did I really consider how being from different generations of old age affected what more senior members of our family could or would do, or the larger social factors that enabled the men's more relaxed, engaged, and fun-loving approach to life. I was three when Granny's husband died, leaving her a widow for the second time. Still relatively young when my great-grandfather died, she had been free to remarry. But the script for elderly widows required that Granny lead a quiet life of occasional outings and family, eschewing exercise, solo travel, and romance. She seemed happy enough in her life and healthy to my child's eyes, yet she made me nervous. She was strict and quick to reprimand, sure of her authority. We had to dress up to visit her, then sit in a "ladylike" pose on her furniture. When once, discussing some athletic event, I described myself as having been sweaty, she told me ladies didn't sweat, they glowed. I felt entirely justified in my mild fear of her and my suspicion that she was as foreign as she was family.

Granny died in her early nineties and her daughter, my grandmother, at only seventy-eight, after years of alcoholism. A family history of a long life doesn't guarantee you'll get one. Granny and Grandpa, her son-in-law, didn't get along. For years they didn't speak, and my grandmother was caught in between, the two central figures in her life each constantly fighting and enumerating the other's failings. Although her children were grown and settled, a woman of my grandmother's background and time couldn't seek out a divorce, job, or therapist for escape, distraction, or fulfillment. Instead, there was alcohol, which worked as most drugs do when abused. It dulled the pain, providing brief, blissful moments of respite, and it ruined her life and health. What I remember most vividly about her is how she would choke at dinner, eyes bulging, face panicked, sweating and unable to breathe. The adults at the table ignored her when this happened. It took me years to gather the courage to ask what was going on and why they behaved that way. She was drunk, they said, and she brought these episodes upon herself. I understood that their refusal to help her was punishment for disappointing them in so many ways, but I could not understand how they could sit so calmly in the presence of her distress. When Grandma choked, the dining room turned to ice. Finally, she would gasp or put a hand to her mouth and leave the room, and dinner would continue as if nothing had happened. A person's age may have little or nothing to do with the ways in which they suffer.

Fewer restrictions existed for men: my grandfather could retire in his sixties from the job he'd done for forty years and begin new, more intermittent work. Because he had health, education, and enough money, his new job could be one that indulged his interests in furniture and travel while taking advantage of his business and social skills. He had the time and resources for all those activities he'd always loved but couldn't pursue in earlier years when supporting his family and building his company. When he became a widower in his late seventies, he continued to enjoy an active social life. Although Gramps had always been charming and interested in everybody and everything, his eighth and ninth decades were the best dating years of his life. Lucky for him: a scarcity of males in the oldest age groups meant that even a short man with little hair could go out with a different woman every night of the week if so inclined—and he was.

There were fewer old people then, and the world paid them less attention. I heard about the Gray Panthers, but the civil rights movement and feminism seemed more visible and relevant. Stories about old-age trials, opportunities, and accomplishments didn't appear daily in the news, and older adults hadn't yet been classified by society as a problem of "silver tsunami" proportions. That metaphor, implying that new human longevity and the aging population would bring tsunami-like overwhelming destruction to society, didn't enter our lexicon until the 1980s. Now it appears everywhere, from *Forbes* and the *Economist* to the *Washington Post,* the *New England Journal of Medicine,* and the National Council of State Legislatures. Its relatively recent ascendance is why I was so surprised—looking back not only at the sixties and seventies but even farther back still, to ancient Egypt and China, the Greek and Roman Empires, and the earliest periods of U.S. history—to discover how much of what we believe is unique to aging in this "tsunami" moment isn't new at all.

### LESSONS

In June 1992 I moved from Boston to San Francisco, my brand-new MD in hand, and began answering to the word *Doctor.* In many ways, this was absurd.

Graduating from medical school doesn't mean a person has the knowledge or skills to independently diagnose and treat patients. That's why new doctors do residencies: the three- to eight-year phase of doctor training that comes after the degree but before adequate competence for unsupervised practice. A primary care internal medicine residency had brought me back to my hometown. At San Francisco General Hospital's Emergency Department, where I did my first rotation, being an inexperienced doctor didn't seem so worrisome because I was surrounded by highly skilled nurses and doctors. More concerning was what happened in a small, fluorescently lit room on the fourth floor of a Parnassus Avenue medical office building each Tuesday afternoon. There, people ranging in age from nineteen to ninety would show up for an appointment with their new internist, and what they got was me.

Every three years, clinics are passed from graduating residents to new interns, and often they have a particular focus, usually a category of disease or type of patient. It's unclear how intentional this is—for example, a future oncologist referring her hospitalized cancer patients to her own outpatient clinic for follow-up—or whether clusters of patients with certain illnesses or traits gravitate toward a particular doctor by some other means. It could be word of mouth, ethnic and linguistic compatibility, or an appointment scheduler's hunch. What was clear for my group of residents was that Arlene had a disproportionate number of patients with diabetes, Sammie's often used street drugs, Rafael's were more likely to speak Spanish or have HIV, Danny's had complicated heart disease, and Gerda's preferred a female physician. Many of my patients were old.

I was in my twenties, and old looked different to me than it does now. Although I cared for more octogenarians than my fellow residents, I also had more patients in their sixties and early seventies, some of whom I would now consider middle-aged. But in those days, "old" was for me a large, fairly uniform category defined by an unspecified but self-evident amalgam of age, attitude, and appearance. Had anyone asked, I'd like to think I would have noted the considerable differences between sixty-five and ninety, but in my day-to-day doctor life, patients at those different ages, although a generation apart, seemed more similar than not.

At eighty-nine, by anyone's definition, Anne Rowe was old.

I met her on a warm Tuesday afternoon about a month into my residency. Perched on the edge of our clinic's tan vinyl, one-size-fits-all chair, Anne's feet dangled above the floor, swinging like a schoolgirl's. She wore what she called her "old lady shoes" and one of what I would soon learn was a handful of cheerful dresses that pulled over her head, allowing her to avoid buttons and zippers that challenged her deformed fingers.

As we exchanged greetings, she studied me from above the bifocal wedges of her gold-framed glasses. She had a humped back and compressed torso, perfectly white hair with a hint of curl, and a smile of crooked teeth.

"What happened to the other doctor?" she asked.

"He moved back east," I answered, trying my best to appear a worthy replacement.

Departing senior residents were supposed to tell their clinic patients they were leaving, but I had already learned that didn't always happen. Losing their primary care doctor could be hard for patients, but, unique in my clinic, Anne seemed to understand and accept the system. That meant we could jump right into discussing her history and current concerns. She had a routine assortment of conditions—high blood pressure, arthritis, allergies, constipation, heartburn—and a long list of medications.

As we shifted to the physical exam, she asked, "What kind of name is Aronson?"

"Jewish," I said. "It was given to my father's family at Ellis Island because theirs was too hard to pronounce."

She grinned. Her family had a similar story, except it wasn't Anne's grandparents who had fled the eastern European pogroms of the early 1900s but Anne herself. She had been three years old in 1906 when her family left Belarus and somehow landed in North Dakota.

Eventually I learned Anne's life story. On that first day, I heard enough to get a glimpse of one of the great pleasures of talking to older people. Anne's life spanned the better part of a century and many continents, and, like all lives, it had included an assortment of personal tragedies and accomplishments. Talking to her was like getting paid to listen to excerpts of a long, captivating novel.

Anne escaped North Dakota by earning a teaching degree and taking a job overseas. I learned later that she'd fallen for and married a British artist-activist, that perhaps she might have been a better mother to their son, and how, after a few years, she had divorced her unreliable husband and supported herself by teaching in Puerto Rico and Michigan. At that first meeting, we did not discuss her years in Mississippi during the civil rights movement or her retirement to San Francisco to be near her four still-living siblings, although I'm certain she told me about her most recent job: caregiver for her sister Bess, a role Anne had acquired gradually and by default. The two siblings, one divorced and one widowed, shared a house.

At the time, I didn't know how hard the job was or how dangerous and damaging it could be to the physical and psychological health of the caregiver. I'm pretty sure this was not a topic covered in medical school, where the social and personal aspects of health are only infrequently mentioned. A doctor's job was to treat disease.

As a first-year resident, I was required to discuss all my patients with a more experienced clinician who would make sure I hadn't missed anything. As I learned more, I could be more selective, presenting only those patients where I knew, felt, or suspected I didn't yet have the necessary knowledge or skills. During these consults, the senior doctor would ensure I was providing high-quality care and also teach me about clinical assessment, reasoning, or treatment. This was almost always a pleasure.

In caring for Anne, I learned a patient's target blood pressure differed in patients over age eighty, and why I should steer clear of common arthritis medications even if they were inexpensive and likely to help her pain. Although readily available over the counter, my teachers said these drugs would put Anne at high risk for kidney failure and internal bleeding. That last, life-threatening side effect occurred only rarely in young and middle-aged patients, but, as I quickly discovered on my hospital rotations, it routinely happened among the old. Drugs that pose serious danger to "adults" in general—no matter the age—aren't available over the counter. However, even today, an obvious oversight in over the counter drug labeling persists: while precautions specify risks to children, pregnant women, and people with certain diagnoses, they do not mention possible harms to older people.

Because my supervisors pointed out differences between younger and older adults and helped me make treatment plans that hewed to the latest standards of care, I thought I was learning everything I needed to take good care of my many old patients. Unfortunately, later that year it became clear that I wasn't, and the consequences of the mistake I made under the close supervision of my outstanding doctor-teachers would not only land Anne in the hospital and endanger her life; it would show me how medicine and society's choices undermine old people. Too often old age itself is blamed for realities created by our choices and policies.

* * *

As we got to know each other, among the things I came to like most about Anne was her smile. Her face lifted, her eyes flashed, and if she found something funny, she'd throw her head back to laugh. Her neck was short by then and the hump in her upper back pronounced, but in those moments of humor and comradery, her face became the embodiment of mirth and joy. At each visit, I would get to see her smile when I entered the exam room, when either of us made a joke, and when we worked together to get her abbreviated self onto the relatively high exam table and out of her shoulder-to-knee slip, an undergarment of a type with which I had no familiarity.

I knew there was something very wrong the day that winter when she didn't smile at all.

"How are you?" I asked, scooting my wheeled desk chair toward her and feeling stupid, since the answer to the question seemed obvious.

"I had to put Bess in a nursing home," she said in a voice so quiet I could barely hear her. Her eyes seemed smaller, darker. Tears traced the creases of her cheeks.

I moved the box of tissues to the corner of my desk where she could reach it.

"I couldn't lift her. I couldn't keep her clean. I'm just not strong enough."

I resisted the temptation to mention that she was nearly ninety and four feet nine inches tall, traits that make it close to impossible to provide total care to a bedbound person. I did point out that she had taken care of her sister for nearly a decade and that most people wouldn't have lasted nearly as long.

A doctor's instinct is always to try and fix, soothe, reassure. In moments like these, those tendencies can be the opposite of helpful.

Nothing I said offered much comfort. Finally, I shut up. I let Anne talk, and I listened. Eventually I asked about symptoms of depression and suicidality. Then I went to consult with my supervisor. We discussed the difference between grief and depression, and I told him that Anne was definitely grieving, but I worried that she was also depressed.

"Do you think she needs medication?" he asked.

I didn't want to medicalize the normal sadness of grief, but I also didn't want to leave major depression untreated.

I decided not to give Anne a prescription that day but to add her to my schedule the following week. At that next appointment, she still wasn't smiling, and she told me she wasn't eating, sleeping, or doing her usual activities. Nothing really interested her.

She needed medication.

I told Anne we were lucky because for years the only drugs for depression had dangerous side effects, but now there was a new medication with few side effects, most of which went away after a few weeks. I relayed this information with great authority, since I had read the latest literature in preparation for a clinic talk and had successfully treated several other patients in my practice with antidepressants. I handed Anne a prescription, scheduled a follow-up visit in a month, and told her I'd give her a call soon to see how she was doing.

When I phoned the next week, I got her answering machine and left a message. I hoped that meant the drug was working and she was out and about again. Even in the moment I recognized my own wishful thinking. In truth, I was relieved, at least as much for my own sake as for Anne's. It was much easier and more efficient for me to reach her machine than to speak to Anne if she was feeling better. Having left a message, the onus for communication moved from me to her. I could take "Call A. R." off my to-do list and move on to my next task. I was on an inpatient rotation that month, and my team was on call from eight in the morning of my clinic day until eight A.M. the next day. Though I usually loved outpatient work, on that day it was an unwelcome interruption in a busy shift that would last at least thirty-six hours. My goal that afternoon was to finish as soon as possible without compromising the care of my clinic patients and get back to the hospital.

You could argue that that setup, a typical one, is a failing of medical training. But it's also prescient training for the realities of primary care medicine, where too often doing the right thing for the patient and getting through the tasks that enable a clinician to complete the workday in just ten or twelve hours are in direct opposition. Tasks such as phoning to check on at-risk patients like Anne, refilling medications, responding to patient queries, and determining whether a patient needs an appointment or if you can spare them an unnecessary trip to the clinic. Tasks like working with hospital doctors or visiting nurses to ensure safe transitions from hospital to home and speaking to caregivers or concerned family members. None of these activities count as part of the scheduled workday, although they can take one, two, or three hours and are essential to patient care. This reality is one of the key ingredients in our primary care and burnout crises, which might be jointly defined as the willful mismatch between what is best for patients and clinicians and what the health care system prioritizes and pays for.

Two weeks later, the clinic medical assistant stopped me as soon as I arrived.

"You have an add-on, and they're already here." She handed me a chart with Anne's name on it. "Her son Jack is with her."

Anne looked even tinier than usual, perched on the vinyl chair as a younger, stockier, and decidedly male version of her paced up and down between the door and far wall.

"I've never seen her like this," Jack said. "She's just not herself."

I turned to Anne. "Can you tell me how you're feeling?" She hadn't looked up since I'd entered the room.

"I just don't see the point," she said, her words emerging at half speed. I had to crouch beside her chair to hear her.

"Of what?"

"Of anything."

She was nearly catatonic. My supervisor and I agreed that Anne needed to be admitted to the psychiatry hospital. I filled out the necessary paperwork, called the admitting psychiatry team, and stayed with Anne and Jack until one of the nurses wheeled her across the street to the hospital.

The rest of my clinic shift was fairly frantic. I was running over an hour late and each patient visit began with their frustration and my apologies. By six o'clock, when the psychiatry hospital extension came up on my pager's flashing green display, every doctor but me had finished seeing patients and the support staff had all gone home. I punched in the number, eager for news about Anne.

The psychiatry resident had been nice earlier in the day. Now he didn't waste time with pleasantries.

"Her sodium is 121," he said. "I can't believe you didn't check it before sending her. You need to arrange her transfer to the medical service."

Anne wasn't depressed—or not *just* depressed. Her critically low level of blood sodium was why she'd appeared catatonic, and for all I knew, it was what had been causing her depression from the start. Shortly before she moved Bess to the nursing home, I had adjusted her blood pressure medications. The new combination can lower sodium levels. Although I'd checked it once in keeping with standards of care, I hadn't thought to check it again when she became depressed because Anne had such a good reason to be depressed.

Horrified and ashamed, I made the necessary calls. As I was doing that, my pager went off again. It was the hospital operator who said a patient's son was demanding that I call him. Jack was furious and questioned whether I knew what I was doing. All I could do was apologize.

In medicine, when something unexpected happens and certainly when patients are harmed, we review the case to identify missteps and learn from them in order to take better care of future patients. After Anne's hospitalization, the attendings, my co-residents, and I discussed the need for blood tests in patients on multiple medications when their health changes, even if there appears to be another plausible explanation. We also uncovered several recent case reports describing elderly patients developing critically low sodium levels on the type of antidepressant I'd given Anne, the then relatively new class called selective serotonin reuptake inhibitors that are now among the bestselling drugs on the market.

But we did not discuss why we had all assumed treating depression in an octogenarian would be the same as treating it in younger adults. Or how it could be that anyone was surprised when a diminutive ninety-year-old developed complications from the same medication dose I had last given to a hundred-and-sixty-pound thirty-nine-year-old.

Fortunately, in this instance Anne and I both got lucky. In the hospital, she steadily improved, and when she went home, Jack was there to help. I remained Anne's doctor until her death five years later. Jack is now himself an octogenarian, and we are still in touch. Some patients give more to their doctor than the doctor could possibly give to them. Anne gave me geriatrics, though I didn't know that for several more years.

# 3. TODDLER

HISTORY

Eight hundred years before Christ and a hundred or so after, leading Greco-Roman and Egyptian thinkers put forth an array of sometimes contradictory ideas about aging. Hippocrates cataloged ailments particular to old people and believed medicine had little to offer them, while a key medical text from Egypt around 600 B.C. included "the book for the transformation of an old man into a youth of 20." Plato's *Republic* opened with the elderly Cephalus describing the variability of old age and how often old people blamed problems on aging even when most older people didn't have those problems. Aristotle advanced his theory of *pneuma*, in which finite life force decreased over time, taking with it vitality and the ability to fend off disease and death. In *de Senectute*, Cicero noted that "since [Nature] has fitly planned the other acts of life's drama, it is not likely that she has neglected the final act." The older man, he argued, "does not do those things that the young men do, but in truth he does much greater and better things . . . by talent, authority, judgement." Galen asserted that aging was a natural process and only disease counted as pathology. He taught that self-care through diet and behavior could slow aging.

Two millennia later, our response to old age isn't so different. Google, the National Academy of Medicine, and a host of other public and private researchers, echoing the Egyptians, have launched campaigns to "end aging forever." Perhaps in agreement with Hippocrates, in 2018 the UK appointed a minister of loneliness instructed to pay special attention to the elderly, and the United States passed the RAISE Act to support family caregivers. Recapitulating Aristotelian fatalism, the medical care of older adults is often unstandardized and unpopular. Although researchers have been required to include women and people of color in their studies for decades, similar stipulations for older adults, a group that uses health services at much higher levels than the young, were only passed in 2018. Meanwhile, in a blending of Cicero and Galen, the terms *healthy* or *successful* aging have become the catchwords for acceptable old age, and thought leaders are competing to coin a word to distinguish the younger, fitter old from the truly old and frail.

And that's only the beginning of the story.


From earliest recorded history, even those who agreed on pathological mechanisms of old age adopted different interpretations of the same findings. Greek doctors considered old people members of the adult group and their age just one factor among many with relevance to diagnosis and treatment. At the same time, while recognizing them as different, they lumped old people of both genders—because they were "too cold"—with children and women, who "exhibited excessive dampness." Everyone but adult men were assigned a status somewhere between health and illness (and a legal status of less than full competence) as a result of their inherent "pathological dyscrasias," or bad mixtures of elements. From earliest recorded history, many societies have considered their oldest citizens less than fully human.

After the fall of Greece, numerous advances in scholarship about the care of older adults came from the Middle East. In Arabia in the tenth century A.D., Algizar detailed ailments of aging, including insomnia and forgetfulness, and wrote books on maintaining health in old age. In the eleventh century, a Persian polymath named Avicenna, often described as the father of early modern medicine, published *The Canon of Medicine*. He advocated health through exercise, diet, sleep, and management of constipation, echoing Galen's *Hygiene*. That classic from over a millennium earlier was rediscovered and became a bestseller in the late twelfth century. It went through 240 printings in European and Middle Eastern languages under the title *Regimen Sanitatis*. Building on Avicenna and *Regimen*, the Franciscan friar and thirteenth-century physician Roger Bacon revived Galen's idea of aging as heat loss, also suggested the still-popular wear-and-tear theory, and advanced the Christian idea that behavior determined longevity. His book *The Cure of Old Age and the Preservation of Youth* was translated into English four hundred years later and well circulated. Little changed over those centuries in Europe, where understanding of illness and aging came primarily from the religious view of humans as immortal and death as the wages of sin.

In the fifteenth and sixteenth centuries, Europeans began taking inductive and empirical approaches to medicine. By observing a range of older adults, philosophers and clinicians concluded that behaviors and interventions could delay and improve but not prevent old age, and also that aging and death were inevitable. In Italy, Gabriele Zerbi's 1489 book *Gerontocomia* described physiological changes of age from skin wrinkles to shortness of breath, illustrating that aging was a physical and physiological process. The Italian octogenarian businessman and philosopher Luigi Cornaro, the "Apostle of Senescence," based his work on self-observation. Although *senescence* refers to age-related cellular damage and biological old age, Cornaro saw old age as a time of promise and fulfillment. He advocated moderation and personal responsibility for health so people could experience its rewards. His *Discorsi della vita sobria* was first published in the 1540s, translated into English in the 1630s, and came out in fifty editions through the 1700s and 1800s. That Cornaro lived to one hundred suggests he was onto something.

In Britain, Francis Bacon studied long-lived people and observed that multiple factors, including diet, environment, temperament, and heredity, influence aging and longevity. Studies in recent years have proved time and again that he was right on all counts. The French physician Andre du Laurens's 1594 text, *Discourse of the Preservation of the Sight; of Melancholic Diseases; of Rheumes and of Old Age*, also went through many editions and translations. Its title alone provides insight, calling out vision loss, depression, and arthritis in old age. At regular intervals throughout the nineteenth century, popular books offered rules for extending life, while others, notably William Thoms's *Longevity in Man: Its Facts and Fiction*, provoked controversy by questioning whether anybody had ever really lived past one hundred.

With the Scientific Revolution in the sixteenth and seventeenth centuries, when physicians began dissecting and analyzing the anatomy and pathology of subjects both living and dead, increasingly accurate specifics about the aging body emerged. The preeminent philosophers of the time, including René Descartes and Francis Bacon, like the scientists of today, believed that humans could prolong life and cure disease through healthy living and interventions uncovered through medical research. The Marquis de Condorcet correctly predicted that science would improve the physical health of populations, while Napoléon believed humankind would eventually be able to engineer its own immortality. A few thinkers questioned this goal in various ways. Thomas Malthus raised concerns of overpopulation, and, in *Gulliver's Travels*, Jonathan Swift imagined the people he called Struldbruggs living the dispirited, purposeless lives of people absent the ticking clock of their own mortality.

Over those centuries, too, some saw old age as a disease in the Galenic tradition, an intermediate condition between health and illness. In France, François Ranchin's 1627 *Opuscula Medica* distinguished between "natural senescence" because of waning heat and "accidental senescence" as a result of disease. In Germany, Jakob Hutter gave away his main point in the title of his 1732 book, *That Senescence Itself Is an Illness*. According to him, people died of old age itself, and he developed a theory to explain the underlying pathology. With aging, he wrote, people developed a "progressive hardening of all fibres of the body," which eventually obstructed blood flow and led to "fatal putrefaction."

Beginning in the eighteenth century, European understanding of the biology of aging rapidly advanced, distinguishing normal aging from disease and recognizing apparently symptomless diseases and organ pathologies in people who appeared to be experiencing healthy old age. This led to the recognition of chronic diseases and of the different presentations of disease in old age. It became clear that death in old age was due not to the waning of invisible humors or heat but to one or many diseases; in other words, it wasn't a disease itself. The accumulation of chronic diseases, which might remain silently asymptomatic for years, was documented in 1761 by Giovanni Morgagni in *De sedibus, et causis morborum*. In 1892 Heinrich Rosin, a German professor (of law, not medicine) wrote, "Extreme old age, with its natural degeneration of resources and the natural decline of organs, is a condition of development of the human body; old-age infirmity is no illness." Meanwhile, in the United States, Benjamin Rush's 1793 *Account of the State of the Body and Mind in Old Age, with Observations on Its Diseases and Their Remedies* noted that old age was only rarely the sole cause of death. Yet even then the messages were mixed. Long-standing preventive regimens for optimal aging persisted even as new ones emerged. Rush also discussed the influence of genetics on aging and the benefits of being married and having a calm temperament.

The nineteenth century brought a significant reconceptualization of aging. This occurred partly as a result of scientific advances, but larger social forces also played a role. Increasingly, the impact of poverty and social policies on health became apparent, and communities and the state were seen as having social responsibilities for their older citizens. In the final decades of that century, the Victorian focus on the behavior of individuals and notions of life as a journey were denounced by modernists as "creating respectable cowards rather than morally empowered individuals." By the early twentieth century, Americans rejected the earlier religious, metaphysical, and cosmologic explanations of aging and began putting their faith in the biological sciences to explain not so much why we age but how. Understand the how, they reasoned, and you could control it. If you could control it, the why was irrelevant.

Despite these scientific and societal changes, the medical care of the elderly garnered relatively little attention. This was largely due to a belief that older adults were doomed and incurable. The focus on pathological changes with age in the nineteenth century and the emphasis on cures in the twentieth put the needs of many old people at odds with the goals of medicine. There were exceptions to this inattention, particularly by German researchers, including Alois Alzheimer and Emil Kraepelin (who named Alzheimer's disease after his mentor), and British clinicians. They produced descriptions of dementia and the impact of early life habits on health in old age, as well as an elaboration of the challenges posed by the coexistence of several diseases in older patients, now known as multimorbidity. Still, by the early twentieth century the lines between normal and pathological aging remained unclear.

Most physicians at the time (as now) deemed old people less worthy of medical attention than younger adults who were easier to treat and more fixable. The common approach to their care was neglect, a relatively inexpensive strategy that required little from doctors and had the added advantage of being a disincentive to malingerers. Old patients were confined to beds in dismal surroundings with few activities and scant stimulation, and provided with little more than food and shelter. This led to depression, obesity, muscle atrophy, and pressure ulcers until the 1930s, when the surgeon Marjory Warren, "the mother of British geriatrics," advocated for the physical rehabilitation of the sick elderly.

Fresh from her residency and given responsibility for 714 patients in a West Middlesex hospital unit, Warren found her new patients "unclassified and ill-assorted." She created the first "block" of exclusively older patients in the UK and began an innovative approach to their rehabilitation with a multidisciplinary team. Very quickly, she noted that even within groupings of older patients, people of the same age might be radically different in function. They did best, she found, when "nursed with those of equal mental capacity." She also insisted that "nothing that a patient can do for himself should be done for him," essentially advocating against the behaviors—still so common today—that breed hopelessness and dependency in the name of expediency, a process so ubiquitous it has a name: "learned helplessness."

Warren modeled her approach on the already fairly well-established rehabilitation of patients after strokes and found that with appealing surroundings, hope, and help, many older patients could return to regular lives: "The number of patients able to leave [geriatrics] wards varies, I think, immensely with the time available and the work done. Many of the so-called 'incurable' cases only need the patience, tact and quiet energy of a staff trained to work with this type of patient to show a considerable measure of improvement."

In that regard, not much has changed over the last century. Our health system penalizes hospitals if they don't fix people and quickly send them home, designates just fifteen to twenty minutes for clinic appointments, and doesn't provide most nursing facility staff with the time, training, or both to help people in ways appropriate to their life stage. This sets up a vicious circle, as age-blind systems lead to bad outcomes for old people, which in turn reinforce people's sense that they are not worth treating.

Although not an official specialty in the United States until the 1970s, medical interest in the care of older adults periodically surged during the twentieth century, sometimes as a result of medical progress and other times in response to social forces. Advances in understanding of pathological anatomy fueled the first surge in the 1910s and early twenties when medicine began its shift from prevention to treatment. In those years, physicians interested in geriatrics began writing popular press articles about health and aging. With these articles describing new therapies, older people turned to doctors to help them with age-related challenges. The second surge began in the 1960s and eventually allowed the doctors interested in caring for old patients to join a legitimate specialty.

Even a brief glimpse at the long history of old age shows that scientists and philosophers have debated the same questions about aging for over five thousand years: throughout history, the experience of being old has been shaped by economics, social priorities, medical knowledge and technology, and our beliefs about life and health. We continue to try to understand aging scientifically and existentially. There are still people trying to find the fountain of youth and others striving to make the most of life within the constraints that have defined it since the beginning of time. The lines between normal and pathological aging and whether science can "cure" aging remain unclear. What is clear is that the history of medicine illuminates the history of old age, and the history of old age shows that approaches currently touted as innovative or transformational are novel only in the specifics of their *how* and *who* and not in their *what* or *why*.

SICK

When I was nine and a half, doctors saved my life . . . twice—I have the scars on my abdomen to prove it.

I was at a sleepaway camp in Colorado when I developed a stomachache. It was my first summer without my parents, so the nurse's initial diagnosis was homesickness. When I didn't get better with attention and reassurance, she thought I might have the stomach flu. Finally, after I could barely eat or walk, my cousins—ages ten, twelve, and fourteen—tearfully made the case that there was something very wrong. The nurse took me to a doctor. After examining my belly, he gave her an intense, concerned look. I remember wanting my mother.

With the nurse riding shotgun, the angel-voiced, no-nonsense camp director's wife drove me and my ruptured appendix over the Rocky Mountains to the local hospital during what would turn out to be that summer's worst heat wave. This took hours. I lay on a navy-striped camp mattress in the back of a station wagon. It was 1972, and the car and its shocks were old at the time, older than me and definitely not what I needed, with my infected, pus-filled abdomen.

Despite its open windows, the wagon was a box of motionless hot air. The outside temperature that day was 102 degrees, and mine was several points higher. I knew the heat-blurred palm trees, pools of shimmering water, elephants, dogs, and green-blue snakes that paraded across the station wagon's faded tan ceiling weren't real and also that there wasn't much point in telling the adults about them. Though the nurse chattered companionably and regularly checked on me, tension hung in the car as heavy and omnipresent as the heat. The director's wife drove as quickly as one can on narrow, curvy mountain roads with a sick child on a mattress in the back.

There are many other moments and "facts" I remember, which might be only memories of the stories I later told about that day. For a while, they made me a more interesting nine-year-old.

I don't recall why the director's wife drove me, a critically ill child, over the mountains to the nearest hospital, but in those days, in medical crises, men made decisions and incisions, and women provided care.

Each time the station wagon drove over a twig or stone or fissure, it felt as if someone had thrust a burning log into my belly. I tried but sometimes failed not to moan or scream. When a mewl slipped out, I pressed my lips together. I felt so hot. It hurt so much.

They said my mother would be there when I woke up after surgery, but she wasn't. There were visiting hours then, even for sick children's parents, and she couldn't get there from California in time. All that night, as I intermittently awoke in my hospital room, scared and sore and wishing she were there, my mother lay awake in a nearby motel, scared and worried too.

Days later, when a kindly nurse announced that she would help me walk, I laughed and said, "I'm nine, I already know how to walk!" Then I stood and my legs gave way and she caught me. That day and the next, she helped me to learn, again, how to walk.

On the Fourth of July, after the sky darkened and most of the doctors went home, the nurses put some of us in wheelchairs and—against the rules—wheeled us out the small hospital's sliding front doors to watch. The summer's fresh night air felt like a balm, and the fireworks seemed as much a celebration of my own brief freedom from the hospital as of our nation's independence.

At the end of that week, people stared at us as my mother wheeled me through the Denver airport. I insisted on walking into the bathroom stall so at least some of those strangers would understand that I wasn't the damaged child I appeared to be, someone they obviously found different and upsetting. I wanted to make clear that I was actually an entirely normal child experiencing a temporary setback. I thought, too, how hard it must be to be a child who would not get up from their wheelchair, who knew people would always stare, and their sympathy and horror would be permanent.

Back in San Francisco, I was happier than I'd ever been to see my younger sister and our house. And I was outraged, fifteen minutes later, when my parents said that I had to go back to a hospital. Apparently it had all been arranged; I wasn't so much going home as moving to a hospital closer to home.

My last two memories of that summer are from the second hospital, ones I wouldn't fully understand until fifteen years later as a medical student.

In the first, I am on a stretcher on my way to surgery. The gurney is surrounded by people in medical clothes: green scrubs, white lab coats, paper hats, face masks. IV bags dangle over my head, and at the foot of the bed, machines flash numbers with squiggly lines.

We are set to go down to the operating rooms. The elevator doors close, and then, before we go anywhere—or so I think now, looking back—there is shouting and the doors open again, and I'm not sure if we have gone up or down or wherever we are supposed to be going, or why we are stopped, and why everyone is so frantic.

After that, there was the hallway outside the operating room and the white ceiling sliding by above. I was given, through an IV, medicine that instantly rendered me and the surrounding world light, wondrous, beautiful, and unbound in ways that might help a person who is not a drug addict understand why somebody could become one.

I didn't recognize that elevator scene for what it was until I was a medical student in a hospital seeing someone else try to die. On that day in the summer of '72, I "coded" in the elevator and was resuscitated. I made it to the operating room, where the surgeon opened my abdomen, cleaned out the pockets of pus that hadn't been adequately cleaned the first time, and put in drains to ensure that this time I got better.

In the second memorable scene, it is evening and my parents are in my hospital room, keeping me company. Although my covers are up, I look pregnant and my stomach hurts with a severity that makes the belly pain I had on the trip across the Rockies seem like a welcome alternative. I cannot get comfortable. I moan and cry. Nurses come in and out, doling out medications. I cry more, though it makes the pain worse.

The hospital and city are dark and quiet when the surgeon appears, wearing neither scrubs nor suit and tie but slacks and a sport shirt. He talks to my parents and me before examining me. The surgeon says my gut is paralyzed. We must get it moving again, he says, and to do that I will need to walk and move around.

I protest, cry more. My mother cajoles. The surgeon insists. He starts me off slowly, has me lie first on one side, then the other. He positions me atop the bed on all fours like a toddler on the verge of pulling up. Then he has me walk the halls with one of the nurses. I begin to fart. I fart and fart. At some point, the adults go home and I go to sleep.

Is it possible that a few key scenes over a month or two in the summer of 1972 made me a certain sort of doctor? I think so. When I first walked into a pediatric ward as a medical student, a body blow of sensory memories time-traveled me from almost-doctor to small-sick-child and that world of cold walls, tall strangers, acrid odors of medications, antiseptics, and bodies, the endless refrains of beeps, moans, whispers, pain, and unknowing and wordless long, lonely nights. My summer of sickness taught me things a doctor needs to know about what care is and is not, and what it's like to be sick and disabled in our ability-obsessed world, and how pain can be so bad that you would do anything to make it go away. It taught me what it's like to be frail and small and vulnerable, and what kindness looks like, and cruelty, and how very much parents love their children, and what medicine can do when its tools fit a problem. And it taught me how wonderful it is to be alive and healthy, and that a great trauma can be transformative in ways both good and bad.

### ASSUMPTIONS

As director of human resources for a large San Francisco medical center, Veronica Hoffman knew a thing or two about doctors. They got up early and they were compulsive. Most likely, she reasoned, they'd get up early on Sundays too.

She waited as long as she could. A little before eight, she looked over at her seventy-nine-year-old mother, Lynne, and picked up the phone.

Across town, I refilled my coffee cup and checked my pager to make sure its batteries were charged. So far, my on-call weekend had been eerily quiet, and I wondered if I'd missed calls. The pager was in my hand when it alarmed, its glowing green display showing a patient's name, record number and contact information, the caller's name, and the reason for the call. In most practices, the caller is the patient. In geriatrics, it's not uncommonly someone else—an adult child, hired caregiver, friend, or visiting nurse. On this particular message, in addition to a daughter caller, the most notable words were: *mother not herself* and *worried*.

After I dialed, Veronica answered almost immediately.

"Thank you for calling so quickly." Her words, although measured and polite, carried an unmistakable undertone of urgency and concern. "I don't know if it's anything. The paramedics were here last night—early this morning—and they didn't think so. I'm probably overreacting."

I said that if something was worrying her, that was a good reason to call, and I asked her to tell me what was going on.

"My mother and I had a special event planned for yesterday. She was looking forward to it all week. We kept talking about it. We'd even discussed what she'd wear and what time we'd leave. And then yesterday morning she didn't get up. She just didn't seem interested in going. It was really strange."

I murmured to signal that I was paying attention and grabbed a pen and scratch paper while launching our electronic medical record on my computer. Already, I knew Veronica was right to have called.

"She did get up eventually, but all day she just didn't seem like herself. I asked if she felt sick but she said no. She didn't even mention the thing we were supposed to be doing. I told her I thought we should go to emergency, but she said no, that there was no need, and she didn't want to go."

At this point, I couldn't resist the urge to interrupt. "What's she like usually? Is she healthy?"

In particular, I wanted to know whether Lynne had any medical conditions that might offer clues to whatever was going on. Given Veronica's response, not only might the potential explanations for her mother's changed behavior differ but so might the treatment options and my follow-up queries and next steps.

"Oh, she's great," Veronica said. "She has some problems but nothing too serious—blood pressure, heart disease, arthritis, that sort of thing. That's why she sees Dr. P., but she's in good shape, mentally and physically. We just live together because we like each other."

That made me smile. Meanwhile, I debated whether to ask for a few more specifics. Sometimes families and doctors have different notions of what constitutes minor and major health issues. In theory, I could get the essentials of her medical history from the electronic record. In practice, getting into the record from afar required making my way through a series of password-protected firewalls, and I wasn't in yet. Still, something new was going on with Lynne, and I needed to prioritize determining its urgency.

I asked Veronica to tell me more. "Is she doing basic things the way she usually does them? Eating? Walking? Talking . . . ?"

"She had a good breakfast and some lunch yesterday. Not too much dinner, but she was tired. We did go out for a walk in the afternoon. I thought it was strange that she wanted to walk but didn't want to go to the event."

I relaxed a little. If Lynne was seriously ill, she probably wouldn't have much appetite or enough strength to go out and walk.

"She's just kind of slow," Veronica added. "And vague."

I unrelaxed. "Has she ever been like that before?"

"Never."

At this point I needed to figure out whether there was a brain problem specifically or if the change more likely represented delirium. Although in everyday life *delirium* is used to mean a state of self-delusion or ecstatic excitement, it has a completely different and very specific meaning in medicine. It refers to a syndrome of mental confusion that is always costly (to both the patient and the medical system), usually leads to other complications, and diminishes the patient's chances of a complete recovery. It prolongs the time a person spends in the hospital, leads to permanent declines in general health and mental function, and increases their risk of nursing home placement and death. A seriously ill person of any age can develop delirium, but it occurs most commonly in older patients, especially if they have underlying dementia. Delirium can develop as a result of something as seemingly minor as catching a cold or taking an over-the-counter allergy or sleeping pill. It can happen because of major or minor infections, surgery, a broken bone, a medication, a new environment, and almost anything else.

I asked Veronica whether her mother's speech made sense.

"The paramedics asked her a bunch of questions about her name, my name, the date and year, how old she is, where we live, and she got them all right. She's communicating, just slowly. Our walk was slow too."

Because of age-related differences in disease presentation, doctors often get more relevant and helpful information from old patients when we ask about changes in basic activities. Such questions resemble those used by pediatricians about eating, sleeping, peeing, pooping, and playing. In geriatrics, we use the same first four and add to them questions about mobility, pain, mood, behavior, and how they spend their days. The point is not to infantilize old people but to recognize the biological reality that at both ends of the life span, diseases are less likely to manifest in the ways we define as "standard" and more likely to show up as a change in basic function.

At seventy-nine, Lynne wasn't in the old-old category chronologically or functionally, but her daughter's answers confirmed a problem in need of attention. Whatever it was, it appeared to be serious and slowly progressing. We needed to act before it became catastrophic.

"Mom got worse last night," said Veronica. "She was getting ready for bed and not wearing her pajama bottoms. She never walks around naked. At around ten, before I went to sleep, I saw the light in the bathroom. When

I got up a little before one, it was still on and mom was just standing there. She seemed disoriented and I thought maybe she'd been there that whole time. That's when I called 911."

She paused as if expecting me to admonish her.

I stopped typing her words into our record system. "You did just the right thing."

"The paramedics didn't think so."

"They were mistaken."

"They checked her out and said they couldn't find anything wrong with her. When I said she seemed confused, they said, 'Your mother's almost eighty years old, it's the middle of the night, what do you expect from her?' I was devastated. They made me feel like I had done something wrong by calling 911."

I had to try and behave professionally, even if what I wanted to do was curse and lament, not just those particular paramedics but our entire health care system with its devastating ignorance about old age. I was also already thinking about who we'd need to contact to provide geriatrics training to our city paramedics and all the reasons they would give for not needing it or not having time for it.

"You weren't wrong."

Shaming a patient's concerned relative is, under any circumstance, unacceptable professional behavior. "What happened next?"

She said they looked through her mother's medications.

That was a good next step. Of the many conditions that can cause delirium, drugs are among the most common offenders. Starting a new medication can do it, as can stopping certain types of medicines abruptly without tapering the dose. Occasionally, people can react to something they've been on for years as their body's ability to process the drug changes.

I scrolled down Lynne's medication list in our electronic record. But what appears on our official logs and what a patient is actually taking often differ, so I also asked Veronica what her mother was on and if there had been any recent changes.

Veronica read me the list, then said, "The paramedics checked all the bottles and said she seemed to be taking everything except the antidepressant. I guess she stopped that three weeks ago, though I didn't know about it. They said that was it. That was the problem. They gave her a pill at two thirty this morning and told us both to go back to bed."

I took a deep breath. Suddenly stopping an antidepressant can cause a bad reaction, but the withdrawal would manifest gradually over days, not suddenly three weeks later.

"How is she this morning?" I asked.

"Sleepy. And still not at all herself."

Since Lynne was a fairly healthy seventy-nine-year-old and because the basic activities questions hadn't led me to any specific diagnosis, it now made sense to run through the review of symptoms, or ROS. After discussing the patient's primary concerns, doctors use the ROS to fill in details and ensure nothing else is missed. The questions progress from head to toe, grouping organs by location, such as eyes, ears, nose and throat, and physiological role, such as cardiovascular or nervous system.

Veronica answered some questions herself but mostly she repeated my queries to her mother. I could hear faint *no*s periodically in the background. No fever, cough, shortness of breath. No increased urination or new incontinence. No chest pain. No weakness in a limb or changed vision, speech, or swallowing. No belly pain, nausea, or vomiting. Some diarrhea for a few weeks, but that happened. No blood in her bowel movements.

But then, there it was: Lynne had a headache, and not just any headache. The worst headache of her life. She described it as a ten on a scale of one to ten, where ten is the most severe pain imaginable. That she said she felt fine while experiencing that kind of pain was another worrisome clue.

I told Veronica that we needed to get her mother to the emergency department right away.

"I wanted to take her yesterday and earlier but she wouldn't go."

"She's not herself and she can't make good decisions. Just tell her what's happening."

We agreed that Veronica would phone for the ambulance and I'd call ahead to the hospital. Before we hung up, I told her how glad I was that she had called, that her instincts were just right, and that her mother was lucky to have such a perceptive and persistent daughter. I also promised to give the paramedics feedback on their care of her mother. At the very least, they needed to know that most older adults are not confused, that sudden confusion always indicates a problem in need of medical attention, and that ignoring a family member's concerns is bad medicine.

After a few hours, I logged back into the medical record. On the CAT scan of Lynne's brain, it looked as if someone had spilled black ink onto a white picture. Sometime between when she'd gone to bed Friday night and when her daughter had gone into her bedroom on Saturday morning, she'd begun bleeding into her head. By Sunday morning, she'd had a large hemorrhagic stroke.

Three months later, I recognized Veronica's name in my e-mail inbox. In her message, she apologized for not writing sooner and thanked me for my help and support. She then gave me an update on her mother, who was finally back home: "It has been a difficult journey, but I was able to come home this afternoon and give my Mom a hug. I was able to ask her what she might like for dinner. I was able to plan her eightieth birthday celebration in September." Lynne was changed by the stroke, but her life still provided pleasure and meaning to them both.

Veronica admitted she was still stunned by the paramedics' comments about her mother. The reality is that they probably meant well. They might even have been following procedures. Across the country, the police are called and often make arrests of people with dementia who get lost and trespass or who fight back when "a stranger" (a caregiver they don't recognize) appears to be trying to take off their clothes or make them go somewhere they don't want to go. In cities and prisons, older people are shot when they are "not cooperating" because they cannot hear commands or can no longer fall to their knees. In some cases, as with Lynne, they are assumed to have dementia when they do not, and in others they are assumed to be fully responsible for their actions when they are not because of dementia. Yet when e-mailed about a course designed to fill in geriatrics education and training gaps among practicing health professionals, a locally and nationally prominent physician leader said he couldn't think of anyone who would benefit. In medicine, clinicians often believe that taking care of older patients is the only necessary qualification for taking care of older patients, a logic they would never consider applying to the care of children or people with cancer.

But change is coming. Many police departments, including ours in San Francisco, increasingly recognize the unintended harms to older adults from their lack of geriatric knowledge and have begun training programs. Their efforts may be paying off. In a recent viral news story, a Southern California police officer called by a bank to arrest an upset nonagenarian instead took the man to renew his expired driver's license, then brought him back to the bank, where he successfully cashed his check.

# 4. CHILD

Growing up, I had a rotating assortment of dreams for my future, but none of them included old people or a career in medicine. In my childhood home, books were everywhere. New and used, paperback and hardback, they overflowed from bookshelves and teetered in tall stacks in the family room and on bedside tables. My mother mostly read literary fiction, social and political histories, and the sorts of writing that eventually would be called ethnic literature—books she passed on to me, shaping my worldview and my ambitions for who and what I might become. My father, a research physician, read novels, nonfiction, and medical journals, and when he made an important point about anything, from politics to sports, he quoted facts and numbers gleaned from those sources in the way others might quote scripture. As a result, scientific thinking provided the pillars and joists in the cognitive architecture with which I interpreted ideas and experiences, even in the days when I planned on becoming an anthropologist, editor, or English teacher.

By my teens my greatest interests lay in people, cultures, and stories, not in figuring out how things worked, testing hypotheses, or fixing broken parts. When my high school college counselor gave me a list of colleges to consider, I crossed off every school with math or science requirements. I didn't have a definite idea of what I wanted to do with my life, but knew it wouldn't involve calculus, physics, chemistry, or biology. Once in college, I focused on learning how to read and think critically and on gaining a better understanding of the world and the people in it, finally settling on a double major in history and an "independent concentration" that included hefty doses of anthropology, psychology, literature, and ethnic studies.

The one group I didn't think about was old people. In young adulthood, they seemed to have little relevance in my life. Once I moved across the country for college, my grandparents were far away, and although I passed older adults on the street, saw them in restaurants, and occasionally had them as teachers, these relationships were by chance, casual, and situational. Children, by contrast, were the subjects of volunteer programs, classes, majors, and career options at my university. Their rearing, education, welfare, and even medical care had also been for many years among the few sectors available to working women, so those fields came replete with female role models, increasing their appeal for me. In college, I tutored kids at an inner-city school, volunteered in a program for autistic children, became a Big Sister, and took summer jobs with psychologists studying childhood development. I thought I'd devote my career to children. After all, by helping them you were potentially influencing an entire life. What could beat that?

Beginning my junior year, I volunteered at a health coordination unit for Southeast Asian refugees and learned two things that would change my life: who you are in the world influences your health, and power sometimes stems as much from position and social expectations as ability. Nurses and social workers did the unit's day-to-day work, but once a month a doctor showed up for an hour or two to make all the big decisions. I wondered whether it might be possible to combine the physician's knowledge and authority with the compassionate, collaborative approach the nurses used with our refugee clients, families who had survived war and genocide only to find themselves in a world that didn't welcome or understand them. It was then that I realized that what I wanted most from my career were the skills and position to make a difference in people's lives. Becoming a doctor was a straightforward path to that end and came with the added benefits of job security, a decent income, and society's approval. For me, it took far less courage than heading to New York to work in publishing or joining the amorphous nonprofit sector, and I have always been a coward.

After graduation, I enrolled in a crash-course, postbaccalaureate, premedical program to complete the math and science classes I'd so carefully avoided. Over the next fifteen months, I applied to medical schools and worked as director of special education in a refugee camp on the Thai-Cambodian border.

In Khao-I-Dang, doctors were consulted about everything: not just medical issues but psychological, social, and existential problems as well. That reinforced my view of doctoring as a human enterprise in the broadest sense. The camp's refugees had lived through bombings, starvation, work camps, displacement, and the deaths of countless friends and loved ones. Their past influenced which illnesses they developed, whether they would believe a diagnosis or follow a treatment plan, and their chances of surviving, much less thriving, in their lives. Knowing that, I entered medical school with a different perspective than many of my peers. I didn't think science and medicine had all the answers or that the same disease affected different people in the same ways. I had seen how proximity to death changed how a person lived, and that fixing the body didn't always alleviate suffering.

I expected those facts to inform my medical training. What I found instead was a divide between the goals of health care and the practice of medicine. My training as a doctor focused almost exclusively on science, relegating everything else to, at best, second-class status. When treatments didn't work, instead of recognizing the impact of societal, personal, cultural, and systemic factors or limitations of our research and care, we blamed the patient or moved on to a better case. *She is noncompliant*, we said. Or, *He failed the treatment*. Also, *It's hopeless; there's nothing more we can do*. Such comments were particularly likely to be invoked for populations and diseases that, overtly or covertly, earned the label of "difficult": the homeless or mentally ill, people with obesity or chronic pain, the worried parents of sick children and the frantic adult children of old patients.

But really, anyone was fair game, particularly if they had different priorities than we did or didn't get better. In medicine, it seemed we preferred certain sorts of people and ailments to others. We were most comfortable with problems—like broken bones and inflamed gallbladders, heart disease and cancer—that we could manage either successfully or with the drugs and procedures we knew best. According to studies, most of us also did a better job when treating bodies and lives that might have been our own. Not that we acknowledged that truth. And not that I recognized it in myself when it stained my thoughts and actions during those early years.

Acculturation to the profession's ways of thinking and doing things is essential in medical training. Still, even after I'd bought into the science-as-king party line, it was impossible to train in medicine in Boston and San Francisco in the early 1990s and not see how medical and social values interacted to affect illness experiences. It was also hard not to notice that, after AIDS patients, many of the people we took care of were old, and that often the things we did to help younger patients either didn't work very well or didn't address what our older patients seemed to care about most. Notably, while most doctors refrained from racist, sexist, and homophobic slurs, few seemed to mind disparaging old people. As Samuel Shem's semi-autobiographical bestselling medical novel, *The House of God*, made clear, old people were "gomers," an acronym for *get out of my emergency room*, and defined as "a human being who has lost—often through age—what goes into being a human being." The book is about medicine and medical training, and has remained popular for over forty years because its story is as essentially true and prescient today as it was in the early 1970s. Looking back at it now, among its most remarkable insights is one lesson the narrator learns from caring for his older patients: if he follows the standard rules of medicine by ordering tests and procedures, they will die. He copes with the horror at this outcome by breaking rules and also, tragically, by learning not to care. "Before the House of God," the narrator tells us, "I had loved old people. Now they were no longer old people, they were gomers, and I did not, I could not love them, anymore." Confronted with medicine's dehumanization of older patients, he and the other young doctors become desensitized and dehumanized themselves, perpetuating the harmful cycle.

From my earliest student days in several of this nation's top hospitals— including the one where *The House of God* takes place—it was clear the lowly status of old people extended to the medical specialty dedicated to their care. Just as gerontology, the multidisciplinary study of aging and older adults by people with master's degrees and PhDs, had been relatively invisible compared with child development during my undergraduate studies, geriatrics, unlike its child-focused equivalent, pediatrics, was barely acknowledged during my medical training. Part of the problem was that geriatrics specialists didn't play by the rules of medicine any more than older bodies did. Rather than give physiology, diseases, and curative treatments exclusive primacy, they also considered other factors that might compromise a patient's health or well-being: where they lived, whom they could count on, what they needed to be able to do to maintain their independence, what was most important to them in their health care and lives, and how they were eating, sleeping, moving, eliminating, feeling, and thinking.

We budding doctors had devoted years of our lives to studying science, learning so many new words along the way that we'd essentially become fluent in a new language. We knew most of what there was to know about organs and diseases, bugs and drugs, and we had mastered a stunning array of technologies and procedures. We only had to look around us in the hospitals and clinics of our training centers to see what medicine was and what it looked like at its best. The low and falling ranking of the United States in patient health outcomes relative to other countries didn't bother us because all over the world everyone knew we had the best medical care. After all, we had the most cutting-edge devices and produced the lion's share of medical studies and innovations. Geriatrics included some of that but focused on all those other things too. Where was the fun in that, we asked, and what was the point of it?

RESURRECTION

Entering my new patient's room, I found him in bed with his eyes closed. Though in his late seventies, Dimitri Sakovich had a head full of mostly dark hair and a model's sculpted cheeks and chin. The day before, he had been admitted to our nursing home's advanced dementia unit.

Having come from home, Dimitri arrived with little more than lists of his medical problems and medications. From those few pages, I learned that Dimitri had end-stage Parkinson's, dementia, and several other common chronic diseases, and that he took ten medications, many several times a day. Irina, the unit's head nurse, told me he'd been living with his wife and adult daughter but they could no longer manage his care at home.

I said his name, but Dimitri didn't respond. Then I touched his arm. Nothing. I shook him a bit, repeating his name in a louder voice, and finally his eyes opened. Irina explained in Russian who I was and why we were there. It wasn't clear he could understand her.

With Irina translating, I asked Dimitri two questions: What was his name? Was he having pain? Because Parkinson's slows people down, we had to give him time to respond. I sang a chorus of "Happy Birthday" in my head to make sure I waited long enough.

In response to the first question, Dimitri's lips moved but no word emerged. He didn't even try to answer the second one, so we skipped ahead to the physical exam.

Although one of his hands shook and his limbs showed the rigidity and ratcheting movements characteristic of Parkinson's, he otherwise seemed quite robust. He had well-formed muscles and joints; all his organs looked, felt, or sounded as they should.

Back at the nurses' station, I studied his medication list. On admission to the nursing home, we usually just continued whatever the person had been previously taking, at least until we got a sense of them and their medical history. Dimitri's medications were all commonly used and each was associated with one of his diagnoses. That was a good start. But two appeared on the Beers Criteria, a national list of potentially inappropriate medications for older adults. The list warns of increased risks for adverse reactions. The hope is that doctors will think twice before prescribing such medicines to patients over seventy and, whenever possible, use alternatives.

I asked Irina whether anyone in the family spoke English.

"His daughter," she said. Her face formed a question, I nodded, and she pulled the chart from me to her, flipped to another section, and put her finger on a phone number. I dialed.

A woman answered. "Alyo."

With Irina on standby for translation, I explained who I was. "Oh, hello, Doctor," the woman said in English. "Thank you for taking care of my father."

I gave Irina the thumbs-up so she could return to her own work and asked Svetlana to tell me about her father. Dimitri had been an engineer in the Soviet Union, she said, and her mother was his second wife. They had been married forty-one years and had been in the United States for eight. I asked her about Dimitri's recent health and care, and she described a fairly typical scenario for a person with late-stage Parkinson's. He didn't move or speak much, was confused and incontinent, and lately had eaten little and spent most of his time asleep. I confirmed his other symptoms, diagnoses, and medications and asked if there was anything else I should know.

"Oh, no," she said. "I think that is everything."

This is where the standard medical interview usually ends, but I had more questions. In geriatrics, the goal is to tailor care to the patient's unique amalgam of health status, abilities, values, and care preferences, no matter how healthy or sick they are. I don't always get all this information at the first meeting, but Dimitri wasn't eating or drinking much, and I worried we might need answers to key questions at any moment. Even if he wasn't dying, I had to know more about him to make him comfortable in his new home.

How people address their lives and deaths varies widely and is deeply personal. I couldn't discuss Dimitri's nursing home or end-of-life care with his family unless they knew how sick he was.

"Can you tell me what your understanding is about your father's condition?" I asked, and quickly learned that Svetlana and her mother appreciated the severity of Dimitri's situation. I hoped she also had a sense of what treatments he would and would not want at this stage of his life.

"Did your family ever talk about what would be most important to your father if he could no longer speak for himself?"

There was a noise in the background on Svetlana's end of the line, and I wondered whether her mother was in the room waiting to hear about the conversation in Russian as soon as we were through. "No," Svetlana said. "We don't talk like that."

This is often the case, so I moved on to proxy questions, which sometimes help families and care teams get a sense of a patient's preferences even if they were never explicitly discussed. Unfortunately, Dimitri's parents and grandparents had all died young and fairly quickly, from what sounded like heart disease or infections.

Because it mattered so much, I tried another tack. "Did your father have any friends or family members who had Parkinson's or dementia or a big stroke?" I asked. Dimitri might have commented on the last years or months of their lives, either positively or negatively, in ways that could guide us.

"Maybe," Svetlana said finally. "I'm not sure. I have to ask my mother."

I told her that would be very helpful and gave her my phone number. She began thanking me for my call.

"Just one more question," I said. Some people in Dimitri's condition die quickly; others live for years. I wanted to get a sense of how quickly Dimitri was declining. I asked what her father had been like two weeks earlier, and two months, and six months, and a year.

Svetlana was only partway through her answer when I stood up and grabbed a pen. Five minutes later, I thanked her, hung up, and immediately called Dimitri's neighborhood pharmacy to ask for the dates of first prescription for each of his medications. When I hung up, Irina, who missed nothing on her unit, appeared out of nowhere at my side.

"What?" she said.

"He was perfectly healthy a year ago. Mind, body, everything. Six months ago, he was still walking, talking, reading the newspaper. This may all be drug-induced."

"Oh my God."

I stopped eight of his medications and tapered the other two. I also asked the nurses to check him frequently over the next few days. I wanted to know sooner rather than later if I was wrong and to make sure he remained comfortable no matter what.

By the end of the week, Dimitri could sit up. He began talking, quietly at first, but each day his voice grew stronger and louder. He ate more and moved better. I ordered physical therapy. His blood pressure went up, and I started him on a different, safer medication. The pharmacy records had been consistent with Svetlana's story of her father's decline. He'd been the victim of a "prescribing cascade." It started when he was given a new blood pressure pill, a good and common one, but—as is the case for almost all drugs—one with side effects. In Dimitri, it had precipitated gout. Instead of changing medications, his doctor treated the gout with a strong anti-inflammatory drug that caused heartburn, earning Dimitri another new medicine. And so it went, each side effect treated with another medication that caused another side effect that was treated with yet another medication, and so on. Just as bad, even when his problems got better, as his gout had, the medications were continued. In just a few months, he'd gone from healthy to bedbound.

Drug cascades like Dimitri's are not the primary causes of Parkinson's, dementia, frailty, or disability in older adults, but it's likely a fair number are never diagnosed. Every geriatrician I know has stories like this one. Some other types of clinicians probably do too. Any doctor or pharmacist who looked thoughtfully at Dimitri's medications and didn't use his old age and apparent advanced illness as an excuse to forgo obtaining a detailed medical history would have come to the same conclusion I did. In a health care system where time is the scarcest resource and care is fragmented among doctors without a clear mechanism for designating a recognized team captain, new symptoms are too often attributed to age and disease rather than to the care or drugs that actually caused them.

Six weeks after his admission to the nursing home, we transferred Dimitri to the assisted living unit. The first time I passed him in the downstairs hallway, I nearly didn't recognize him. He wasn't even using a cane. Although he could have moved home, it seemed that he'd found a new life that suited him. He began painting, was elected to the Residents' Council, and acquired a new female friend. Since Dimitri was still married, this caused a small scandal, but he didn't care.

CONFUSION

Before I became a doctor, I thought senility was a normal part of aging. Live long enough, I figured, and memory fails. I didn't realize that *senility* was the lay word for *dementia*, and this syndrome had more than seventy medical causes. Nor did I know that as long as you didn't contract one of those conditions, you could live without dementia into your eighties, nineties, and hundreds. These days, we hear much more about dementia and its most common type, Alzheimer's, but twenty years ago, that wasn't the case. Still, I should have known better based on a sampling of old people in my own family. Granny, my great-grandmother, lived into her nineties and at no time was there anything wrong with her mind. Ditto my maternal grandfather, who died at age eighty-six, and my two grandmothers, who died in their seventies. Incredibly, despite personal experience to the contrary, I thought dementia and aging were synonymous.

I wasn't the only one with that erroneous belief. The word *dementia* appears nowhere on a report from the Centers for Disease Control (CDC) listing the top ten causes of death for all ages in the United States from 1933 through 1998. The word *Alzheimer's* showed up on that listing for the first time in 1994, as the eighth leading cause of death among women. It did not appear on the men's or combined lists until 1999.

The explanation for its appearance late in the twentieth century was not, like AIDS or Zika, that it was either a newly discovered pathogen or newly affecting our populace. Nor can Alzheimer's ascendance be entirely a result of people living longer, though that surge clearly affected not only disease prevalence but public and medical awareness of it. Part of the change reflected the fact that doctors who fill out death certificates are products of their culture and training. In their civilian lives, if they heard about the topic at all, they heard of senility, not dementia. In most medical schools, dementia warranted only a passing mention. In textbooks, it wasn't featured nearly as prominently as similarly common, life-altering diseases. That might have made sense if it was a normal part of aging, although one could argue that any condition that affects a person's body, function, and well-being is a health issue.

Conditions that doctors have not been trained to adequately evaluate or manage are unlikely to appear on death certificates. Certifying clinicians, and even CDC scientists, also may have believed that dementia and aging went hand in hand, that it didn't matter in the same way as heart disease and cancer.

Since 2007, Alzheimer's has been the sixth leading cause of death in the United States, and for people eighty and over, it's now in fifth place for men, third for women. But even that isn't quite right. For the most part, the causes of death that have led the CDC listings for the last century are broad categories of disorders such as "diseases of the heart," "malignant neoplasms," and "accidents" (unintentional injuries). As a result, many diseases fall under each heading, and the numbers of deaths counted are high. If we list heart attacks, heart failure, arrhythmias, and other cardiac conditions separately but cancer as a single entity, for example, heart diseases would not top the list; cancer would. But cancer would also drop lower down the list if we separated out the different types—listing breast, lung, skin, prostate, colon, blood, and each of the many others individually. Yet the CDC considers Alzheimer's a separate disease on its own, rather than grouping the many dementias together. A more taxonomically consistent approach would be to have a dementia category that included vascular, Lewy body, frontotemporal, and all the other dementias. This matters because where a condition appears on this and other lists affects all aspects of medicine—from doctor training to money for research and departments within health systems, as well as the public's imagination and our political and social priorities.

Serious disease always transforms. My father looked like my father until his death at age eighty-four, but in his last years he acted less and less like the dad I had known for the first forty-eight years of my life. That change in a person with dementia is why the condition is sometimes described as a double loss for families. First, the recognizable face and body become those of an unfamiliar character, and then in death, often many years later, everything is gone. In *Elegy for Iris*, John Bayley, who cared for his wife, the writer Iris Murdoch, as she advanced into the late stages of dementia, described the years of her illness this way: "Alzheimer's is, in fact, like an insidious fog, barely noticeable until everything around has disappeared. After that, it is no longer possible to believe that a world outside fog exists." It seems intentionally unclear whether Bayley is speaking for his wife, for himself as her caregiver, or for them both.

My father did not live into those final stages. Until the last year or two of his life, he could still fool people who didn't know him. Once, as he and I sat in an emergency department cubicle with my mother, who, light-headed from a stomach bug, had fainted and hit her head, the nurses had my father sign papers he could no longer fully understand. Later that day, when it was clear the cut on my mother's head was the worst of her injuries, one of the emergency physicians tending her—a man who had won multiple awards for his thoughtful, knowledgeable teaching—said the paperwork would take time and I should feel free to go back to work. Apparently, he hadn't put my father's vague, sometimes irrelevant comments and his appearance—sloppy without my mother's oversight that morning—together into a likely diagnosis. I had to tell him that I needed to stay for my father's sake. Without help, my father was unable to find the bathroom, or the cafeteria one floor up, or his way back to my mother's cubicle.

Dementia's early stages can be subtle, discernible only to the trained or watchful eye. In describing her mother in the months leading up to an Alzheimer's diagnosis, the French writer Annie Ernaux says this:

> She had changed. She started laying the table much earlier . . . She became irritable . . . She was inclined to panic if she received a circular from her pension fund . . . Things started happening to her. The train she was waiting for on the station platform had already left. When she went out to buy something, she discovered all the shops were closed. Her keys kept disappearing . . . She seemed to have to brace herself against invisible threats.

The most common dementia, Alzheimer's disease is, by definition, gradual in onset. Symptoms generally begin several years prior to diagnosis. Early on, its manifestations are subtle and often attributed to old age or inattention. "I'm having a senior moment," people say of their normal brain's normal lapses, laughing and at the same time terrified. Americans fear dementia more than any other disease except cancer. Aging changes the brain, and diseases cause dementia. People with dementia struggle to do things in their lives they previously found easy: managing finances, handling their medications, shopping, cooking, driving. Slowed processing, delayed recall, and greater sensitivity to distraction are inconveniences, not major impairments. They are fundamentally different from not being able to roughly copy a simple drawing or name more than a few animals when given a minute to think about it. An older person with a healthy brain may do things more slowly or differently for reasons that have more to do with their hands, their eyes, or their aging brain, but they can do them.

A lot of Americans have dementia: 5.3 million in 2015, which is four and a half times more people than have AIDS—and some estimates suggest that only about half the people with dementia have been diagnosed. While most older adults do not have dementia, age is a key risk factor. Over 80 percent of people with dementia are over seventy-five years old. But just 14 percent of adults in their seventies or older have dementia on average. Dementia is more common among black Americans than whites, with Latinos falling somewhere in between, and it's least likely in Asian Americans, but there is significant variability among ethnic group subtypes. Even after a diagnosis of Alzheimer's, the average person lives eight to twelve more years and dies of heart disease or cancer, just like the majority of their peers. Dementia is almost always progressive, but sudden and significant drops in function are usually from drugs, infections, or strokes and can be treated. There is no single truth with dementia, and the reality of living with it is complex, fraught, funny, infuriating, gratifying, tragic, and profound.

Until recently in medicine, even though patients with dementia needed care from most types of doctors, only neurologists, psychiatrists, and geriatricians learned much about the disease during their training, and what each specialty learned differed. Neurologists prioritized diagnosis by brain pathology and treatment with medications. Psychiatrists attended to dementia patients' anxiety, depression, and psychotic symptoms. And geriatricians, new in medicine and few in number, focused on managing a patient's health, social situation, and physical environment to maximize their and their caregivers' well-being. These days most doctors know something about dementia, though it still falls far below the standards for other common, devastating diseases.

Studies published at regular intervals from the 1980s on have found that doctors frequently miss the diagnosis of dementia, at least until its middle stages. At the University of California, San Francisco (UCSF), where I work and have spent most of my career, just 3 percent of patients over age sixty-five were documented in 2018 as having some kind of cognitive impairment—way lower than you'd expect in patients at that age. Recent research has asked why that is. Some clinicians don't have the relevant knowledge or skills. Others report they suspect it in patients but feel there's no point in making the diagnosis, since they have little to offer by way of treatment. Still others admit to feeling they lack both the time and wherewithal to make a diagnosis so existentially abstruse.

Dementia forces us to think about what makes us human. If an accurate definition included people with dementia along with the rest of us, we might find it easier to cope with a disease that currently strips the living of their basic humanity. We also might have broader notions of what counts as "medical" treatment, more clinicians with the necessary care skills, and greater flexibility in our health system to respond to highly varied patient needs.

In 2010 I was asked to give the "Geriatrics Year in Review" lecture for a continuing education course. Each presenter had to select and interpret the most important published studies in their specialty from the previous twelve months.

The day after I submitted the brief initial description of my talk, the course director told me there was a problem. "You can't do dementia. Somebody is already giving a whole talk on that."

The somebody was a prominent dementia researcher and head of a major memory institute. Under his leadership, a small program had become a vibrant center for research, teaching, and clinical care.

"I bet we'll be talking about different things," I replied, reasoning that neurologists focused on science, while I would be discussing clinical care.

The course director wasn't convinced. "It's really important that we don't have the same material covered twice."

Given our different emphases and the fact that over seventeen hundred articles had been published that year on the dementia, I suspected we could avoid duplication.

"How about this?" I offered. "I'll ask for his outline or slides, and if there's any overlap, I'll take dementia out of my talk. But if we're covering different studies, it stays in."

He agreed, and I sent the researcher an e-mail.

A few weeks later, a friendly note and his slides appeared in my inbox. Most of his slides focused on molecular changes and drug targets in different dementias, particularly the rare types. His images included electron microscopy photos and PET scans of diseased brains taken from journals like *Nature*. It looked like a terrific talk that would bring the audience up-to-date on the current understanding of dementia biology.

For the dementia portion of my presentation, I had selected three studies from top clinical journals. One established diagnostic criteria for the dementia precursor condition known as mild cognitive impairment; the second offered guidelines for evaluation and management of driving risk in dementia; and the third was a large study of quality of life and hospitalizations in patients with late-stage disease.

I sent the continuing education course director a note, assuring him that my talk and the researcher's had no overlap.

Science is essential for understanding and advancing medicine, but it doesn't always have direct utility in patient care. Seeing via electron microscopy the helical filaments in the brain of a person who died from frontotemporal dementia helps doctors understand how and why that disease differs from other dementias; however, it tells them little of what they need to know to diagnose or treat patients with that condition, and does not help their caregivers manage the often socially unacceptable behaviors common in that particular dementia. By contrast, learning that the survival of patients with advanced dementia is similar to that for metastatic cancer or end-stage heart failure provides doctors with critical information about how to help patients and families with end-of-life planning and how to minimize patients' distress and physical suffering as death nears.

The researcher's talk reflected not just his own interests but medicine's more generally. In the wake of their huge contributions to twentieth-century medicine, lab tests, radiologic studies, procedures, and drugs began to be viewed as the primary and, often, the only constituents of medical care. That's problematic when it comes to diseases like dementia. Despite diagnostic advances and a handful of minimally helpful drug treatments, most of the knowledge and skills needed to take good care of patients comes from a different toolbox. The needed expertise includes helping patients manage the practical challenges and existential distress of a dementia diagnosis; techniques for communicating with people with different types and stages of cognitive impairment; the ability to recognize and manage caregiver distress; mastery of not just drugs but also less toxic and more effective social, behavioral, and environmental approaches to symptoms; and prowess in navigating the difficult terrain of life planning, family grief, conflict, and tough decision-making as the disease progresses.

A few years later, I learned I'd underestimated the researcher. His center now studies, teaches about, and provides some of those geriatrics-based approaches to dementia care while still doing cutting-edge science and neurological evaluations.

\* \* \*

The dementias can't currently be prevented or cured, though some of the more common types can be delayed by minimizing the same risk factors associated with heart disease, stroke, and certain cancers: regular exercise, healthy eating, avoiding obesity and cigarettes. These things are harder to do if you're poor and lack the access, education, resources, or hopefulness about your own life to support healthy living, facts that account for at least part of the ethnic variation in prevalence. They are harder still if your community has been poor for a long time and developed traditions, including favorite foods and family activities, that are simultaneously deeply meaningful and unhealthy. Some poor health comes down to individual choices and behaviors, and some of us are better set up to succeed than others. In dementia, as in most of medicine, social inequality leads to bad health and unnecessary health care expenses.

In many ways, dementia is the prototype of the American approach to old age, and also its metaphor. When and how we talk about it, what we do and don't understand about its impact on lives, and how we have and haven't dealt with it both societally and medically in recent decades perfectly exemplifies our attitudes and modus operandi to the larger topic of aging. The questions so often asked about dementia apply equally well to old age itself: Who is this changed self? What is our place in and relationship to society and other people? There is an important difference between an older person who can no longer run a 10K race but who can still work a register, sit on the Supreme Court, provide afterschool grandchild care, drive for a ride-share company, be a museum docent, or run a medical center, and one who can no longer find her way home or remember his children. What's not different is that both are human beings worthy of attention and care. The former may become the latter, and the latter was once the former. They are the future "us," and we are the past "them."

## STANDARDS

As CEO and chief medical officer of Denver Health, Patricia Gabow transformed a large safety-net health system by introducing systematized

approaches, called clinical pathways, to specific medical problems. Such
pathways are among the most effective ways to take cultural biases and physician idiosyncrasies out of patient care. They encourage or compel doctors to
follow standard approaches and practices by providing unambiguous goals
and essential, evidence-based steps. Gabow's pathways resulted in unprecedented health outcomes in Denver Health patients who had often
received lesser care for reasons ranging from little education, low income,
hunger, and skin color to mental illness, addiction, and disease burden. She
was rightly proud of her work.

But when her mother—a frail ninety-four-year-old with advanced
dementia—injured herself in a fall, Gabow realized the standard care she
had put into place, while transformative for many patients, was not what
her mother needed. It wasn't just that Gabow feared the clinical pathways
wouldn't help her mother; she knew they would hurt her. Her mother's
designated decision-maker, she said no to a long list of procedures: a neck
brace, a heart monitor, an IV, a CT scan, orthopedic surgery, and a hospital
stay, but yes to sewing up a forearm gash, a splint for her mother's multiply
broken wrist, and nonoperative treatment at home for the hip fracture.

The hospital doctors were uncomfortable with this last choice, arguing
that the surgery was quick and minor, but Gabow—more in her physician-
daughter than physician-CEO role—saw it differently:

> I pictured the intravenous line, which she would try to take out, leading
> to soft restraints that she would also struggle to get out of. Then sedation
> and a downward spiral. Every part of this would seem like torture to
> her—and I would have to watch this torture.

Instead, after calling the vacationing head of orthopedics on his cell phone,
Gabow and her mother went home. Within a week, her mother was walking
thirty feet with a physical therapist. Not only had Gabow saved her mother's
life; she'd saved the health system approximately $156,000. It was a win-win,
but only because Gabow had the knowledge, authority, and money to circum-
vent our usual medical and social care systems.

Gabow derived the cost-savings figure from the services that would have
been unhesitatingly provided by the hospital and paid for by her mother's

insurance had Gabow not refused them. In the past, she hadn't seen how the standards she herself had put into place did not address the needs of all patient populations. Clinical pathways assumed all patients with the same condition would benefit from the same treatment. Standards are helpful, but they almost always focus on individual diseases without considering that a person might have multiple interacting diseases, or that both disease and treatment behave and are experienced differently by the young, old, very old, and by people who are otherwise healthy, chronically ill, or dying. Equally important, as the physician-anthropologist Arthur Kleinman pointed out in *The Illness Narratives*, for patients of all ages, our health care system still too often treats *diseases* rather than attending to *illness*—the unique expression of that disease in a particular human being.

In Gabow's mother's case, our health care system also saved money for two other notable reasons. Years before the fall, Gabow helped her mother determine and express her health and end-of-life wishes while she still could. The decisions Gabow now made on behalf of her mother reflected her mother's values and preferences; they were as close as the older woman could come to retaining control over her own life and dignity, as well as relieving her daughter of difficult decision-making without guidance. Absent such information, Gabow might have been tempted to say yes to surgery or a host of other costly, standard procedures more likely to harm than help her ancient, frail mother. Many people err on the side of biotechnologically aggressive care, and doctors in our current medical culture rarely explain how cruel and injurious that can be or adequately present alternatives better matched to the person's situation. Last but not least, our health system saved money because the Gabows paid out of pocket for most of the at-home care needed after the fall.

Families often assume doctors know best. But most medical professionals are the products and purveyors of a system that pays for only certain sorts of care, even when it's more likely to prolong suffering than to restore health and even when, in report after report, most state they would not choose that care for themselves or their loved ones. Among the reasons clinicians cite for not liking to take care of old patients is the moral distress they feel when they are asked to provide futile treatments that cause significant suffering. People shouldn't need to have parented a physician to get the care that suits them best in old age. But the problem goes beyond doctors.

Our current care system rarely questions the need for procedures, and unquestioningly pays for the complications they routinely cause frail old patients. It does not, however, reimburse for the care that might allow those same patients to return home safely and comfortably, as Gabow's mother did. The child of another patient with similar health problems would have been forced to choose between hospitalization and a downward spiral for her mother, or her own loss of job and income. Gabow's calculation of $156,000—a prolonged hospital stay, subsequent nursing home stay, and readmissions—is the rule, not the exception, for most people at some point in old age.

A common argument against such initiatives is that most people can't afford the sort of care Gabow's mother received. Such arguments forget that we are already paying for extremely expensive care that doesn't help.

OTHER

Since most of us reach old age, you might think old people would engender fewer "Not me" and "Not my problem" reactions than many categories defining our social identities. After all, old age is not like gender or race. For the most part, people remain what they were at birth. Nor is it quite like cancer or heart disease: although many people get those diseases, not everyone does, and you don't know which camp you'll be in until you get one. But unless you die, you will become old. Beliefs and appearance, nationality and religion, also differ from old age. Although you might not make changes in your politics or hairstyle, throughout life you have that option. Perversely, then, it seems likely that part of the reason why we band together so universally and effectively against old age is precisely because it's indiscriminate. It doesn't matter who you are.

Early childhood aside, youth comes with increasing strength, social, and sexual power, each defined in ways that make them inevitably temporary and, therefore, all the more precious. This wasn't always the case. In Puritan

America, older people represented the highest in human achievement and were duly venerated. Nowadays, the public celebration of young models, actors, and athletes exceeds the rewards and accolades offered everyone else, even the billionaire techies who now shape so much of our daily lives. But there may be an even more elemental explanation for our othering of old age. By definition, social identity is relational. Human beings figure out who they are by comparing themselves with others. As Simone de Beauvoir explained, "Otherness is a fundamental category of human thought. Thus it is that no group ever sets itself up as the One without at once setting up the Other over against itself."

Spending our first many decades with old as Other has consequences. The octogenarian poet turned essayist Donald Hall offered one of the best articulations of old age's essential dilemma:

> When we turn eighty, we understand that we are extraterrestrial. If we forget for a moment that we are old, we are reminded when we try to stand up, or when we encounter someone young, who appears to observe green skin, extra heads and protuberances. People's response to our separateness can be callous, can be goodhearted, and is always condescending.

Clearly, being old comes with real challenges, but those challenges are only part of what makes old age difficult. The critical ingredient is our response to it. The biological facts of life alone don't shape our experience of old age, or Puritan elders wouldn't have received the best seats in houses of worship. The personal, societal, and cultural constructs we build around our biology are no less important in shaping our old age. We age at the intersection of nature and nurture.

When it comes to age, othering is not confined to old people. It begins early, happens often, and is usually but not always negative. As Sarah Manguso says in *Ongoingness*, "From the point of view of a child, a mother is a fixed entity, a monolith, not a changing, evolving human organism [that is] similar, in many ways, to a young person." Her comment can be read as a limitation of the young brain, but also represents our earliest sense of otherness and our first almost instinctive reduction of the other to something distant and abstract. Across history and geography, we humans have done this to those who differ from us in tribe, nationality, race, religion, gender, sexuality, ability, politics, class, caste, priorities, company, industry, region, dress, comportment, and so much more. The individual other is seen not as a unique human being but as a group representative, and the group is not so much made up of real human beings as it is a notion—simplified, singular, and essentially different. The phenomenon includes traits we can control, ones we can't, and, more often than I would have ever expected, the life stages we don't currently inhabit. If younger people are inclined to call someone "over the hill," it seems the older among us are equally liable to express exasperation about "kids these days."

Given the ubiquity of othering, our tendency toward it seems part of being human. And like many of our other unjust, unkind, and self-defeating social tendencies, recognizing it is the necessary first step toward a more thoughtful approach, though no guarantee of such moral progress. When it comes to aging, that different approach should somehow account for the fact that while much of who we are doesn't change over time, our age group does. On the *Today* show, at age seventy, Cher said, "I look in the mirror and I see this old lady staring back at me. And I have no idea how she got there!"

In discussing race, Claudia Rankine has talked of how, in trying to account for the world around them, people often want "to write about the other without investigating their relationship to the other, and that, I think, is what became or becomes problematic." She points out that until we understand that much of whiteness and blackness—and, I would add, much of youth and old age—is fabricated, we end up "resorting to stereotypes that are made by the culture." Even about ourselves.

Said the poet Molly McCully Brown, who was born with cerebral palsy and has spent much of her life in a wheelchair, "Language has so much to do with how we explain ourselves to ourselves and to others . . . I'm grateful to have had these scientific and concrete explanations for why and how my body works and my brain works, or doesn't work, the way that it does. But I will say that it does shape your sense of yourself. You know, the earliest language I had for my body was a list of the things that were wrong with it and a list of the things that people were doing to make it, quote unquote, better. And I think that does really shape your sense of who you are."

Othering and stereotypes allay our anxieties about how little in the world and even in our own lives we can control. They give us shortcuts "embedded in larger archetypes, ideals, or myths that societies use to infuse experience with shared meaning and coherence" by which to understand ourselves, others, and the world. They allow us to see a type or trope, to look rather than to notice—a critical distinction. When we look at something, we merely direct our gaze. When we notice it, it's known to us in an intimate and particular way. Thus, in the late nineteenth century, when Americans began viewing the body as a machine and not a divine gift, their sense of old age changed too, in ways that encouraged looking over noticing. Having previously seen old people as closer to God, Americans now saw them through an industrial lens, lacking function and efficiency. Old age began to seem "less than" compared with youth, and aging came to be associated with decline and obsolescence—conditions people distance themselves from even today, invoking that same singularly mechanistic definition of human worth.

# 5. TWEEN

NORMAL

According to our medical school doctor-professors, we would not be able to recognize and understand disorders unless we knew what normal looked like. Normal, we learned, only days into the first year of medical school, was a healthy 70 kg male. Although no one said so, this "Norm" fellow was also obviously white, heterosexual, and, in the spirit of Goldilocks's three bears, neither too young nor too old. The transmission of those last three traits was not explicit, but they were easily deduced. With the exception of human embryology and certain conditions related to youth or old age, our textbooks focused almost exclusively on adults.

In case studies, on the rare occasions when Norm didn't have those "basic," "normal," "healthy" traits, he always had a pathology that tipped us off to his demographic deviation, conditions such as pregnancy, sickle cell anemia, AIDS, or stroke. In those pre-obesity days, 70 kg Norm was never a child. Kids were a different species that we would learn about later.

I didn't question the framework that portrayed the vast majority of human beings as something other than normal—none of us did. Fortunately for me, there was no question that children mattered at least a little in medicine, despite being fundamentally abnormal.

Starting with fertilization, we spent weeks listening to lectures, discussing cases in small groups, and looking at tissue under the microscope, moving chronologically from embryology through to physical maturity. We learned about bodily changes and psychosocial development in neonates, toddlers, children, and adolescents, topics touched on again in our second year, when we were introduced to childhood diseases and deformities, congenital and acquired. If you added those weeks of classroom learning to our required third-year pediatrics rotations—a month in the hospital and a weekly session or two in a pediatrics clinic during the outpatient block—all medical students spent several months learning about children. That sounds like good training for future doctors, unless you consider that childhood constitutes a quarter of most lives, and a few months was by no means a quarter of our education. In those days, it never occurred to me to wonder how priorities were selected in medicine or why an age group's health care needs and health service use didn't affect how much time we spent studying it.

Scientific knowledge is considered objective, but it operates within the same social structures and biases as those who conduct it. For most of the history of Western medicine, no distinction was made between the treatment of children and adults. That approach paralleled the societal approach to childhood. Kids were not essentially different from adults, just smaller. Accordingly, they were put to work as soon as they could walk, as they still are today in many parts of the world. Over centuries, they were portrayed in paintings as adults of small stature, with clothing and bodily proportions the same as those of grown-ups and thus anatomically inaccurate. In the mid-1800s, England and several European countries passed child labor laws, and soon thereafter childhood became a more distinct period of life. The specialty of pediatrics emerged in response to those larger societal changes. Since the best medical literature of the day came from across the Atlantic, physicians in the United States were aware of the new specialty but weren't much interested. Children were the purview of women, and medicine the purview of men. Although the first pediatrics organizations were founded in the late 1800s in the United States, pediatrics didn't get much general attention until the lead-up to World War I, when the powerful realized our country would have more soldiers if fewer children died. Like so much history, pediatrics owes its existence both to some people doing the right thing for the right reasons and to advantaged others doing that same thing because it also helped preserve their power and supremacy.

When the numbers of women entering medicine transitioned from token to near parity, women's health emerged as an area of scholarship and care worthy of clinics, departments, research grants, and centers of excellence. The class ahead of mine, the class of 1991, was the first at Harvard

Medical School to be half female, half male. That's nearly thirty years ago, yet we still speak of "health" and "women's health," implying they are distinct entities and that health is a mostly male condition. Concern for the health of brown- and black-skinned people, who make up a majority of human beings worldwide and a significant proportion of the U.S. population, followed a similar trajectory. By the start of the twenty-first century, with the student bodies of many schools beginning to resemble our diverse population, the marked racial and ethnic disparities in health care began receiving attention and funding. Now medical schools have diversity deans and the National Institutes of Health operates a National Institute on Minority Health and Health Disparities.

These efforts, helpful and needed as they are, also paradoxically reinforce the status quo. They are overlays, not essentials, focused on "minorities," even in places like California, where so-called nonwhites are a majority. When people are defined by what they are not, we are in trouble.

Social forces and cultural rationales determine what doctors study and value. Throughout medical history, this has played out in brilliant discoveries, lifesaving treatments, and better health, but also in worse health, injuries, and deaths. The negative outcomes have been unintentional—sometimes. Other times, there have been overt travesties and pervasive conditions of nefarious neglect. Among the glaring blemishes on the tip of the iceberg of my profession's not-so-distant past are the Tuskegee syphilis experiments on black men, the blaming of mothers for their children's autism, and the sterilization of poor and disabled people without their consent. In science and medicine, as in the rest of life, bias infiltrates our thoughts, actions, emotions, and priorities in ways we can only partially control, and then only if so inclined. Without exception, most types of human beings haven't received the focus, funding, respect, and care they needed for good health until they were associated with a pressing national concern or could advocate for themselves.

In medical school, we occasionally encountered Norm's 60 kg sister, "Norma." The reason for her infrequent appearances was another unstated but easily ascertained curricular lesson. What mattered most about Norma by far—indeed, what warranted her place in our studies—were her sex organs, hormones, and reproductive abilities, which apparently didn't pertain to most of medicine. We sometimes discussed diseases with racial or ethnic predilections—terminology that almost always referred to anyone who was not of European descent. We learned that the differences between Norm and Norma, and between Norm and people who were black or brown, both complicated medical research and created problems in patient care. For example, black people didn't respond to certain first-line medications for high blood pressure the way Norm did, and this "unresponsiveness" put them at an especially high risk for strokes. Similarly, Norma had failed to read the heart attack manual and regularly presented with "atypical" symptoms—ones different from Norm's—thereby causing dangerous delays in her diagnosis and treatment. It turned out that differences in gender, race, and ethnicity affected disease course, drug effectiveness, clinical care, and health outcomes, including mortality. Fortunately for me, by the time I entered my clinical years, some people had begun suggesting that excluding a majority of the population from trials that help us understand and treat diseases might not be such a terrific idea. Norm's norms weren't universal after all.

Thirty years later, medicine has made incremental, not fundamental, progress. In recent years, as I have traveled the country giving a talk that mentions Norm, medical students nod and smile in recognition. Despite the increased attention to most forms of human diversity in medical schools today, future doctors still learn little about older patients, and most of them rarely question why that might be. I don't like that unreflective bias, but I understand it. My classmates and I were exactly the same. Had I been asked whether I had learned enough geriatrics in medical school, a question that once appeared on the Association of American Medical Colleges' (AAMC) annual graduation survey, I would have said yes. Three-quarters of recent medical students give that same answer, though few get much more training in the physiology or care of older adults than I did. The problem with knowing very little about a topic is that you don't know how much you don't know, and the problem with valuing one social group less than others is that your ignorance about them doesn't bother you. In the classrooms, clinics, and culture of medicine, even a small dose of geriatrics strikes most people as more than enough. Perhaps that's why the words *geriatrics, elderly,* and *old* are entirely absent from current AAMC surveys, which dutifully list so many other specialties and populations.

We in the class of 1992 considered ourselves open-minded, thoughtful, and compassionate. While we lobbied for better care of underserved and vulnerable people and more attention to women's and LGBT health, it never occurred to us that we might be leaving out an entire social group. Working with old people either didn't occur to or have much appeal for anyone.

At the same time, illness in old age wasn't entirely ignored during my medical school years. Like women, old people often presented "atypically" when experiencing common conditions, and, like children, they routinely developed life-stage specific conditions. Children and adults each had specialized doctors, hospitals, and clinics because they needed them. Old people only had nursing homes, which weren't really medical facilities at all, as their name made perfectly clear. Besides, nursing homes had been around for ages—you could tell by looking at many of them—and clearly served a purpose. People moved there when they couldn't really do much, and—close as they were to death—it didn't seem surprising that we couldn't do much for them. The residents we worked with in the hospitals often pointed out that medicine's usual goals of saving lives and curing disease seemed misplaced or ill-advised in many older patients. There being no apparent alternatives, they focused on sending older patients back to their nursing homes as quickly as possible.

For years after I became a geriatrician, if I'd been asked whether we were taught much about conditions particular to old age, I would have said, *Very little.* Several of my medical school textbooks argue otherwise. Those thick volumes contain detailed information on common geriatric syndromes, including delirium, incontinence, and falls, and occasional mention of unique disease presentations and needs. Yet such topics didn't get attention proportional to their effect on patients' lives or prevalence in hospitals and clinics. Even when they were covered, their impact was undermined by what's known as the "hidden curriculum," a "set of commonly held understandings, customs, rituals and taken-for-granted aspects in the clinical setting." The second-class citizenship of older patients in medicine is entrenched and systematic.

Among my accumulated professional texts is the maroon 1987 edition of a medical book long considered the bible of history-taking and physical examination. Curious about its contents, given my recollections of medical school, I looked up the most common disorder associated with old age. Cognition and dementia received just two and three lines, respectively, in the index, while heart disease, which occurs in both middle and old age, had over ninety lines and multiple subheadings, such as *causes*, *assessment of*, and *techniques of examination*, none of which appear under *dementia*. Near *dementia*, another D condition also got three listings. *Drusen* are yellow or white spots of extracellular material that accumulate in the back of the eye with age. Although now known to sometimes occur along with macular degeneration, a serious eye disease, that was not the case when the book gave drusen and dementia equal attention. Also notable is a "D word" that's missing altogether. Even then, *death* was an exceedingly common diagnosis that warranted a careful physical examination.

Those omissions were typical of twentieth-century medicine. The fifty major textbooks from across medical specialties were organized into disease-oriented chapters with little or no end-of-life care content. We all die of something, mostly diseases, and death from those diseases rarely occurs all of a sudden. A fifth of the way into the twenty-first century, most books have chapters on death and dying, yet the different physiology and pathophysiology of older bodies and late-stage illness and lives continue to get short shrift.

A key reason for this is historical. Medical advances led to cures of diseases that for millennia had killed people, surely and usually rapidly: infections, childbirth, and blocked bowels, then high sugars and high blood pressure, failing hearts and kidneys, as well as certain traumas and tumors. By later in the twentieth century, doctors could unclog arteries to prevent heart attacks and forestall strokes, replace failing vital organs via transplantation, and treat certain cancers with targeted therapies. The phrase "miracle of modern medicine" felt apt.

As people lived longer, it became clear that those cures had consequences. They developed chronic and more slowly lethal diseases, as longer-lived cells had more time and opportunities for replication errors and toxic exposures, and as damage accumulated in organs like brains, hearts, lungs, livers, intestines, and kidneys. Parts like ears, eyes, joints, and feet sometimes wore out even when essential internal organs held on.

Although American medicine now recognizes the "epidemic of chronic disease" and "aging epidemic" as among health care's main challenges, chronic ailments and the often older or aged patients who suffer from them, along with the professionals who focus on them and the tools and techniques for treating them, remain relegated to second-class citizenship.

### DIFFERENT

In an essay he asked me to read, a resident physician described how he had allocated just fifteen minutes for the admission of a dying patient, figuring it was "yet another dying old woman." After admitting another patient, he went to see the dying woman, who turned out to be in her forties, though physically and mentally in exactly the condition he expected. Suddenly, the time he'd allotted for her care seemed wholly inadequate. In the last part of the essay, he wrote about how bad he felt and how he had ended up confessing his mistake to several other residents. Most of them had had similar experiences. The young doctors agreed the takeaway lesson of the experience was that they needed to list age more prominently on handoffs to each other so the receiving physician could plan their time appropriately.

"Have you written the ending yet?" I asked via e-mail. "It's done," he replied. "It ends with the lesson. I thought that's what the journal wanted?" Apparently neither he nor his co-residents had noticed that, given two people in identical medical condition, they ascribed greater time and value to the final care of one over the other. It chilled me, though not as much as the alternative: that they did notice the differential but thought it morally justifiable.

Over a half century ago, in his seminal book, *The Nature of Prejudice*, the Harvard psychologist Gordon Allport pointed out, "People who are aware of, and ashamed of, their prejudices are well on the road to eliminating them." In contrast are those who are neither aware nor ashamed. In medical settings, grossly prejudicial comments about old people are uttered without shame or with obliviousness to their blatant bias. Such comments are acceptable in medicine because they are acceptable in life. The devaluing of old people is ubiquitous and unquestioned, a great unifier across the usual divides of class, race, geography, and even age.

In the 1960s, the U.S. physician Robert Butler coined the term *ageism*, which he defined as "a process of systematic stereotyping of and discrimination against people because they are old, just as racism and sexism accomplish this with skin color and gender." Butler helped establish the National Institutes on Aging in the United States and founded the first department of geriatrics at an American medical school. He won the Pulitzer Prize for General Nonfiction for his 1975 book, *Why Survive?: Being Old in America*. Many of the book's observations are as on-target today as they were forty years ago.

"Aging," wrote Butler, "is the neglected stepchild of the human life cycle. Though we have begun to examine . . . death, we have leaped over that long period of time preceding death known as old age." He ascribed this neglect to ageism, noting that older adults are often viewed as universally sharing certain negative attributes, including senility and rigid thoughts and beliefs. In fact, old age is the most varied time of life; there are the eighty-year-olds who hold public office, work in factories, and run marathons, and there are those who live in nursing homes because they can no longer walk, think, or care for themselves.

Why, then, might people ascribe such uniform negativity to old age? Butler had the following explanation: "Ageism allows the younger generations to see older people as different from themselves; thus, they subtly cease to identify with their elders as human beings." While this makes sense, it doesn't fully explain the widespread need to hold older adults apart. It's also true that we feel sympathy for people with malaria, lung disease, or cancer, but most of us don't and won't have those challenges. We are safe. Not so for old age. Barring an early death, old age is every human's fate, and generally not one met with eager anticipation. In some ways, even death is more attractive. It's more clear-cut, more definitive; we are either alive or dead. For many, it is the way in which life might be compromised by advanced age, limping slowly rather than leaping toward death, that brings the greatest dread.

A few years ago, the National Council on Aging released a public service video about flu prevention featuring an attractive sixty-five-year-old actress being denied the vaccine at her doctor's office because she looked too young. A week later, the million-dollar Palo Alto Longevity Prize was announced as "dedicated to ending aging." While the flu video provided important information, it implied that attractiveness and being sixty-five or older are mutually exclusive. The Longevity Prize may inspire important advances, but it also raises questions about whether we should be trying to "cure" one part of normal human development or reward exclusively biological approaches to existential challenges.

While well-intentioned efforts, both examples illustrate a common way that age bias adversely affects our approach to aging. We tolerate negative attitudes about old age to degrees that we—at least publicly and officially—no longer tolerate racism or sexism. We treat old age as a disease or problem, rather than as one of three major life stages. We approach old age as a singular, unsavory entity and fail to adequately acknowledge its great pleasures or the unique attributes, contributions, physiology, and priorities of older adults.

Our age bias is so profound that actions viewed as outrageous when applied to other groups are considered acceptable when it comes to older adults. It's virtually impossible to imagine release of a video in which a health professional refuses to give the flu vaccine to an attractive patient because of her skin color, or a prize with the goal of accelerating childhood so parents are less burdened by years of dependency and expense.

Sometimes when teaching, I ask the assembled students or practicing health professionals about what proportion of older Americans live in nursing homes. The answers usually range from 20 to 80 percent, exponentially higher than the actual figures of about 3 to 4 percent overall and 13 percent among the oldest old. In reality, most people over age sixty-five are content, active, and living independently. But we rarely acknowledge how well old age can and often does go, with years and decades offering new opportunities for work, fun, family, leisure, learning, and contributing. Instead, in everyday life, our attention is directed at baldness, stooped posture and slowed paces, wrinkles and canes and hearing aids. In medicine, we work with a biased sample. When older people are doing well and when they are ill but otherwise fairly well, we think of them as middle-aged, if we think of them at all. That leaves "old" associated with the common, disquieting extreme: old people who are ill, disabled, or almost dead. Perhaps it is because the effects of age are visible in even the healthiest older adults and most people do become ill or disabled in some way before death that we reduce the last, decades-long phase of life to a single, noxious state, despite clear evidence of its joys and variety.

The English literary humanist William Hazlitt described prejudice as "the child of ignorance." This comment rings true for certain sorts of prejudice. But we all have parents and grandparents, or friends and mentors, who are old. Sometimes, it seems, prejudice is born less of ignorance than of fear and dread. I am inclined to go with Voltaire, who said, "We are all formed of frailty and error; let us pardon reciprocally each other's folly." Obviously, we must do better.

While elimination of prejudice is utopian, recent advances in the rights, achievements, and medical care of systematically marginalized groups offer precedents for how we can reduce bias and improve care. The first step toward a less ageist health system is acknowledging the problem. As Allport pointed out: "If a person is capable of rectifying his erroneous judgments in the light of new evidence he is not prejudiced . . . A prejudice, unlike a simple misconception, is actively resistant to all evidence that would unseat it." Medicine has a problem, and so does our larger culture.

No one disputes that older adults differ physiologically from younger adults, and abundant evidence shows that older people vary widely in their health, functional status, life priorities, and medical preferences. Yet, in the UK, health policy sometimes assumes old age inevitably brings incapacity and denies care known to preserve health and independence on the basis of age, not functional status. This phenomenon is known as "undertreatment," which means depriving someone a treatment with a high likelihood of health benefit. In the United States, the opposite, called "overtreatment," is the norm. Older patients often are cared for as if they were just like younger patients; drugs and treatments developed in studies of middle-aged adults are given to old patients irrespective of age, other medical conditions, incapacity, or life expectancy. Neither approach makes sense. One discriminates on the basis of age; the other denies the impact of age. Both lump all older people into a single monolithic category in complete disregard for the diversity of health and function that increases with advancing age. Both are forms of ageism. The old may differ from the young, and the care of older patients may differ from that of younger patients, but older people are no less deserving of high-quality medical care.

Ageism within medicine is a manifestation of a larger problem. It is well known among those who care for old people that you endanger a center or program if you use the words *aging* or *geriatric* in its title. If you want patients, funders, institutional support, and referrals from colleagues, you must replace those terms with *wellness* and *longevity*. In other words, old people themselves, individual and institutional donors, medical centers, health systems, and health professionals all demonstrate a strong preference for euphemisms over terms that are more precise, more inclusive, and not inherently negative. Within geriatrics, we entertain ongoing debates about changing our name (to "complexivists" or "transitionalists"), largely because *geriatrics* has "negative connotations." But surely a profession dedicated to the care of old people should not reject association with old age! Imagine pediatricians changing their specialty name so as to distance themselves from children, or surgeons starting to call themselves interventionalists. It's absurd.

At the same time, age phobia is understandable. Even people who remain healthy and active as they age will experience changes in strength, endurance, and appearance, and a significant proportion, though not all, will have increasing illness and disability. But these facts belie the more complex reality of the longest, most varied period of our lives. Some people become frail in their sixties while others remain healthy past their centenary. Much of what we accept as fact is actually a "glass half-empty" interpretation, an assumption that all age-related changes are for the worse. To be sure, the aging body disappoints and frustrates. Yet each stage has pros and cons. After all, it's those of us between youth's substandard thinking and judgment and old age's physical frailty who pour billions of dollars into stress-relieving activities and products.

Part of what makes old age hard is that we fight it, rather than embracing it as one stage in a universal trajectory. We also fail to properly acknowledge its upsides: the decreases in family and work stress or the increases in contentment, wisdom, and agency that accompany most years of old age. Sometimes people—from those working in medicine to families of older adults—attribute the bad outcomes of our flawed, biased approaches to old age in medicine and society to biological destiny. Sometimes that's true, but at least as often, it's not.

# 6. TEEN

In a 2016 interview about his memoir, Bruce Springsteen, age sixty-six, was asked by fifty-six-year-old *New Yorker* editor David Remnick, "Why now?"

Springsteen let out a long breath, making an "oof" sound, and chuckled. "I wanted to do it before I forgot everything, you know."

Remnick laughed heartily. The audience watching the live interview cheered and clapped.

"So it's getting a little edgy with some of that," Springsteen added, "so I thought now was the time."

When that interview took place, Springsteen was coming off a sold-out tour, playing exceptionally long sets—over three hours of continuous, highly physical singing and cavorting. Night after night, he played in cities around the world. When his book came out a month later, it topped bestseller lists, and Springsteen launched a new tour, or rather two tours: one book, one concert. By virtue of either his age or stamina, a case could be made for Springsteen as still decidedly middle-aged, but the artist himself clearly felt that whatever *old* was had begun for him, and he saw, or thought he could see, where it was headed. Somehow neither he nor the *New Yorker* editor, ten years his junior, recognized the irony of positioning Springsteen partway down a nefarious spiral when the career details they were discussing suggested not just a new high point but a remarkable addition to his artistic skill set. After decades of renown as a musician, he was now also recognized as a talented writer, a fact that introduced new options and opportunities for his future.

A writer doesn't have to jump up and down or dance along a stage and into an adoring crowd. Then again, not all musicians do that either. Springsteen could sit at a piano, or on a chair cradling his guitar, or with just a microphone and a small spotlight, the audience's entire focus on his face, words, song. That would not be a traditional Springsteen concert, but would it be worse, or just different? Would it tarnish his legacy and shrink his audience, or expand it, showing range and adaptability? He's had ballad albums before (*Tunnel of Love*). The point is Springsteen has options, as many people do, though his are significantly different from most people's. A different sort of concert, perhaps playing a modified or different sort of music, is just one of Springsteen's options. He also could sit at home with a mouse and keyboard, or a pen and paper, or a voice recorder, or an assistant taking dictation, and he could write. Such transitions are often framed as devolution, but that's only the case if the frame is constructed from static expectations. Build it instead with an understanding of the human life cycle, and it looks more like evolution: a gradual process in which something develops into a different form.

If not quite three score and ten, Springsteen was certainly within the long-accepted territory of "old." For two thousand to three thousand years, from the time of Socrates and the Athenian Empire in the west, and much earlier in the Middle East and Asia, old age has been defined as beginning around age sixty or seventy. In the United States, sixty-five became the federal demarcation line between middle and old age with the launch of the Social Security program in 1935. The group that developed the program, the President's Committee on Economic Security, chose sixty-five partly because it was consistent with data on prevailing retirement ages at the time and partly because it was the age already selected by half the existing state pension systems (the other half used seventy). Although retirement norms, longevity, and actuarial outcomes have changed since the 1930s, sixty-five has endured in many minds as either a strict divide or a marker of having entered the transition zone headed toward old.

For most people, early, middle, and advanced old age are significantly different. In our current conceptualization of *old*, physical degradations and lost options are its sine qua non. That's why, until those things become overwhelming, many people don't think of themselves as old, even when most younger people would swiftly and definitively put them in that category. When people arrive at the stereotypical version of old, they sometimes no longer feel like themselves, although for most of us the transition to old happens gradually over decades beginning at age twenty. The changes are both positive and negative, though we tend to focus on the latter. Those losses and diminutions are imperceptible at first, then easy to disregard, then possible to work around, and, finally, blatant.

Springsteen signaled that he was aware of the negative changes in his own mind and body. Once you reach a certain age, it's hard not to ask: Will my mind go first, or my body? Will they both go, or will I get lucky? When will it happen and how quickly?

Aging begins at birth. In childhood, the changes are dramatic. In those early decades, the fact that living and aging are synonymous is lost, couched first in the language of child development and then forgotten in the busyness and social milestones of young adulthood. After a friend moved to another state, I didn't see her infant for nine months, at which point I found myself with a toddler, not a baby. Stages of child development are predictable and universal across cultures, except in cases of grave illness or disability. As we move through the life span, the boundaries between stages get blurred. Although people debate whether life begins at conception or birth, childhood starts with a big breath upon emergence from the womb, its beginning uniform. Its end is less clear. A ten-year-old is always a child, but eighteen-year-olds can be teenagers or young adults, depending on their behavior. Some people achieve physical, emotional, and intellectual maturity in their teens, others in their twenties. Females tend to get there before males. Still, most people become adults in the same several-years-long window of time.

With the arrival of the twenties, development seems to abate, taking on the imperceptible pace of hair growth or melting glaciers. The changes that defined us as we moved from infant to kid and teen to adult appear to stop. But unseen or not noticed are not the same as not happening. Changing continues throughout life—physically, functionally, and psychologically. At some point, we cross into the territory of "middle age" and discover aging isn't just a characteristic of that mythical land called old. Sometimes the evolution is welcome, bringing a greater comfort with self, a deep-seated confidence and greater security about what is and has been. At the same time, accumulating physical changes collude in ways that can complicate, distress, and impoverish. A person's identity can feel challenged.

Even in the decades when change seems slow, almost irrelevant, it is present, significant, ongoing. In my thirties, I had the straight white teeth of a person fortunate enough to have had braces in her teens and dentistry throughout life. By my early forties, my little front bottom teeth began to overlap as if so much time had elapsed that they'd forgotten their training at the hands of metal braces, headgear, neck gear, rubber bands, and retainers. As they overlapped, I saw along their edges the imprimatur of decades of morning coffee, the occasional glass of red wine, and the erosion of daily eating and drinking. Yet my dentist says my teeth look great. She can tell I faithfully brush and floss. What she really means, I know, is that they look great for someone in her fifties, not that they look as good as they once did or great in the absolute sense. At some point the caveat, the conditional clause, goes unspoken.

At the age of apparent aging, the once distant land called "old" no longer seems foreign or exotic to me. Daily, my joints offer protests. Sometimes one has a solo; more often there's a noisy blur of voices, the new background music accompanying my every movement. I regularly switch among my three pairs of multifocal glasses, each with a different function. I have a faulty gene, a history of cancer, and seven visible surgical scars, and am now missing several nonessential body parts. These days, when something goes wrong in my body, I don't just consider how it might be fixed; I worry that fixing it won't be possible and that my new debility will not only endure but beget a cascade of injuries and additional disabilities. In my head, I hear the child-hood song about how *the foot bone's connected to the leg bone, the leg bone's connected to the hip bone,* and so on. Although it's not yet clear how it will go down, I can now imagine me = old, even if I still sometimes register my relentless progress toward citizenship in that vast territory with surprise.

Those physical changes are real but tell only part of the story. For me, the rest of the saga goes something like this: though I have yet to take up perma-nent residency in old age, I have acquired an intimate familiarity with its culture and customs, and I'm looking forward to it. I imagine its early years, and if I'm lucky, decades, much like the best parts of midlife: the solid sense of who I am and how I want to spend my time, the decreased volume of the sorts of ambitions easily confused with the hollow vanity of social recognition, the greater time and energy for generosity and attention to others, the confidence to stick to my convictions, the exciting new goals and profound sense of life satisfaction. Similar sentiments are found with aging the world over.

It may be that after the great celebrations of childhood milestones, we feel surprised and uneasy about our quieter progression through later turning points. A friend in his late thirties thought it absurd that his peers didn't want him to refer to himself as middle-aged when he so obviously was. I looked at him and agreed; he's far from old, and also clearly no longer young—he's somewhere in between. Out the other end of adulthood, my mother says aging isn't really that bad until you hit eighty, then there's a nosedive. She said this as we had dinner at the assisted living facility where she moved because of my now-deceased father's needs, not her own. Seconds later, frustrated because we hadn't been brought water, she jumped up, grabbed our glasses, and darted across the dining room to fill them. She wasn't her old self, but she didn't seem to me like a person in a steep downward plunge. Yet, to her, a threshold had been passed into a territory of greater risk and vulnerability.

By far, the least fixed dividing line separates adulthood and old age. With good health and good luck, some people don't seem to be or see themselves as making that transition until their late seventies and occasionally later still. By contrast, major stressors such as homelessness, poverty, or incarceration can cause accelerated aging, making others "old" in their fifties, with cellular changes and risks of chronic disease and death akin to those of more fortunate people many decades their senior. And still, use of the word *old* for fifty-somethings requires quotation marks. We define age as a definite place in life's chronology, other times as a bio-psycho-social state, and mostly as an amalgam of the two. Using that logic, a frail seventy-two-year-old is called old while a marathon-running seventy-two-year-old executive is not. In reality, both are old, and even if the executive continues her current activities in her eighties, she'll be "old."

Because aging is a long, stealthy process, a person's arrival at old age is less a switch thrown than a series of ill-defined thresholds crossed, the transition often first noted by others. Most people over thirty, and certainly those forty and older, will recall the first time "mister" or "lady," "ma'am" or "sir," meant them. As our third decade of life cedes to our fourth, aging seems to accelerate. By the time the fifth decade fades into the sixth, the resulting accumulation of physical changes that define adult development transitions from inconsequential to subtly manifest: the crow's-feet or balding pate and tricky right knee, the friends with cancer, the talk among your peers about ill and dying older relatives. By the ebbing of the sixth decade, if not sooner, the changes are undeniable. Not long after that, they transition to conspicuous, each decade seemingly more profoundly marked than its predecessor. On a daily basis, nothing seems to change, but look back a year or five or ten, and the transformation is pronounced.

There have always been old people. Egyptian hieroglyphs from 2800 B.C. depict a bent person leaning on a staff. For over nine hundred years beginning in 775 B.C., the Greeks put forth an array of theories about aging. As their ruins attest, the ancient Greeks had systems, roadways, and efficient processes for sewage removal. Hygiene was good and most hard labor was done by slaves. Aristotle may well have noticed that the slaves, with their long hours of physical work, poor access to food, and constant exposure to the elements, aged more quickly than the citizens in his circle. He suggested that aging occurred because of the loss of *pneuma*, an internal heat or vital spirit that was gradually consumed over time. Because there was a finite amount, older people had less, which made them more vulnerable to disease, and although slaves spent theirs more quickly than scholars, everyone eventually ran out.

For most of human history, people didn't expect to grow old, and those who did often outlived their children. Because old people made up just a small fraction of the population in societies rich in children and younger adults, there was little point in considering them when building houses, making laws, designing cities, developing a workforce, or training doctors. Now most people born in developed countries can expect to be old, and there are more old people than at any time in human history. Old age also lasts longer and includes many more healthy years. Unprecedented numbers of us are or will be doing in old age most of the things younger people do, though sometimes in different ways, as well as many other things that aren't possible earlier in life or in shorter life spans.

In societies that identified themselves by their traditions, their past, and their religion, "the elderly, closer by birth to the sacred past and by death to divine and ancestral sources of power," had prestige and a clear, important social position. Today, when the past is viewed as irrelevant and death is more often seen as an ending or abyss than a chance to be with God, being old lacks both those charms. Even middle age is dreaded. Lydia Davis captured this sentiment perfectly in a one-line short story called "Fear of Ageing":

At 28,
she longs to be 24 again.

Meanwhile, in my fifties, I find the idea of returning to twenty-four horrific. I don't miss the stress or insecurity or posturing, all those things that at the time often felt—deceptively—like potential and strength and opportunity.

Old age has boundaries and landmarks that are both real and subject to interpretation. We reach *no longer young* decades before becoming old, and what different people and cultures count as *a long time* varies widely.

Like pornography, we know advanced old age when we see it. But the exact inflection point between middle age and old age is hard to pin down. It might even be impossible, both in an individual life and for our species, given the plethora of biological markers and their unpredictable behavior and interactions. Nor is culture the only other notable piece in that elusive equation. The traits that signal emergence from the liminal zone where *adult* gives way to *old* vary in the eyes of beholders. Diagnosed with cancer at age sixty, my mother resigned herself to dying, saying it was okay because she was old and had had a good life. A quarter century later, she looks back on her thoughts then, amazed at how both her perspective and old age itself have changed in the intervening decades.

PERVERSIONS

Stocky and not quite six feet tall, Clarence Williams Sr. was a recently retired seventy-two-year-old attorney who always had a book in his hand or lap. One week he'd been active and healthy, and the next he was my patient on our hospital's cancer service. Although he didn't have the worst kind of cancer, in 1992 all the treatments we had on offer earned the word *brutal* as one of their descriptors.

I looked forward to seeing Clarence on morning rounds and in the afternoons when I needed to give him test results or check how he was handling his many treatments and their side effects. He was brave and kind in many small but important ways, not the least of which was his attitude toward me, one simultaneously avuncular and respectful, even though I was a novice doctor, young, and female—three states that put off some patients. I'd like to think his generosity of character is why I remember him so well all these years later, but I suspect it's because of what we put him through.

The oncologists started Clarence on chemotherapy within hours of his arrival. I gave him medications for nausea and pain, antibiotics to protect him from infections, and diuretics to remove the excess fluid that built up all over his body. Most days, after his labs came back, I ordered infusions of potassium and phosphorus; some of the treatment drugs, as well as some of the medications for the side effects of the treatment drugs, led to loss of essential elements. The kidneys, those small, paired organs tucked under the rib cage on the lower back, serve as the body's garbage disposal system. When properly functioning, they remove toxins and waste from the blood and excrete them out with the urine, sending cleaned blood back into the body. If you imagine the kidneys as filters, the effect of the chemo was to enlarge the holes in the mesh such that certain molecules like potassium slid through. With low potassium levels, people have fatigue and painful muscle cramps, and their heart can slow to a life-threatening rate. With lethal potential, various minerals poured out of him, and I poured them back in, trying to keep up.

Meanwhile, ulcers formed in Clarence's mouth and intestines, causing them to bleed. Despite the medications, he had nausea, diarrhea, and pain. His skin blistered and peeled. Antinausea drugs weren't as good then as they are now, and he vomited so often that we used intravenous fluids to keep him hydrated. As days turned into weeks, his eyes dulled, his glasses became smudged, and his skin looked more tan-gray than brown-black. Despite his bloated body, the bed seemed to engulf him.

That was when the cancer doctors decided he needed a colonoscopy. They wanted to see how his intestinal lining was holding up and how much more chemotherapy they could give him. As reasons for ordering a test go, this was a pretty good one, since it would provide information to guide our next steps. As the team intern, my job was to make the test happen. The problem was that by this point in his treatment Clarence had trouble sitting up, and he wasn't eating or drinking much of anything. He needed the help of an aide or two to get to the bathroom only five yards from his bed. To clean out his colon for the test, he would need to drink four liters of a liquid that looked clear but made people gag, then endure hours of running to the toilet. I looked at him, and I looked at the huge plastic container of bowel cleanser, and I thought: *This won't work*.

The oncology fellow came to the same conclusion. His solution was to order a feeding tube through which the liquid could be injected directly into Clarence's stomach. On the surface, this was a good plan. Usually a patient had to drink sixteen eight-ounce glasses of the prep liquid, one every ten minutes for nearly three hours. Clarence sometimes took a few sips of juice or bites of soft food, but even as the worst of the side effects from his first round of chemo subsided, his decimated appetite and ongoing throat discomfort made drinking large quantities of anything impossible. With the tube, we could put the bowel cleanser straight into his body without him having to drink it. Such tubes are used fairly routinely in hospitals. I had already inserted several and cared for many patients who had them. I understood their uses and benefits, and I hated them. To get to the stomach, the long, hollow cylinder of flexible plastic first had to be inserted up through Clarence's nostril, then make a 180-degree turn and drop down the back of his throat. There, it would need to enter the right opening, the one for his esophagus, rather than the adjacent one that led to his trachea. In Clarence's case, this was particularly important, since the lungs are a place where you definitely do not want to put four liters of fluid. Most people find both getting the tube in and the reality of having it in their nose and throat quite uncomfortable. Still, sometimes it goes in quickly and easily enough.

Sometimes. Not surprisingly, many patients also hate these tubes. During insertion, the tube doesn't know it's supposed to make a downward turn and often tries to keep going up, digging into the soft tissues in the back of the patient's nose and throat. Even when it goes in smoothly, people often gag or hover on the brink of gagging. People who are confused just pull it out . . . unless their arms are tied to the bedrails, in which case their existence is reduced to something that looks suspiciously like torture. There is, after all, a plastic rod where it doesn't belong, so the body says: *No*. That was Clarence's body's reaction and also mine when I saw what the tube was doing to him.

Worse still, the tube insertion was just the beginning. Clarence's nostril itched, swelled, bled, and dripped. His eyes watered. He had a choking sensation and searing pain as the tube pushed against the chemo-ravaged back of his throat. He was torn between wanting to swallow the irritant and not wanting to swallow ever again because it hurt so much. When a nurse began pushing the fluid through the tube to his stomach, his belly bloated and churned. His nausea worsened. He retched. She slowed down but kept going. An hour later, the fecal urgency began. If you're fairly healthy and recently turned fifty, earning yourself a screening colonoscopy, such urgency is manageable. But when you're seventy-four and have been in the hospital for weeks, when your cells have been under siege from chemo-therapy, when your muscles have shrunk from disuse, and when, because of all this and more, your cancer and its treatment are getting the best of you, well, then, even getting to a commode placed beside your bed can seem about as possible as running a marathon.

When the pressure built inside Clarence's belly, he pressed his call button. When no one came, he called out with his weakened voice. And then? Rarely does anyone come quickly in a hospital. Everyone has too much to do, and nurses and aides can't abandon whomever they are caring for at that moment unless someone else's life is in jeopardy.

Clarence knew what was about to happen, and he hated it. He considered getting up, but knew he would fall, and also that if he hurt himself badly enough by falling, the chemo and all his suffering would have been for nothing. So instead he lay there as a warmth seeped around his lower torso. His chemo-raw skin stung. He closed his eyes, though less from the discomfort as from his shame. Only a small child shits himself, he kept thinking, and if that was where he was at, then he had come full circle. At least, that was how it looked to me when I checked on him. His eyes and expression said he knew his life was almost over, and this was how it was going to end—alone, miserable, and undignified.

In medicine, a colonoscopy is a "minor" procedure. Although major procedures are major for everyone, the same is not true of those labeled minor. That designation, based on the procedure's difficulty for both doctor and patient, does not take into consideration the particulars of the patient receiving it. It also encourages the use of such procedures in people and circumstances where they do more harm than good, most often in the very sick or very old. When doctors do discuss the risks and benefits with patients, too often it's to meet a legal requirement rather than to inform, inquire, and collaboratively conclude. The focus, other than getting it over and done with, tends to be on side effects and adverse incidents. We don't have language or record-keeping mechanisms for the experiential facts of procedures, the in-the-moment trauma and its subsequent distress.

Clarence Williams entered the hospital as a "young-old" person who clearly enjoyed his life. In his few weeks on our cancer service, he became a prototypical old man, sickly and frail, his coming death writ on both body and spirit. Witnessing this horrified me, but like so many of us I said nothing and continued doing my job. Sometimes he and I would simply look at each other for a few moments after completing our usual tasks and conversations. In those moments, we discussed all that was never said aloud in a wordless universal language unrecognized by my profession.

That month, I watched the oncologists save many lives. All ages and cancer types. I also watched them ruin many lives. All ages and cancer types. That is medicine, and that is life.

Clarence's existential suffering never came up on rounds. Instead, we talked about his chemo cycles and potassium level, his symptoms and next procedure. Eventually, we began talking about when he might leave the hospital, headed most likely to a nursing home, given his weakness and poor prognosis. We hoped that he would gain weeks or months of life from the chemo—an unlikely scenario, seeing how sick it had made him, though we couldn't know for sure, since the regimen hadn't been studied in patients his age. We didn't discuss the obvious: that he was unlikely to spend any gained time feeling well and doing the things he enjoyed. Maybe he would have wanted the treatment anyway, as some people do and in case it helped. This was years before we knew that some people, particularly older adults, live both longer and better without treatment for certain clearly fatal cancers. Or maybe Clarence wanted the chemo and then, once it was clear how bad it would be for him, changed his mind but couldn't find a way to get off the high-speed treatment train. Perhaps it didn't occur to him to ask about other options.

It didn't occur to me to offer any. Partly this was because it wasn't my place; the oncologist was his primary doctor and I was his lowest assistant. But the real reason was more fundamental. I didn't know what the alternatives were or how to arrange them. On the cancer service, we learned only about chemo and radiotherapy. Although age is the greatest risk factor for cancer, and cancer is the second most common cause of death, geriatrics and palliative care were not part of oncology training programs. With few exceptions, they still aren't. A doctor is unlikely to make assessments and recommendations she doesn't know how or when to make.

It is our right as Americans to demand care that makes no sense. To insist that our bodies be crushed, disfigured, and disrespected, that what once was sacrosanct be intentionally and systematically desecrated. That American right asks doctors to do the impossible, the ugly, the appalling. Some enjoy the sport of their procedures and expertise; for others, motivated by a desire to heal and help, doing such things erodes the softness of them, leaving wounds they cover with callus and corruption. It is the war zones of our body politic and the vast wastelands of our health care system that allow us to commit such travesties and label them care.

## REJUVENATION

The woman behind me in exercise class was pretty, maybe even beautiful, one of those women whose face looks better at eighty than mine did at twenty. Yes, I could tell she was well into old age—dyed hair, plastic surgery, and makeup notwithstanding. But she looked good, and I became even more impressed as she lifted weights and did planks and push-ups, squats and crunches. I noticed she couldn't fully straighten her arms or legs and thought: *She's so fit and still she has contractures.* The youngest she could be, I decided, was late seventies; more likely, she was in her early eighties. I wondered if she'd taken up exercise late, or whether tendons hardened and shortened in some people despite regular exercise. But I also had a moment of shock about forty minutes into the workout when we lay down on our mats. As her hair flowed away from her forehead, pulled by gravity toward the floor beneath, the contrast between the lustrous blonde-brown of it and her translucent skin seemed wrong. Worse than wrong, it was disturbing. Without the hair's protective framing, I saw where her skin had been pulled and tucked and how it fought with itself, surgical residua pulling one way and gravity another. Suddenly, she didn't look pretty. She looked like a mannequin in a horror film. At some point, when you take one thing and try to make it another, you run the risk of the grotesque. Probably they didn't tell her about this risk; maybe she didn't care. Almost everyone values the present more than the future.

An Internet search of the term *anti-aging* yields over forty-six million hits. The first of many items that come up are lists of tips, secrets and routines (some "recommended by doctors"), beauty products, and clinics that promise to help minimize the impact of aging on skin, body, and mind. The most frequently used words include *prevent*, *reversing*, and *corrective*, followed by *age spots*, *hormones*, and *wrinkles*, though *younger-looking*, *refreshed*, *lively*, and *robust* are also popular. Much of this language is borrowed from science— smart marketing that lends legitimacy and an aura of truth, rigor, and objectivity to what is mostly cosmetics. It also reinforces, overtly and insidiously, the idea that aging—even though we are all doing it all our lives—is bad, that old is ugly, and that evolution over a lifetime is evidence of failure. They offer the hope of an old age absent all that leaves us feeling unattractive and all that we fear.

In the twenty-first century, many scientists have concluded that tackling human health one disease at a time makes little sense. Incredibly, even if we cured all of today's big killers—cancer, heart disease, dementia, and diabetes, to name just a few—we would only gain a few extra years of life. Our parts would still wear down and out. (As Oedipus said, "Only for the gods / Is there never old age or death! / All other things almighty time confounds.")

According to this relatively new "geroscience hypothesis," since aging is so closely linked to illness, debility, and death, the best way to address those problems is by interrupting the aging process itself. That approach could allow simultaneous prevention (or, more likely, delay) and treatment of multiple aging-related diseases and functional impairments, from osteoporosis to diabetes, heart dysfunction, and frailty. In the pipeline already are treatments like resilience therapies for high-risk older patients, making them less frail and vulnerable to disease, and medications that would remove inflammatory protein-producing cells that harm nearby tissues. The goal of most such treatments is to increase our healthy years, or "health span," rather than our life span. Of course, some people would like to do both.

The search for eternal youth dates back to at least to 3000 B.C. in Babylon, when Gilgamesh stated that a long life could be achieved by pleasing the gods with prayer, heroism, and sacrifice. Ancient Chinese emperors sought an elixir of youth, and ancient Hindu writings, the Vedas, hinted at alchemy that offered not just the promise of ongoing vitality but an actual return to youthfulness. In Europe, the idea gained and waned in popularity over centuries. In the fifth century B.C. Herodotus wrote of a people who all lived to 120 years old and claimed their secret was bathing in a particular fountain. In medieval times, a Golden Age or Place of eternal youth was sometimes presented as having once existed and other times as still existing but hidden, so it or the secret to it needed to be discovered.

Others focused less on youth and more on longevity. In thirteenth-century England, Roger Bacon drew on ancient texts and Christian beliefs in the natural immortality of humans before the Fall to posit that proper behavior could extend the human life span to 150 years. If future generations continued the same beneficial practices, he also suggested, human lives might reach three, four, or five hundred years. The same themes recurred over time: seeking youth, living longer, and restoring (sexual) "vitality." Approaches often echoed earlier periods and beliefs about aging. A long-standing view, derived from Galen's waning vital force theory, held that an element or humor— breath, blood, semen—from the young could be used to improve the health, energy, or beauty of the old. Invoking that reasoning, some recommended living or sleeping with the young to draw warmth from their proximal bodies. (The latter option may have been popular for reasons other than health . . .)

In 1888 Charles-Édouard Brown-Séquard, a famed French physician, claimed to have rejuvenated his septuagenarian self with injection of extracts of animal testes. Around the same time, Élie Metchnikoff, a Nobel Prize–winning Russian father of modern immunology, believed hormone injections were among the essentials for the prolongation of life. In 1907 his book *The Prolongation of Life* made hormone injections popular in many countries, most prominently Germany and the United States. Serge Voronoff, while disdained by his French medical colleagues in the first half of the twentieth century, achieved great public popularity for his work on glandular grafts and injections of monkey hormones for rejuvenation of older people.

In the twenty-first century, it's the specific techniques we plan to use to achieve longevity that have changed, not the goal itself or even many of the scientific strategies.

In organisms from yeast and roundworms to mice and nonhuman primates, caloric restriction has markedly improved health and extended the life span. It lowers body fat, delays immune system changes, improves DNA repair capacity, and much more. In one article, in addition to the usual graphs, there are photographs of two sets of monkeys, both twenty-seven years old. The monkeys fed a usual diet look old, with wrinkles, sunken faces, and lost muscle mass and hair, while their calorie-restricted peers appear young and healthy. The restricted ones also had better blood sugar and cholesterol levels, and lived longer. At age thirty, fewer than a quarter of the control monkeys were alive, compared with 70 percent of the calorie-restricted ones. The long-lived (human) Okinawans, with their twelve-hundred-calorie-a-day diet, suggest something similar happens in humans. Some people are giving it a try. An international calorie restriction society claims thousands of members, although its physician founder died at age seventy-nine. Preliminary human studies haven't lasted long enough to affect longevity but show positive hormonal changes, such as lower insulin levels and higher maintenance levels of the steroid hormone DHEA, similar to those seen in the calorie-restricted monkeys.

That's great news, except most of us have trouble restricting ourselves to so-called normal amounts of food. Most Americans are overweight, and many in normal weight ranges still regularly eat more calories than they need, just for the fun of it—I do, and I love it, even though I know I shouldn't and even as I live to regret it. Most scientists also like to eat, so they began looking for the biological mechanisms of calorie restriction. Maybe, they hypothesized, it worked via a molecule that they could copy, manipulate, or manufacture so people could get the benefits of calorie restriction without having to deprive themselves so drastically.

Enter resveratrol, a plant-derived compound that activates sirtuins, a class of intracellular proteins that regulate important biological pathways related to aging and other processes that influence aging, including inflammation, energy efficiency, and stress resistance. Resveratrol induces cellular changes associated with longer life spans, extends the life span of multiple lower species, including fruit flies and fish, and improves both health and survival in mice on a high-calorie diet. It can also be credited with the increased popularity of red wine. People are most likely to adopt dietary changes they enjoy.

Scientists are also investigating other molecules that the body makes in response to caloric restriction, such as the ketone body beta-hydroxybutyric acid (BHB) created when people eat a "ketogenic diet" high in fat and low in protein and carbohydrates. A recent study in aging mammals demonstrated positive effects of BHB on memory and life span. The results suggested that BHB affected gene expression. As the senior scientist involved in the project stated, "We're looking for drug targets. The ultimate goal is to find a way for humans to benefit from BHBs without having to go on a restrictive diet." Those who want the benefits now can exercise, a natural way to create ketone bodies. In fact, ketogenesis may be why exercise improves brain function, health span, and life span.

There are many different paths through which scientists believe they can affect aging, health, and possibly longevity. Cell-based strategies include therapies such as "senolytics," clearing senescent cells with certain aging-associated markers. Other therapies under investigation to slow or stop aging include antioxidant supplementation and a compound called rapamycin, which was first discovered oozing from bacteria on Easter Island. Rapamycin influences the immune system (it's already used in transplant medicine) and has been shown to prolong life in flies, worms, and rodents. Last but not least, and putting a modern twist on the humoral approach, several start-ups now replace the blood of older people with blood from young volunteers, hoping to transfer a variety of youth-related compounds all at once.

Some therapies, however widely touted and seemingly sound, aren't remotely ready for human trials. Stem cells, for example: although they have proven uses in regeneration, in 2018 there is no evidence they work at achieving longevity.

The language and arguments of "anti-aging" have evolved, but the underlying message isn't new. Nor is the participation of physicians in the anti-aging business. Throughout history, some have entered that arena with the intent of improving human lives, while others have exploited people's endless appetite for self-deception and false hopes. Market-driven manipulators have invoked the same militaristic terms used by medicine in reference to cancer, drug abuse, and AIDS, simultaneously suggesting that not to "fight," "battle," or "defy" aging is foolhardy, and that to do so is to avail oneself of the full armamentarium of modern medical science. Never mind that only a tiny minority of these products and procedures are considered medical enough to warrant the investigation, impartial review, and safety and efficacy oversight we accord actual medical products and devices. And the field is made confusing by the overlap between real and pseudoscience in the use of hormones, blood, and other bodily substances that were no less popular in the 1880s than they are today. It's also gendered. Men aim for ongoing sexual vigor and, among the supremely wealthy and powerful, more time in which to enjoy their money and power. Women strive for beauty and all that feminine beauty carries with it in our society—namely, visibility, relevance, allure, and worth.

In scientific circles, *anti-aging* usually refers to efforts to delay or "cure" old age, not to the multitude of discriminatory beliefs and policies related to aging. In coining that term, proponents hoped to align it with words like *antibiotics*, one of the most significant medical advances in human history. But this *anti-* is primarily used in relation to *aging* as it is used in the words *antiestablishment* or *anti-immigration*, meaning opposed to or against part of the natural life cycle. Worse still, it's a tiny leap from that usage of *anti-aging* to being against aging people and traits.

The American Academy of Anti-Aging Medicine, unlike most medical organizations, has a .com and not a .org address—the difference being a profit goal versus a mission goal. In 2002 fifty-two of aging's most prominent scientists—including Leonard Hayflick, who showed the finitude of cell divisions, "the Hayflick limit," and Jay Olshansky, who has worked on discovering the upper limits of longevity—issued a statement that "the business of what has become known as anti-aging medicine has grown in recent years in the United States and abroad into a multimillion-dollar industry. The products being sold have no scientifically demonstrated efficacy, in some cases, they may be harmful, and those selling them often misrepresent the science upon which they are based."

For at least the last century and a half, humans have had great faith in our ability to affect aging in ways superior to those of our predecessors. In 1905 the immunologist Arthur E. McFarlane wrote in "Prolonging the Prime of Life" that science will bring fitness and health to old age. Over a hundred years later, science has yet to deliver on that prediction. The leading researchers say the prospects are promising, although that has been said by leading researchers for centuries. That they haven't succeeded yet doesn't necessarily mean the concept is flawed; perhaps the failures come from the methods rather than the goal. (Never mind the various nondisease issues, including overpopulation, climate change, pseudo foods, social policies, and tech use that have negative impacts on human health and longevity.) For many, science and technology have become the only hope, the only way. As a result, clear and present suffering gets ignored, as do the many noncurative strategies that might diminish or alleviate it.

Also largely ignored are the late effects of cures. Fixing one problem often creates new ones that might be avoided or mitigated if only all people and problems counted and we were willing to invest in the full range of tools and skills at our disposal. For instance, survive your cancer and you're liable to develop delayed side effects ranging from other cancers to diseases of any organ in the body. Survive your heart attack or infection and you're likely to become old.

That will mostly be a good thing, except that the longer we keep you alive, the more likely you are to reach the phase of old age when most of modern society and medicine have nothing for you, not even dignity or compassion.

Innovation comes with trade-offs. Our ingenuity and technical skills have nearly doubled the human life span, but now people who previously would have died shortly after birth, or after devastating war injuries, or in extreme old age, remain alive. Draw the line too close, and lives are unnecessarily sacrificed; draw it too far, and we cause systematic suffering. To further complicate matters, looking at the same set of circumstances, people draw the line in different places. Generally, we tend to err toward life. Some of this is likely instinct, but part may be learned, a sociocultural habit adopted in the early years of modern medicine when antibiotics and surgeries offered what would have seemed like miracles in earlier eras. Our current advances have very different consequences than the ones of earlier generations— consequences that millions must live with but that are barely recognized or addressed by the medical institutions that produce them, especially if the current best approaches to improving human health and lives don't require science or technology so much as shifts in attitudes, priorities, and values.

Someday, iterations of one or more of the "anti-aging" approaches are likely to succeed, maybe not in reversing aging altogether but in eliminating some of its downsides. Meanwhile, there are two paths we can take that would be transformative in the near future: justice in policy and kindness of attitude.

GAPS

Before clinic one day, our administrator informed me that my new patient was ninety-eight years old and went by the name of Kid. I began reviewing his old records with a smile on my face and high expectations for our first meeting.

Seconds later, I stared at my computer in disbelief. Although by and large American health care puts its money and efforts into treatment, prevention is unequivocally the better approach economically, medically, and morally, since it keeps people from getting sick and needing medical care in the first place. Usually, I am all for prevention. But the most recent entry into Kid's electronic medical record was a note from a neurologist prescribing daily aspirin for stroke prevention, and I was not at all sure about aspirin for Kid.

Aspirin has risks that increase considerably with age and include internal bleeding, hospitalization, and death. A 2011 study found it was one of the top four drugs associated with emergency hospital visits in people over age sixty-five.

Kid had been older than sixty-five for over thirty years. What does prevention mean, I wondered, when a person has already outlived 99.99 percent of his fellow humans?

Trying to take good care of Kid, my neurologist colleague had applied the only evidence she had—evidence from younger patients—in deciding on a plan of care. That calculation had two important flaws. First, we do not know whether aspirin prevents stroke in ninety-eight-year-olds, as that has never been studied. Second, we do know from outcomes data, common sense, and scientific studies that the body's response to drugs changes and the risk of drug side effects increases in old age. Basically, we could not know that aspirin would benefit Kid, but could be confident that the medication put him at significant risk for internal bleeding, kidney failure, and other adverse effects.

The routine prescription of medications with proven benefits in younger adults and only proven harms in old people happens with all kinds of drugs. Old people, excluded from the trials that show benefit, are prescribed the drug, and sooner or later the reports of adverse events start coming in—except, of course, when patients, families, nurses, and doctors attribute the symptoms to disease, age, or the relentless decline they expect in a sick old person.

On call one sunny, spring weekend, I received a message from the caregiver grandson of a patient in her nineties with atrial fibrillation. Her cardiologist had started her on a newly approved blood thinner that had been shown to be safer and easier to manage than the one she was on. The potential benefits to this mostly homebound nonagenarian were huge. She wouldn't need to have her blood drawn to check drug levels. Getting this very old woman into the lab for blood tests was an ordeal, and finding veins was hard, causing bruising. Equally important, since what and how much she ate varied widely and certain foods interfered with her past blood thinner, she had been at risk for having blood that was either too thin, which could lead to dangerous bleeding, or not thin enough, increasing her chances of stroke. That risk would be eliminated on the new drug.

On the phone, her grandson said that she was confused. She didn't seem sick or different in any other way. While there might have been an illness brewing, medications commonly cause confusion in old people, and the timing was just right for a reaction to the new pill. I stopped it, and she got better. On Monday, the cardiologist said the medication didn't cause delirium and restarted it. On Tuesday evening, she was confused again. We again stopped it, and she got better. Here's the worst part of this story: it's mostly older people who have atrial fibrillation, yet there were no requirements to include them in trials of the drugs to treat that or other age-related conditions. (The Inclusion Across the Lifespan Policy starts in 2019.) Even when not excluded based on their age, old people are frequently rejected from studies because of their lab results, organ function, or chronic diseases. Once the studies are published, other older patients with the same conditions are prescribed the "trial proven" medications and told they are safe and helpful.

In clinical medicine, we are supposed look for "Occam's razor," or a single unifying diagnosis that explains all a patient's symptoms, physical exam features, and test results. This strategy often works well in young or mostly healthy people. In older age groups, it's more often the exception than the rule—as it is for younger and middle-aged people with multiple chronic diseases. And still most guidelines, "standards of care," and quality metrics are developed one disease at a time. Relatively few guidelines address what happens in the real world: people who have two, three, or multiple conditions. For them, guidelines can offer contradictory advice or lead to so many recommendations that an inordinate amount of a person's time, efforts, and money are going to their medications and health behaviors. In that situation, their risk of adverse consequences is high. Medications interact with one another, leading to numerous or synergistic side effects, or the regimen becomes impossible, undesirable, or unaffordable. Maybe the person stops the most expensive drug or the one that makes them feel bad, not knowing until it's too late whether it was a minor one or a critical one.

Age changes the organs that clear medications (mostly the kidney and liver), and old people are particularly susceptible to adverse reactions that can affect anyone. Older bodies also have reactions that younger bodies generally don't. An old person taking more than four medications has a significantly increased fall risk, one factor that puts falls in the top tier of problems that cause illness, disability, and death in old age.

In real life, what's going on with a person's heart or lungs or mood never occurs in isolation. In science, you need to isolate what you want to study to ensure your results are relevant to your topic. Because medicine leads with science, we have organ and disease specialists, and they form professional groups and societies that produce guidelines about the care of their organ or disease. In an article for the *Journal of the American Medical Association*, doctors illustrated what a guideline-adherent hypothetical seventy-nine-year-old patient would have to do if she had diabetes, hypertension, arthritis, osteoporosis, and chronic obstructive pulmonary disease, conditions that commonly coexist. Following guidelines, this person would take twelve medications in nineteen doses at five different times of day on average. She also would receive fourteen to twenty-four daily (depending on how you count) recommendations for diet and exercise. Her grand total of twenty-six to thirty-six health activities per day would constitute a near full-time job and put her at jeopardy for many interactions and adverse events. If she failed to do those activities, she would run the risk of being labeled "a non-compliant patient."

The exclusion of old people from studies is ridiculous. Osteoporosis—and the sometimes treatable, sometimes debilitating fractures it causes—is largely a disease of old people, with the majority of cases in both men and women occurring in people in their late seventies or eighties. Yet a study looking at all the randomized control trials on the management of osteoporosis entered in the rigorous Cochrane Library Database found that the mean age of participants was sixty-four. For this condition with a mean age near eighty-five, a quarter of all trials excluded patients on the basis of age. This is like studying menopause in thirty-year-old women.

High-quality care for the decades of life beginning at age sixty-five often requires different approaches and metrics than those developed for younger adults. Paradigms based not on chronological age but on more dynamic variables that also include illness burden, functional status (a real-world marker for physiological fitness), health goals, and life expectancy have been proposed in areas of medical care from cancer screening to surgery.

Currently, we don't know enough about how the substages of old age differ biologically, immunologically, or in health risks because we haven't studied them the way we've studied subphases of childhood and adulthood. In part, that's because in the past the relative rarity of old people made it hard to enroll enough of them in trials and would yield results of use to fewer people. But our population has been aging for over a century, so that's not the whole story.

Studying very old people poses unique practical challenges, from demands that are more onerous for older participants to the impossibility of getting informed consent from people with dementia. It also can be hard to distinguish age effects from those of the many diseases and medications most of us acquire in our later years. Last but not least, many people have argued that studying old people is a less-good use of resources than studying younger populations. But life is rarely a zero-sum game. Most Americans are or will become old, and all of us benefit from a healthier populace. Frequently, research on older adults helps younger people, too. In one recent study, young and middle-aged adults who received more aggressive treatments for colon cancer fared worse than the older adults who received what some clinicians would call "less care." You can't distinguish age from disease or better from worse if you don't look at all the options. And you can't safely prescribe medications for people if you haven't studied those medications in those people's bodies.

I met Arturo seven months after he had been hospitalized for diverticulitis and then, two weeks later, for pneumonia. When he was finally home and healthy again, his dementia worsened, and he had trouble sleeping. Part of this was likely the dementia, but another part was situational. Except when the physical therapist came and helped him out of bed, he lay on the same mattress in the same room, day in and day out. There was a window and a TV and his daughter, Teresa, who brought food or sat with him chatting when she got home from work, but come bedtime, he was in the same place and position he'd been all day and sleep eluded him.

In the weeks after he came home, Teresa did everything she could think of to help him sleep. She gave him warm milk. It didn't help. He suggested a slug of bourbon might be more effective, but she thought that would be a mistake with his medications and the forgetfulness and confusion that had gotten so much worse during his weeks in the hospital.

The less Arturo slept at night, the more he dozed during the day. By nighttime, he was wide-awake. Sometimes he hallucinated, calling out to people who weren't there. The apartment was small, so if he was up talking or watching TV, Teresa slept poorly. She'd already missed days of work when he was sick, and now she was showing up exhausted and impaired. She reasoned that if he could sleep at night, they'd both be in better shape.

On her way home one Wednesday, Teresa stopped at the pharmacy and found an entire aisle devoted to sleeping medications. Always dutiful, she read the warnings. The cautions were mostly about things her father no longer did: driving a car or operating heavy machinery. Many had cautions about use in children or pregnant women as well. At home, she gave him the pills, and they seemed to help a little.

In the months that followed, Arturo complained that his vision was getting worse. His family assumed that it was old age. His grandson bought him a larger television. Then one day he couldn't pee and ended up back in the hospital. They said he had an enlarged prostate blocking his urine and putting him into kidney failure. They put in a urinary catheter and told Teresa he would need to have a catheter for the rest of his life.

I met him the next month. He'd actually been referred to us after the first two hospitalizations, but we always had a long wait list. Sometimes people died or worsened before we could get to them. There weren't enough of us, and since people who are homebound and their 24/7 caregivers tend not to have the time or wherewithal to make a fuss, either no one noticed how many old San Franciscans had inadequate access to the health care they needed even when they had perfectly good insurance, or it wasn't the sort of thing they cared about enough to take action.

Four to six million older Americans are homebound, and homebound old people have 22 percent more emergency department visits and 57 percent more hospital admissions than nonhomebound old people. Housecalls reduces those numbers, sometimes considerably, saving the health system money, and patients and families much pain and hardship. This is partly because the cost of one emergency visit equals the cost of ten housecalls—numbers that demonstrate our system's skewed and counterproductive reimbursement and priorities.

During my history and physical exam of Arturo, Teresa said something about the blindness and urine problems being new and fairly sudden. That made me look up from my computer. I asked her a question I had asked earlier, but this time I had her show me any medication she had given him over the last few months.

The culprit was on top of the refrigerator, not with the official medications, the ones with labels from the pharmacy as a result of a doctor's prescription. Like most people's, Arturo's over-the-counter medications were neatly organized in a pillbox, with separate compartments for each day's morning, noon, afternoon, and nighttime doses. Like most people, Teresa had assumed that medications she could get over the counter without a prescription were safe if taken as directed, weaker than those that required a prescription.

"Why are so many medicines so easy to buy if they're so dangerous?" she later asked me, as the pieces came together.

It's a good question. Her father's sleeping medication was sold over the counter, and its side effects and toxicities weren't mentioned on the packaging. Because of Arturo's prostate disease, the pills shut down his urinary tract, leading to kidney failure. They worsened his glaucoma. While the medicine helped him sleep at first, eventually it worsened his confusion and that made him more likely to hallucinate, so neither Arturo nor Teresa were getting much sleep.

At the hospital, when asked about medications, she had even mentioned the sleeping pills. Yet no one had said anything. Maybe they, like Teresa, assumed the medication was safe.

"We used to give patients that all the time," said a friend of mine who's a retired nurse. "I only stopped taking it myself when my daughter read online that it was dangerous."

Current over-the-counter medications harm older adults and current warnings value certain lives over others. When an old person gets sick, we assume it's par for the course. A quote often attributed to Hippocrates offered sound geriatric advice on this topic: "Leave your drugs in the chemist's pot if you can cure the patient with food."

### CHOICES

In the third year of medical school, doctors-in-training moved out of the classroom and into hospitals, spending two to eight weeks in each of the core medical specialties. At its start, the only thing I knew for sure was that I wouldn't be a surgeon. I was born nearly blind in my left eye, so I lack depth perception, and no one wants a surgeon who can't tell for sure where her scalpel is in relation to their colon or artery.

Of course, my first rotation was surgery. Within hours of arrival at the hospital, I watched with fascination as a resident and senior surgeon opened a patient's abdomen, removed its faulty parts, made additional improvements, and—after hours of concentrated, painstaking work—closed it again. Later that evening, the patient woke up, sore, groggy, and considerably healthier. It was amazing.

On the second day, I scrubbed in on several cases, one surgery with each of the three residents on my team, all male, all over six feet tall. By midday, I realized that we all look more or less the same inside, and the slow process of cutting, cauterizing, and reattaching, while terribly important, wasn't very interesting to me. "It's way better when you're doing it yourself," explained the kindest member of my supervising quartet. In the final days of my rotation, Ahmad would guide me through an amputation, the rare sort of surgery where my lack of depth perception didn't matter, and I would realize that he was right.

In the interim, I learned many things about surgery, making it clear that even with perfect vision it wasn't for me. Most mornings, my team of residents would discuss our patients in the cafeteria. The only times in fifteen or forty hours that we would eat, these sessions were also where I learned in person what some men sound like when women aren't around. As a female medical student *not* going into surgery, I achieved a unique state of being simultaneously present and invisible. They "pimped" me about my cases, aggressively testing my knowledge while listening to my patient updates. The rest of the time, they spoke in ways I've otherwise only ever overheard. By the end of the first month, I could pretty accurately guess the rating on a scale of one to ten each resident would assign any unsuspecting women who passed through their sightlines. I assume that had my own looks warranted a higher rating, this might not have happened. I also assume that Ahmad's kindness stemmed in part from his having suffered similar insults. Further, I realized that making repairs on a sleeping patient wasn't too different from making them on a hard drive or a vacuum cleaner. While cognitive skills are essential, much of the actual work is physical and technical. I wanted a specialty where the challenges were more intellectual and relational.

Pediatrics remained at the top of my list for the first five months of my third year. In the sixth month, I did my required rotation on the toddler ward at Children's Hospital. Very quickly, I realized that sick kids saw doctors as mean and scary—and that included me. Like the nursing staff, some doctors had long-standing, affectionate relationships with families, but theirs were more formal and skewed by a power differential. They also spent less time with the children. These little patients had heartbreaking stories of genetic bad luck, parental abuse, or horrific misfortune. At every procedure, they cried and screamed, too young to understand what was being done to them. Meanwhile, my classmates on our outpatient rotation reported that in clinics most kids were healthy, therefore medically "uninteresting." By winter break, I knew I would not become a pediatrician.

Over that vacation, I began reading books on mental illness. Psychiatry was my next rotation, and I liked the idea of a specialty where talking to patients was paramount. I was eager to learn the medical take on such human basics as mood, behavior, identity, and sanity, and gain the skills to translate these concepts into better lives for patients. On my first day, after an orientation, I was told to join a therapy group already in progress. I entered a room of young to middle-aged adults arranged in a large circle.

Trying not to be disruptive, I scanned the room to pick out one of my supervisors. When I couldn't, I moved quickly toward one of the two empty chairs and tried to figure it out from the discussion. On an inpatient psych ward, I reasoned, that should be easy. Thirty minutes later, other than the doctor leading the session, I still wasn't sure who was who. More disturbing still was that when I began tending the sickest patients, I would sometimes have thoughts like *This person is completely crazy.* That could have been funny, considering where I was, if it weren't so clearly morally reprehensible. By the first week's end, I had to admit that I didn't have what it took to be a good psychiatrist. To my surprise, I found that although I considered myself less science-oriented than the average doctor, I wanted a specialty that would allow me to use more of my newfound biological knowledge and technical skills.

Next came neurology, then obstetrics and gynecology. Those weren't for me either. I began to worry that the years and substantial expense of my medical education had been wasted. I was running out of both time and specialties, and concerned that I'd made a terrible mistake. Maybe I didn't want to be a doctor. I considered my remaining options. I was drawn to fields that recognized people as more than the sum of their parts and ailments, valued considerations of context and culture, and acknowledged life's inherent ambiguities. Those preferences ruled out dermatology, pathology, radiology, and anesthesia, with their focus on a single organ, cells, images, and machines, respectively.

That left two options: family or internal medicine. Over spring break, I read John McPhee's *Heirs of General Practice* and John Berger's *A Fortunate Man*. I loved the idea of family medicine, but neurotic as I was about ever knowing enough medicine to do right by my patients, a specialty that required expertise in kids and adults, medical, surgical, and obstetric care might leave me in a state of perpetual anxiety and insecurity. I wanted breadth, but maybe not quite that much of it.

Internal medicine was my last rotation. Right away, I knew I'd found my niche. It included everything about the care of adults except major surgery. Patients could have physical or mental illness, or both. They could be eighteen, one hundred, or anywhere in between. You could talk to them, and most could choose the treatment course that would work best for them. I loved its range and possibilities. Also, the internists I worked with that month were smart, thoughtful, and kind to each other and to their patients—traits not present on many of the teams I'd worked with in other fields.

Internal medicine allowed a honing of specialized skills while offering an array of career opportunities: primary or intensive care, hospital or clinic, global, preventative, or occupational health. I would know how to take care of most internal organs and diseases and many different populations. For me, this was the perfect option.

# ADULTHOOD

*We don't imagine that we, who strive to be and view ourselves as well-meaning and competent, might be neither.*
—Balford Mount, MD

# 7. YOUNG ADULT

TRAUMA

It is summer, 1992. I am a new doctor in the emergency department at San Francisco General Hospital, standing in a chaos of crash carts and swarming, shouting men and women in green scrubs. The trauma room is rectangular, windowless, and whitewashed in bright, artificial light. Life-support equipment occupies one long wall and chrome cabinets line another.

I am female, white, and young. The patient is male, brown, and younger still. I have just moved across the country to start my residency training in primary care internal medicine. He has suffered multiple critical wounds from a gun or knife. Both of us are new to this hotbed of urban urgencies and emergencies—a relentless montage of bleeding, breaking, nodding, gasping, screaming, and dying humans.

At one end of the room is the bed; at the other, two opposing doors aligned so a person could race with a gurney in a straight shot across the room's width. He is in the bed, of course, and I am standing in that race path.

In those early days of being a doctor, I am surprised again and again to find myself the healthy, clothed person in the doctor-patient relationship. I ask people questions that would be considered rude in other circumstances and touch them in places their closest friends never will. To this patient, I look like everyone else in the blur of professional faces. But there I am, just standing and watching, fully cognizant that the patient and I are the only people in that busy, crowded space not moving in purposeful ways.

Around us, doctors, nurses, residents, and medical students assess the patient's airway, breathing, and circulation, do the head-to-toe survey, and locate and quantify his visible injuries and other, less obvious sites of damage, the vital organs and easily nicked arteries along the trajectory traveled by the blade or bullets. They put in IVs, order fluids, X-rays, and CAT scans, set up for a central line, page the senior trauma surgeon, and call up to the operating room and intensive care unit, setting other crews of competent people into action.

I have been taught each of these steps and have some idea of what needs to be done, but "some idea" seems dangerously inadequate and abstract. I have no experience with serious traumatic injuries and little idea how to actually do what needs doing. I don't know how to decide what happens when, who should do what, how to figure out what has already been done or begun, or how to jump usefully into the fray. I also don't know how to get answers to any of those questions in this moment when the patient needs everyone's full attention. I am far more afraid of doing something harmful than doing nothing at all. After all, the bottom line about what is going on in this trauma room is that the patient is, to use a vernacular in which I'll become fluent later that summer, *trying to die.*

"You!" someone yells. "Prep the chest wall!"

Relieved, I position myself on the patient's left at torso level. There are tables of supplies on either side of me and countless people clustered along each of the bed's four sides. I recognize the tall form and short ponytail of a woman I like who had been a year ahead of me in medical school. She's training in general surgery.

A bottle of antiseptic appears in my hands. I find gauze, rip open the packets, and soak them. I have read about chest tubes and once saw one inserted, so I know where to clean. Equally reassuring, I know from other procedures that the antiseptic effect will be maximized if I apply three layers, allowing each to dry before adding the next. I don't consider that the method of application might vary contextually.

I spread the tawny liquid at the patient's armpit, below the thick, dark hair he probably didn't have just a few years earlier, moving the gauze in long, circular sweeps and overlapping the wet lines so no skin is left vulnerable to infection. An injury has torn his lung, and the air it can no longer hold is filling the thin pleural space between the lung and inner chest wall, compressing the damaged lung and making it harder and harder for him to get the oxygen he needs. Once the outer chest wall has been cleaned, the surgeon will insert a thick tube into that space, draining the misplaced air and allowing his lung to properly inflate. I appreciate the urgency of the situation and am moving quickly, but I'm also focused on doing it well and getting it right.

As I wave my hand near his chest wall to accelerate drying, I look around, noting that the bed and floor are littered with medical detritus: plastic and paper wrappers and sheaths, as well as pieces of the patient's cut and ripped-off clothes, remnants of which dangle from his body amid catheters, leads, and blood. I am surprised by how little blood there is and how much of it appears iatrogenic—the result of his medical care rather than his injuries.

Just then, near my right ear, a female voice says loudly, "What are you doing?"

It's the surgeon, the woman I knew from medical school.

"Give me that." She rips the antiseptic bottle from my hand, pulls off the cap, pours the liquid onto the patient's chest, and drops the bottle. Color soaks the sheets and drips onto the floor as she reaches for what she needs from the open chest tube insertion tray on the table behind us. In emergencies, time matters more than some protocols.

"Hold him still," she barks, and I do.

Blood appears instantly along the neat line she makes with her scalpel. She moves her gloved fingers and a clamp into the space she has created, lifting and separating the skin and subcutaneous tissue from the structures beneath. The patient's insides are strikingly pale. A red trail of blood flows out from the wound and down his side, creating a small pool on the sheet below.

She works quickly. An instrument goes in, she leans forward, and there's a visible give as the metal shaft enters the pleural space. She puts her long finger into the aperture she's just made, inserting it as far as the knuckle, then moves it around. I do nothing but watch. Her motions are ones I might use when preparing a Thanksgiving turkey, but she's working on *a living human being*. I am not disgusted so much as mystified and appalled by the things one person can do to another.

I remember the patient bucking, which seems questionable in retrospect, though not impossible. In truth, the trauma I recall most vividly from that day is my own.

A quarter century later, I remember that as I painted our patient's chest wall using the same deliberate technique I now use before injecting a patient's knee or shoulder, the surgeon was looking at me with disgust, not disappointment—professionally, in other words, rather than as a friend or acquaintance. Her glance, as much as the trauma room events themselves, seared this moment into my uneven memory of that long-ago summer.

For days and weeks and years after that day in the trauma room, I couldn't discuss what had happened with anyone. I felt ashamed by my incompetence and discomfort, and by something else I couldn't name.

In medical school, there had been those who couldn't wait to do the audacious things doctors do in and for human bodies, things that would be considered preposterous or criminal in other circumstances. Those students weren't by any means all future surgeons, though I suspect most, if not all, future surgeons fell into this category. Without hesitation, and with what seemed to me uncanny instincts about what was required and how to do it, they made themselves useful. They fit right into medical culture, and I did not. Terrified of hurting patients, I awaited guidance and permission.

As disturbing to me as my own failings was the fact that a woman I had known as nice could violate another person's body so casually and with such brute force. I could not think of how to politely phrase a question about what made that possible for her, or how to ask it with genuine curiosity. I also recognized that a portion of my discomfort had to do with gender, since she, like me, was female, and female violence is less likely to be physical. That thinking, I knew, was not entirely fair to either her or most men, even if I thought it for reasons based on abundant social, biological, and historical truths.

Here is a summary of what went on in that trauma room: the patient needed a chest tube. The surgeon did what needed doing the way it needed to be done, quickly and accurately. I neither understood nor adequately accomplished my own small task. We kept the patient alive long enough to make it to surgery and then walked away, acting like it was just another day at the office, because that's what it was.

These are facts.

But so, too, are these: metal, plastic, and fingers were shoved into most of the patient's orifices and through his flesh to create new holes in his endangered body. In his first moments in the trauma room, when he cried out or tried to complain or resist, he was forced into submission. At no time in the process did any one of the many people not doing something critical at that moment tell him what was happening or why, in case he could understand. At no time after did anyone pull the team together to discuss what we saw, and what we did, and what we might have done differently or better.

In situations like that—settings and circumstances where at least some people deem the violence necessary—there are so many facts. And many opportunities to do, and be, better.

I know this because I have seen doctors who are equally skilled in compassion, communication, procedures, and crisis management. Most of us are better at some of those than others, yet too often the first two are considered added bonuses, while the second two are seen as essential. This perspective is a defining trait of medical culture, though few recognize it as the ethically charged selection of priorities that it is. They see only the benefits of procedures and only the challenges of teaching, encouraging, and evaluating compassion and communication. Such valuing of certain sorts of knowledge over others is also a choice.

MODERN

The twentieth century was a period of rapid growth and progress in medicine, the highest of high points in medical history. Pathologists discovered causes and mechanisms of diseases and age-related changes, and researchers developed new diagnostic and therapeutic options, from EKGs and surgery to antibiotics, hormones, and other lifesaving medications. Medical advances in areas like cardiology, oncology, dialysis, and joint replacement in particular saved lives of people over fifty. Humans stopped dying when they once would have, gaining years and sometimes decades of meaningful life. They lived into old age with more "treatable" medical conditions—approached with the same fix/cure mentality that had reaped such great rewards earlier in their lives.

But treatment that had been beneficial in younger adults could be problematic in old age. Patients were increasingly kept alive in warehouses, either those called "skilled nursing facilities" or nursing homes or others, scarier still, where machines breathed for them and fed them, where they lay day and night, unable to move or talk and receiving few, if any, visitors.

For most of the century, the majority of research to elucidate specific diseases and their treatment was done on young or middle-aged people. Of course, old-age specialists studied old people, but they focused on the oldest and frailest patients and on geriatric syndromes, conditions such as falls and frailty of critical importance to old people but of little interest to most doctors. That left much of old age and most people in their later sixties and beyond languishing in a no-man's-land between standard adult internal medicine and geriatrics.

In the late 1930s and 1940s, panic about declining birth rates and increasing longevity fueled an interest in the study of aging and geriatrics in developed countries. By the 1950s, gerontological societies and journals existed in at least seventeen countries, mostly in Europe, and by midcentury geriatrics was at least an unofficial specialty in most of those countries, though nowhere with large numbers or high prestige. In 1953 the United States had three geriatrics professors, and Glasgow appointed the first UK professor in 1964.

Unfortunately, those developments did little to improve the experiences of older patients. Not only were old-age specialists few in number, but their efforts were often stymied by the medical establishment. In the 1950s, American geriatricians complained about the unwillingness of general hospitals to admit older patients and the paucity of geriatrics-trained nurses. Similarly, a 1956 British government report noted that "the old age group are currently receiving a lower standard of service than the main body of consumers and there are also substantial areas of unmet need among the elderly." They cautioned that doctors should not be writing off ailments in old patients with "the facile explanation as being due to 'old age.'"

This still happens. The best response to this combination of social prejudice and medical laziness came from a nonagenarian who went to see a doctor about knee pain. After a history and exam of the knee, the doctor said, "What do you expect? The knee is ninety-five years old!" To which the old man replied, "Yes, but so is the other one, and it doesn't bother me a bit."

In the wake of World War II, improved diagnostic and treatment methods led to increased awareness of the roles of functional and psychological factors in the health of older adults, and some expansion of special institutions for people with dementia and other age-specific conditions—at least in some countries. Many national health systems in Europe, Japan, and elsewhere combined medical and social care to effectively allow older adults to remain at home (as almost all wish) and to prevent costly hospitalizations and nursing home placements. The United States bucked this logical and socially responsible trend.

The line between medical and social care is created by politics, not biology. Most European countries began providing glasses, hearing aids, walkers, and dentures as part of national health care. Not so in the United States, where they continue to be viewed as "nonmedical," leaving individuals or families to pay for them. Today, the very poor can sometimes get them through Medicaid or charitable organizations, and the well-off can easily buy them. Everyone else is out of luck. The thinking behind this is that medical problems require drugs or surgery; a condition that doesn't need one or both of those isn't medical, even if it is a bodily dysfunction that affects well-being and health. In the United States, you can get laser treatments that might not help your eye disease, but not the glasses that will enable you to keep active despite your visual loss. And you can get a cochlear implant but not a hearing aid. By calling costly, "sexy" interventions medical, and cheaper more functionally focused devices nonmedical, American health care supports the high-profit pharmaceutical and device industries (that fund political candidates from both major parties) at the expense of the far larger numbers of citizens who would benefit from assistive devices (the people many politicians would like to represent but cannot because not supporting big health means not getting reelected).

## INDOCTRINATION

PubMed is the search engine for the National Library of Medicine's comprehensive biomedical and life sciences journal article database, an online resource where doctors look up almost everything. Put in the word *violence* and dozens of key phrases pop up. However, none of them address the violence doctors inflict on patients. Searching *violence* by *doctors* yields articles on violence *toward* or *against* doctors.

At this moment in American history, violence figures daily in the news, the perceived need for violence is highly subjective, and certain people are more likely to be its victims than others. Police and prosecutors, policymakers and the public, are all examining how they contribute, consciously and unintentionally, to our society's explicit and structural violence. Yet, in my profession, we are not reconsidering our own violent acts from new or varied perspectives.

It's not that we're avoiding current events, but doctors look at violence as we look at everything: from a position of power and privilege on our turf (conceptual as well as concrete). These days medical professionals are talking more about race and racism and how violence affects the lives of our patients, trainees, and colleagues. But we aren't looking at the unnecessary violence of our own work—in particular, those instances when we say we have no choice, claiming there's no other means to our unquestionably laudable ends and that people who question our violence in those moments, when lives or organs hang in the balance, clearly do not understand what we're up against. In medicine—as in law, policing, politics, and education—we labor under the delusion that our challenges are unique, our coping mechanisms justified, our fundamental assumptions accurate, and our moral imperative sacrosanct.

When my PubMed search came up empty, I e-mailed a renowned academic, a person well versed in the medical literature, to ask whether I was missing some key search phrase or literature. Her reply made it clear that no one is studying violence from this particular angle, at least not directly. It's also worth mentioning that her speculations about the people who might know about violence by doctors all studied the topics of *problem patients* and *problem doctors*. While these groups matter, I am at least as interested in violence by those of us who are *not* problems, we who are by all measures just doing our jobs and doing them well.

A 2002 World Health Organization report notes that violence lacks a singular meaning, since both acceptable behavior and harm are culturally influenced, subjective, and fluid. Then it offers this definition: *the intentional use of physical force or power, threatened or actual, against oneself, another person, or against a group or community, that either results in or has a high likelihood of resulting in injury, death, psychological harm, maldevelopment, or deprivation.*

Strictly speaking, by this definition, violence in medicine is inherent and ubiquitous. In most doctor-patient encounters, the physician holds the power. We have license to use some types of physical force. Many medical decisions, discussions, procedures, and prescriptions carry a high likelihood of harm or trauma, as does our deprivation-filled, hierarchical, and psychologically demanding training process. As we move through our days, violence is a constant threat and frequent reality.

But this definition neglects the issue of intent, as in the person's primary goal in the act. In medicine, force or power are generally exerted with the goal of improving a patient's health or saving a life, not with the intention of harming or killing, though those things regularly happen as well. As a child with a ruptured appendix, when I nearly died in an elevator on the way to the operating room, people jammed needles into me, shoving parts of my body, yelling, and thrusting a tight oxygen mask over my face. As a teen, when I dislocated my shoulder playing volleyball, a tall, muscled orthopedist yanked at the arm in order to put it back where it belonged, using a maneuver that felt medieval and, if only briefly, shockingly painful. The first medical violence saved my life; the second restored function in my dominant arm.

Yet there are many other instances where I'm left wondering about where and how we determine what violence is necessary or acceptable. For example, does being in the trauma room offer license to do things as expeditiously as possible, providing a pass to doctors who are stressed and afraid of performing badly or failing their patient? And if so, what about doctors who have too much to do and need to get through this procedure or that admission, and this call night or that clinic, so they can move on to the next one? Where do we draw the line of acceptability, and where should we? Should the line's location vary by circumstance or specialty, or by individual acts versus systemic and structural ones? At present, we count only a small fraction of medicine's harms, prioritizing those suffered by patients over those to staff and systems, and counting almost exclusively the harms that visibly affect the body or its function while ignoring the scars of violent words, actions, and policies on psyches and relationships.

I'm also thinking here of the damage done by harms inadequately acknowledged. A friend whose husband has cancer sent me e-mails in which she described his treatment, meant to induce remission of his disease. In the less likely but ideal scenario, his treatment would also cure him. Three months in, she wrote of his chemo: "It halts—reverses, more like—his recovery progress from the surgery. He's skinny skinny—it feels like an inadequate word to describe his physical condition."

Two months later, she explains that he stopped the chemo early. "It was just so grueling. Since he stopped, he's been gaining some strength and weight and eating with somewhat less suffering."

Those last three words haunt me. The chemo didn't have just *a high likelihood of resulting in injury, death, psychological harm, maldevelopment or deprivation*; it was undeniably causing all those things except his death, and it was pushing him toward that terminal precipice as well. Equally telling, the violence had been such that my friend and her husband couldn't even imagine the end of suffering; the most they could hope for was less of it.


Anyone who has been through medical training, and most people who have been in medical settings for other reasons, particularly as a patient or as a person who loves a patient, has witnessed violence. Often it is necessary but sometimes it is not, or it is questionable, or more of a potential than actuality. I should explain that I'm using the word *potential* here as we do in anatomy, to signify a space that exists but isn't always apparent between two adjacent structures . . . until it fills with inflammatory fluid or blood as a result of injury or disease. Thus, even now, when violence can be felt everywhere in our divided body politic, it's entirely possible for certain sorts of people—a middle-aged white female doctor like me, for example—to go weeks and see it only if I choose to.

So much might be questioned or questionable in the minute-to-minute practice of medicine, but we have been conditioned to assume its necessity. In both medicine and society, when it comes to violence, we haven't done enough to negate the negative, or to adequately explore the line between necessary and unnecessary. If we were to find that line, I suspect it would be like the line between water and land in a tidal zone, where what is expected varies with seasons, weather, time of day, and who is looking—a local, a tourist, a fisherman, a naturalist, or a poet.

Numerous exposures to violence shouldn't necessarily affect how we respond to the distress of others, but they seem to. In this regard, it seems that violence functions a bit like smell and opiates, stimulating a phenomenon called tachyphylaxis, in which a person's response rapidly diminishes with repeated exposure. We stop noticing the perfume, or need more narcotic, or we no longer register another person's suffering. Some people argue that the last of those insensitivities is an essential adaptation to an environment replete with danger and misery. That may be true in part, but studies also show a near universal decline in empathy during medical training. Some of what we classify as healthy adaptation may be toxic acculturation. We stop perceiving patients as people and see them instead as tasks, impediments, or problems—as other or less than. When a plurality or even a visible minority of people in one setting or profession become insensitive to the essential humanity of others, the culture itself is unwell.


In almost all situations, context matters and stress erodes empathy. Both influence not only what happens but what we see and how we understand it. When I was a resident, the hospital was my home. There are 168 hours in a week; most months, I worked 100 hours a week. That sort of immersion is known to ease and speed acculturation. When combined with restricted access to basic life functions, including drinking, eating, urinating, sitting, and sleeping, it begins to resemble indoctrination. We saw our colleagues far more and more often than our families or friends. The norms around us became our norms, especially when we felt most stressed or frustrated, scared, angry, overwhelmed, or exhausted. By my second and third years of residency, I was very competent at my job. In all contexts, I felt like a doctor. It's only now that it occurs to me that when I felt like a doctor, I felt important, powerful, and (mostly) benevolent, and I noted the violence less or accepted it more easily; it was just part of the work. Only as I emerged from training and began resuming more of what might be called normal life activities was I able to see, in unquestioned ubiquity, medicine's violence and the threat of it.

But that isn't quite right either. I keep thinking of the concept of conscience and remembering situations in which I submitted to cultural norms even when I suspected or knew they were wrong. Throughout my residency and occasionally since, my patients have sometimes needed procedures only a different sort of specialist could do. In many of those instances, the other doctor forged ahead without allowing me enough time to draw up local anesthetic or order and administer premedication. They didn't seem to care when a patient was moaning or holding the side rail in a grip so tight their knuckles blanched.

Violence is easy for people without empathy or a conscience, but even among nonsociopaths, some are more inclined to it than others. In medicine, we tend to see surgeons as more violent and their subculture harsher. While there is evidence for the accuracy of such generalizations, they blur the more important truth that most of us have done little to question or reform the violence we so often encounter.

"Empathy," writes Rebecca Solnit in *The Faraway Nearby*, "is first of all an act of imagination, a storyteller's art, and then a way of traveling from here to there." In all interpersonal relationships, and so in all medical care, the *here* is me and the *there* is you. Physicians have produced an extensive literature about empathy. There are scales to measure it and interventions to increase it, and still it plunges downward as people become doctors, and the innovative new curricula we come up with every decade or so make no difference. I see this year after year when teaching reflective writing to doctors and doctors in training. With medical students, shock and horror at witnessed medical violence bubbles up in their stories, sometimes inadvertently, often insistently. They identify with the patient. When I teach the same material to practicing physicians, it is evident that by residency, and certainly thereafter, the horror largely vanishes, replaced by other topics, such as mortality, suffering, affection, impotence, or disillusionment, in which the violence is at most the main event's unacknowledged backdrop.

There are also countless articles by doctors about doing things they instantly or later regret, and about standing by or laughing or helping while other doctors say or do reprehensible things. These stories often lead to shame so profound that people don't talk about the events for decades. One article of this sort that caused controversy a few years ago involved a male doctor's admission that during medical school he had played along with a male physician's indefensible behavior while the latter's hand was inside an unconscious postpartum patient's vagina. Very notably, the article's content was not the primary reason it got so much attention both in the medical blogosphere and in publications from *Cosmopolitan* to the *New York Times*. The fuss erupted because the medical journal had insisted that the author remain anonymous. Its editor in chief stated that this unprecedented action was taken to "prevent the identification of others in the story, most importantly the patients involved," but because years had elapsed and names had been changed, and because unconscious women having life-threatening bleeds following delivery of a baby tend to remember things other than the name of the medical student standing by during the day's traumatic events, many found it hard to believe that the patient was the journal's primary concern.

There are so many ways in which a culture of violence is built and reinforced, and so many ways, direct and indirect, that all of us become part of the aggression and its consequences.

## MISTAKES

Now and then, like all doctors, I make mistakes.

In medical school, we had been taught to ask about sexual orientation by saying, "Do you have sex with men, women, or both?" Asking about a stranger's sexual practices does not come naturally to most people. If you are in your twenties, asking a fifty- or eighty-year-old "grown-up" what they do in bed or in bathroom stalls or in dark alleys or on business trips feels wrong. The afternoon my class spent practicing that question included a fair amount of sweating, terror, flushing, humor, awkwardness, and anxiety. You had to remember that you were asking solely to ascertain whether the person's practices posed health risks. You weren't prying or being rude or engaging in voyeurism. You were going to be a doctor, and a doctor needs to know such things to keep her patients healthy and safe. You had to prepare your mind and face and voice for answers that surprised, disgusted, or intrigued you. You had to listen without preconceptions or judgment, searching only for something that might raise concern about your patient's safety, health, or well-being. Then you could gently offer advice from your expertise. As in normal life, unless it involved a child or abuse, the rest was none of your business.

By the time Kate came to see me in the early spring of my intern year, I felt completely comfortable with the question and thought I pulled it off quite well. Kate was just out of college, new to the West Coast, and very healthy. She had long brown hair and wore a miniskirt over green tights and retro pumps. When we got to the sexual history part of the interview, I asked the question, certain I knew its answer.

"Women," Kate said. "Only women." She had her head tilted down slightly, but her eyes were looking straight at me. The surprise showed on my face. I had made faulty assumptions based on stereotypes, and we both knew it. I scrambled to recover, asking subsequent questions in an even, reassuring tone. Though we continued as if nothing had happened, the truth hung like a stench between us.

Mistakes come in many shapes and sizes. When patients aren't sure whether they can trust their doctor, they are less likely to be honest when questioned, and less likely to bring up personal concerns. I had hurt Kate's feelings that afternoon and damaged our relationship. If I were Kate, I would have changed doctors. She didn't. She was young, so maybe she didn't know she could. Or maybe she thought all doctors were prejudiced, a bias she might have acquired through the same channels that I had acquired the biases that made me wrong about her. Every time Kate came to see me over the next couple of years, I felt guilty, and every time she left my office, I knew I'd missed another opportunity to bring up what had happened.

My failure to apologize to Kate was the first instance of a pattern. I would do *or not do* something that was less outright error than a misstep falling short of obvious ideals—seeing normal test results, then getting busy with clinic and forgetting to let the patient know; a follow-up call a month or two after the immediate aftermath of a spouse's death. Later, I would feel horrible, think obsessively about my lack of consideration, tell myself to phone, to say something. And, too often, I would do nothing. Recurring mistakes tell a doctor so much about who she is, especially when intuitively she knows better.

Even well-trained doctors with the best intentions make mistakes. What matters are the kinds of mistakes they make and how often they occur. Some come as a result of sincere efforts to address complex situations, and others signal professional incompetence. The former are more common than the latter. Almost without exception, recognizing my errors, apologizing for and learning from them, has not only made me a better doctor but also brought me closer to my patients and their families. Apologies join patient and clinician in shared humanity.

Studies also show doctors who apologize are less likely to be sued. There are few things more insulting and infuriating than knowing something went wrong and having a doctor or hospital pretend it didn't, essentially ignoring your distress while filling their circled wagons with lawyers and jargon. That's the sort of response that transforms disappointment and sadness into anger and litigation. I suspect doctors who apologize usually feel better too. Apologizing doesn't eliminate my regret, but it renders it more tolerable and that makes it possible for me to learn from my mistake.

In our second year as residents, we got more responsibility and independence. I led teams of doctors and medical students in the hospital and in my clinic. I could decide whether to walk down the hall to consult with a supervisor.

I needed the senior doctors less often, but I consulted them that winter about Maria Calderon. I knew I was missing something; I just couldn't figure out what. As it turned out, neither could my supervisors, though in fairness to them their impressions would have been tainted by what I told them. It was only when she was correctly diagnosed that I realized I'd been looking for the symptoms that "Norm" would have had, not what I should have been looking for given her eighty-six years.

In the biological science of aging, *normal* is defined as "due to the natural course of events rather than a pathologic process." That can be hard to determine without also knowing all the causes of diseases and aging, and perhaps even quixotic, given that how humans define aging and disease has varied by culture and over time. But it's even more complicated than that. Many diseases are age-related, and with scientific progress, changes initially attributed to aging can turn out to be the consequence of disease. Conversely, aging can mimic disease, which further muddles the picture. There is also the question of whether what's normal changes with age. Normal is often considered inevitable and universal, while pathological implies a deviation—but is it fair to compare patients who are twenty years old to octogenarians? If disease is common in old age, does that mean it's normal? It gets confusing, and the best answers to many of these questions come from philosophy, not science.

Such debates notwithstanding, doctors have noted the unique norms of old age for millennia. Hippocrates commented that "the fevers of old men are less acute." Aristotle discussed an increased vulnerability to disease among old people and how even minor diseases might result in death. In Britain in 1863, Dr. Daniel Maclachlan considered what is now known as "multimorbidity," noting that older adults often had several diseases simultaneously, complicating diagnosis and treatment. Around the same time, the most famous nineteenth-century French physician, Jean-Martin Charcot, also noted the "special characteristics" of older bodies when sick. In 1866 he wrote that even the "gravest disorders manifest themselves by slightly marked symptoms." In the early 1990s doctors were often aware of these special characteristics, but they contributed little to the lens used to assess and manage older patients.

\* \* \*

Maria Calderon had a long list of diseases, the worst of which was trigeminal neuralgia, a facial nerve pain so severe that sufferers sometimes kill themselves. I had been her doctor for a year and a half when she complained of feeling unstable. When a patient uses the word *dizzy*, most clinicians will tell you that something inside them clutches, if only for a second.

People mean so many different things when they use that word. It can express vertigo, a general feeling of unwellness, feeling faint, or feeling out of sync with the world, physically, mentally, or spiritually. It could be caused by specific conditions of the ear, heart, nerves, brain, eyes, or psyche, or be a sign of a stroke or an abnormal heart rhythm, anxiety, or a drug side effect. It could simply signal the need for new glasses. Given all Maria's diagnoses and medications, I came up with a handful of plausible causes. I cleaned her impacted left ear, adjusted her drug regimen: Was her blood pressure low? Were her sugars high? Was the dizziness from the pain medicines for her trigeminal neuralgia? I repeatedly checked her heart and nervous system. Nothing helped.

Then I went on vacation, and after Maria fell at home, she was seen in clinic by one of my co-residents. Sunny made the diagnosis of Parkinson's disease as Maria walked down the hallway toward the exam room. I hadn't seen it before in the early stages or in someone as old and frail as Maria, but Sunny recognized it right away. Maybe, not knowing Maria, she hadn't been distracted by Maria's existing diagnoses and medications, any one of which could cause dizziness. I confessed my missed diagnosis to my supervisor, and he told me he'd made the same mistake a decade earlier; it was far easier to spot Parkinson's in an otherwise healthy sixty-year-old than in a frail, arthritic eighty-six-year-old.

When I saw Maria a few weeks later, two of her daughters were with her. Given the new diagnosis and all her other problems, they were going to move her to Sacramento with them. I apologized for not seeing the Parkinson's, and the three of them looked at me with surprise. The daughters had brought me presents to thank me for my very good care of their mother. Maria said she would miss me, took my face in her hands, and blessed me. We hugged good-bye in the exam room doorway, and then she was gone. Some days being a doctor can fill you in equal measures with joy, satisfaction, sadness, and chagrin. Sometimes you know you have the best job in the world.

## COMPETENCE

One morning on a routine housecall, I climbed steep brick steps and rang a doorbell. After a brief wait, I rang again. The doorbell, visibly in need of repair, drooped from the stucco wall. You had to hit it just right for it to chime. I made sure I heard it ring and restarted my waiting clock. Millie moved very slowly. Often, before she opened her door, I could read and sometimes answer an e-mail. After I'd responded to several messages, I called our office coordinator to make sure she'd spoken to Millie the previous afternoon and confirmed the appointment. She had. I thought: *This isn't good*. Millie had dementia, alcoholism, and a marginal home situation supervised by a nephew who lived an hour away. I was fairly sure she wouldn't have gone out; she hadn't for years, and there was also the practical challenge of her front steps. I punched in her number and heard the phone ringing inside the house. I was debating whether to call her nephew or 911 when I heard a noise. It stopped, then started again. It sounded like it was coming closer, so I waited.

Finally, the door moved inward from the frame, though without fully opening. When Millie still didn't appear, I carefully pushed it. She was leaning against the wall, looking awful: disheveled, sweaty, pale, weak, and breathless. I grabbed a pillow off the sofa and lowered her to the floor. After a quick assessment and a few key questions, I knew she had spent the many hours with chest pain and several other symptoms of a heart attack. I found an aspirin in the bathroom and put it in her mouth while phoning her nephew. I started with him, not 911, since her advance directive said to avoid hospitalization.

He and I agreed Millie should go to the emergency room to confirm the diagnosis and get her comfortable at the very least. That would give us a better sense of severity and care options, and time to arrange visiting nurses and home help. Millie couldn't weigh the pros or cons but she was amenable, which she wouldn't have been if she had felt well. The last time she'd gone to the hospital, years earlier and before I'd met her, she'd suffered through alcohol withdrawal, then a rehabilitation unit stay where of course they wouldn't let her drink. She didn't see the point in any of that. I called 911 and finished my assessment while we waited.

Ten minutes later, the paramedics had taken over, and I phoned the emergency department to tell them what to expect. I was way behind schedule and had an urgent add-on appointment. When I was told there'd be a wait before I could speak to the doctor in charge, I said I couldn't wait. I gave the clerk the essential information and continued to my next housecall.

A few hours later, I called the hospital to see how Millie was doing and learned she was still waiting to be seen. That made no sense. I told the doctor in charge what had happened that morning, and immediately she set in motion the wheels of appropriate care. Later, we pieced together what had gone wrong. My message had been abbreviated beyond recognition through a series of hand-offs that began with a nonclinician taking notes and ended like a child's game of telephone. The paramedics had been summoned to another emergency just as they arrived to drop her off, accidentally taking their paperwork with them, and the emergency department was overwhelmed with critically ill patients. When the triage nurse had asked how she was doing, Millie had said, "Much better, thank you. How are you?" The paramedics had treated her en route, and without chest pain or shortness of breath to report and unable to remember recent events, she'd invented a stomach flu to explain why she was there. She had been parked in the hallway ever since.

In the trauma room, an EKG revealed a largely completed heart attack. It had probably happened overnight, but it might have still been partially treatable if I'd waited to give a report to a doctor or nurse, or if the paramedics had left their documentation. Millie also would have received the prompt care her symptoms warranted if someone in the emergency department had noticed the disconnect between her appearance and story of an unbothersome minor illness. Since more than a third of people over age eighty-five have dementia, those discrepancies should have provoked a brief cognitive assessment and then a call to me or the paramedics to find out why she was there. While most older people do not have dementia, it's common enough that checking should be the norm, especially in a patient like Millie, who was neither homeless nor mentally ill but had the dirty fingernails, skin, clothes, and feet of a person unable to care for herself well enough to meet usual social standards.

\* \* \*

Like coins, the common challenges of old age have flip sides. If Millie's experience in the emergency department was tails, then Ray's stay upstairs on the medical wards was heads.

At age one hundred, Ray was admitted to the hospital with a blood clot in his leg. On the third day of his hospitalization, the hospitalist—a doctor specialized in the care of hospitalized patients—called me to discuss how they should decide among outpatient treatment options, since Ray's partner had died years earlier and he didn't have other family.

"What does he want to do?" I asked.

The hospitalist laughed awkwardly. After a pause, he said, "We thought his mental status put him beyond decision-making capacity for something like this."

In medicine, when it comes to a patient's ability to make decisions about their own care, we consider two distinct but related states: *competence*, a legal status decided by a judge and rarely revoked without evidence of dangerously impaired judgment; and *capacity*, which is situation specific and can be assessed by any clinician, though many call psychiatry consults, a situation that makes many psychiatrists roll their eyes. Capacity comes down to the person's ability to accurately assess the implications of each possible course of action. If they can do that, they're entitled to decide however they want, even if their decision differs from what their doctors recommend and seems to go against their well-being or best interests.

Ray was fully competent and perfectly capable. "Is he delirious?" I asked. When I'd spoken to the intern earlier, he hadn't mentioned that.

"No," said the hospitalist. "We think he's pretty much at his baseline."

At this point, I was feeling confused. "Sorry if I'm not following. What would he like to do?"

There was a pause, then the hospitalist asked, "He doesn't have dementia?"

Suddenly, I had an idea of what might be going on. "He's profoundly deaf. Is he wearing his hearing aids?"

Although more than 80 percent of people over age eighty-five have at least mildly disabling hearing loss, the team hadn't considered the patient's hearing and the hospitalist couldn't answer that question. It's the rare centenarian whose ears are still working normally.

The inpatient team thought Ray had dementia because whenever they asked him a question, he gave nonsensical answers. Ray's brain was just fine. That was why he'd left his costly hearing aids at home, so they wouldn't get lost in the hospital, as had happened to him once before. Later he told me he'd tried to get by reading lips. "I guess that isn't my forte," he said, and we laughed.

I suggested the hospitalist borrow the pocket talker from the nurses' station.

"The what?" he asked.

Although an associate professor well into his career, this doctor didn't know about the little devices that enable communication with hard-of-hearing patients. Pocket talkers consist of small, over-the-ear earphones for the patient and a sound amplification microphone for the speaker. They are primitive, only making speech louder without mitigating the sound distortions of impaired hearing or muting background noise the way good hearing aids do, but they help.

With the pocket talker, Ray easily made and communicated his own decisions. The nursing home bed the team had ordered for their "demented patient" was canceled, and he went home, where he completed his six months of blood thinner medication without any trouble.

### SHAME

Here is another scene from my training years that I cannot forget. It's early evening in San Francisco on the sort of cool, clear fall day when you can turn a corner and see a long, horizontal line where the flat expanse of Pacific Ocean meets the glow of creeping dusk and understand why humans thought the world was flat. But instead of walking out the hospital's sliding double doors into a satisfying night of exercise and dinner, friends and sleep, I am a second-year resident in the days before duty-hour restrictions, on my way to see the sole patient on my service whom I don't particularly like.

His room is midway down the hall, not far from the nurses' station. It is dimly lit, less because of the time of day than because he prefers it that way. He is full of demands. I rarely dislike patients, yet I'm struggling to find something in this endlessly dissatisfied man from which to create even a thin laminate of affection or respect. I sincerely hope that I will be able to make it through the procedure he needs without saying as much to my team.

Of course, the patient is only part of the problem for me this evening. Our team is on call. For the next twenty-four hours, we are responsible for all admissions to the medical service, our significantly sick current patients, and those of the several other teams who get to go home. Also at play are one solid but not stellar intern, another enduring her year of medical training before she can sink with relief into the words and milder rhythms of a psychiatry residency, and three medical students, including a third-year I am working hard to help but who, barring a miraculous transformation, will fail his core medicine rotation.

We will not leave the hospital until we have done everything that needs doing for both our new admissions and all the other sick patients on our service, work that generally takes an additional nine to eleven hours after we hand off on-call responsibilities to the next day's team. At this point in my training, I have been on call every third or fourth night for the better part of four years. I do not expect to have much of a life and have put aside not only thoughts of the world outside the hospital but also images of the garden burger I like to order for dinner at this hospital, the lumpy mattress in the medical resident call room, and the one not completely revolting water fountain a few floors down. Strangely, I don't feel tired; working despite chronic exhaustion has become as natural as breathing, even if it is not without its impact on my physical, intellectual, and emotional well-being. Efforts on behalf of patients and my endurance during this arduous young adulthood of medical training often fill me with the smug warmth of righteous self-satisfaction. Nevertheless, this particular call day is testing me. To use proper residency lingo: we are getting slammed. This is better than "getting killed" or "getting slaughtered," but our growing tallies of admissions, or "hits," and the large burden of other patient tasks, or "hurts," mean we might yet achieve an even less desirable status.

I am thirty years old. The patient in question is older than me by ten or fifteen years, also white, but male. He has AIDS, as so many of our patients do in this San Francisco hospital in 1994. He is not a new admission. Those acutely ill patients are gathering elsewhere in the hospital: in a handful of other rooms along this same hallway, in the intensive care unit two floors below us, and in the emergency department on street level awaiting the availability—via discharge, transfer to another service, or death—of a free bed upstairs.

He has a fever. We have already sampled the usual sources: sent his urine and blood to the lab, X-rayed his lungs, surveyed his skin and looked in his ears and mouth, pressed on his belly, and tested his nervous system. Since we cannot adequately explain or treat his fever, protocols require that we pull from his spinal cord a few tubes of the hopefully clear—but, because he was ill, perhaps cloudy, straw-, orange-, or red-colored—fluid bathing his brain and test it for bacteria, fungi, and mycobacteria.

The subpar medical student and I collect the lumbar puncture supplies, have the patient sit up so we can identify the correct level of his spine for needle entry, position him on his left side in the fetal position facing the pulled shades, and clean and disinfect his skin. Before we entered the room, I had run through all these and the subsequent steps with the student, and now I stood back and let him take charge. Except for the patient's demeanor, this is a perfect student case because the patient is relatively young and has terrific bony landmarks.

The student is slow but appears to be doing everything just right. I hover while pretending not to and he frequently looks up at me for confirmation. We silently confer about entry place and direction, and he inserts a local anesthetic and then the thick lumbar puncture needle, pushing first through the skin and next toward the slim space between vertebrae. The needle goes in smoothly. All three of us release breaths we didn't realize we were holding. Then the needle stops. From the way it stops, I know it's hit bone. We had discussed this. My student looks at me, I nod, he makes an adjustment and tries again. And again, and again.

I step in without tipping off the patient that the student had failed, assessing the patient's position and adjusting the needle until it's just right: angled slightly toward the patient's head and aimed at his belly button. I am good at lumbar punctures. In over two years of residency, I've never missed one . . . until now. I pull back slightly, shift the needle upward a fraction of a centimeter, and push it forward. When you find the right spot, the resistance feels rubbery. If you push a little harder, the needle successfully pops through and then you pull the stylet out of the needle and the syringe fills with fluid. I hit only bone, solid and impenetrable.

I smile apologetically at my poor student. His situation was like mine the day before I took my driver's license test, when my mother took me out for what we were sure would be my last practice session. I couldn't even start the car. I tried and tried. Nothing. Exasperated, she insisted we change places. But the car wouldn't start for her either. We called a tow truck.

I again try the lumbar puncture. Each time I move the needle, our patient tenses. He asks if I know what I'm doing and doesn't believe my answer. I march along the seemingly endless hard surface of his spine with the needle, feeling for the slightest change in resistance indicating I have reached the soft space between bones. His already curled body is coiled with tension. Goose bumps cover his skin. Now and then, he gasps. At the needle's tip, I encounter bone, and bone, and bone. Each time the metal hits the highly sensitive periosteum, he protests.

I look at my medical student. He can't take a coherent history or do a competent physical exam, but he has well-developed muscles and can hold in place our patient—thinner than he is, sick, and twice his age. Sweat forms dark stains on the armpits of his blue scrubs, but if he is disturbed by what we are doing, I can't tell by looking at him. More obviously present in his eyes is the unwavering desire to please me. On academic thin ice, he will do whatever I ask.

"Try to relax," I say to the patient in as gentle a voice as I can manage. But what I'm thinking is: I've never had a problem doing this procedure, even in patients whose landmarks were obscured by obesity or whose ancient spines were distorted by arthritis, but of course with this patient, who is unpleasant and often dramatic under the best of circumstances, I can't get in.

I am usually vigilant about premedication, pain control, bringing bedpans, and whatever else patients require to feel as comfortable as they can in a hospital. This evening, I don't care. I suppress a desire, an almost physical urge, to stab the patient more and harder. I need this procedure over and done with. My pager keeps alarming. My interns need supervision. I have no idea where the other student is and hope she isn't still with the new patient I asked her to admit three hours ago. All over the hospital there are other patients with my name on their charts. I would rather be doing anything else other than dealing with this particular person. I am hungry and have to pee and my desire to flee this room is like an itch I can't reach.

Time to heed my own advice. I take a deep breath. I reassess the situation. I pull the needle all the way out and start from the beginning. I speak little and move quickly, intent on success. The patient's breath becomes audible as the needle slides in. He groans as I feel the pop. The medical student hands me tubes and we collect the fluid we need.

The patient remains in a fetal position, his back to me, trembling. We lower his thin gown to his waist for the procedure and the air in the room is cool, but I know his shaking isn't just a matter of temperature.

"Okay," I say. "Okay. It's over." I cover him. The room is quiet, though beyond its closed door we hear voices and a beeping machine. He looks frail beneath the sheet. Looking at him, I realize that for a doctor, for me, there may be a fate far worse than failing at medicine's necessary violence. I have just hurt someone I am meant to help.

When I put my hand on his shoulder in a lame, late gesture of comfort, he flinches. The answer to what's making him sick may be in his spinal fluid, and the sooner the fluid gets to the lab, the sooner we'll be able to give him the medication he needs to get better. He knows that as well as I do, but both of us also know that's not the reason for his submission. In becoming a doctor, I have become a monster. Instead of taking time to ensure his comfort, physically and psychologically, I have used my power, position, and physical strength to get the procedure over and done with. I have defeated him, and I have never felt so ashamed.

BIAS

In *The White Album*, Joan Didion quotes a transcript from the Alameda County grand jury in which a nurse describes the day the Black Panther founder Huey P. Newton showed up at the Kaiser emergency room with a bullet in his stomach from an encounter that left one police officer dead and another wounded. Newton became a political martyr as a result of this incident and received a (subsequently reversed) prison sentence of two to fifteen years for voluntary manslaughter. During the quoted exchange, Newton asks for a doctor, and the nurse, who describes Newton as "this Negro fellow," repeatedly asks whether he's a Kaiser member. She insists that he sign the admission sheet while he yells that he's bleeding and needs medical attention. The year was 1967.

Didion, who is white, offers the excerpt to illustrate a "collision of cultures." By *cultures* she seems to mean not so much the cultures of black and white Americans as those of the sort of person Didion thinks would be a Kaiser member and the sort of person she believes would not. When she discovers Newton was indeed a Kaiser member, she feels that her theory of him as a historical outsider confronting the established order has been shattered.

Since this story is at least partly medical, it might be useful to borrow a medical concept to better understand it. In medicine, the "differential diagnosis" is the list of possible explanations for a patient's condition. Items that might appear on the differential diagnosis for Newton's encounter with the Kaiser nurse as Didion presents it include:

- The supremacy of bureaucracy over human decency and good medical care.
- Racism, conscious or unconscious, on the part of (a) the nurse, (b) the system, or (c) both.
- Differences in points of view, namely, how the same amount of blood can appear quite different from different perspectives: Huey says, "Can't you see all this blood?" and the nurse says, "It wasn't that much."
- A collision of cultures, version 1: "He didn't appear in any distress," said the nurse. It's now well known that people from different backgrounds and demographic groups express distress in different ways, whether they're contending with a gunshot wound, a heart attack, childbirth, a broken bone, or the death of a loved one. It's also well established that doctors and nurses respond differently to people in pain depending on their gender and skin color.
- A collision of cultures, version 2: "He called me a few nasty names," continued the nurse. Though rude behavior is rarely if

ever called for, it's also true that there are individuals who curse when frustrated or otherwise upset—Newton and me, to name just two examples. Newton, in pain, bleeding, and being given the bureaucratic runaround, had reason for frustration, if not for rudeness.

- A collision of cultures, version 3: A white nurse saw a black man with a bullet wound in a city and country where poverty and violence are ubiquitous in most black lives and bullets regularly penetrate black skin. A black patient saw a white nurse in a white institution saying *Hold on a minute*, saying *Calm down*, saying *I need to know that you belong here*, saying *I know better*, saying *We have rules and procedures that need to be followed and have nothing to do with the color of your skin*.

- Evidence that medicine is not outside or above the fray of social issues.

- Evidence that James Baldwin was right: the story of "the Negro in America" is the story of America, and it is not a pretty story.

In medicine, a doctor generates a differential diagnosis in hopes of identifying all possibilities and arriving at the right one. That approach works best if one looks only at disease, not illness. If we look instead at the individual patient as a human being in a larger social context, single explanations rarely tell the whole story. In Newton's case, it seems likely that each of the explanations on the "differential" of his Kaiser encounter fit. Certainly, it's hard not to suspect that an entirely different conversation might have ensued on both sides of the equation if a white man had presented with the same bleeding gunshot wound and, equally, that it might have been a different conversation regardless of whether or not he was a Kaiser member.

But maybe that's just my bias.

Forty-two years and 14.1 miles from the hospital where Huey P. Newton showed up with his gunshot wound, a patient of mine arrived at the emergency department of our university hospital. Mabel was confused, with slurred speech and a fluctuating level of consciousness, meaning she was alert at some times and sleepy and hard to interact with at others. Tests were done to determine what was going on, including a toxicology, or "tox screen," for certain legal and illegal drugs, which is a fairly routine test when patients have what clinicians call "altered mental status."

So far so good, right? Except that Mabel was ninety-four years old and had been bedbound and fed through a tube for nearly five years after a devastating stroke. While she was too confused to be able to relay the details of her condition, it could have been diagnosed from the doorway of her emergency department cubicle: the ancient face, the unnatural kink of her neck and left arm, the feeding tube puckering her gown where it jutted up and dangled from her abdomen. Alternatively, the doctors and nurses taking care of her might have glanced at her chart that prominently listed her age and underlying conditions, or they could have asked a few basic questions of her concerned daughter, who stood at the bedside stroking her mother's forehead and murmuring soothing words, or her two sons in the waiting room. Any one of those approaches, all such routine parts of the initial patient evaluation that they have standardized labels—"general appearance," "chart biopsy," and "past medical history," respectively—would have made clear that by far the most likely cause of Mabel's altered mental status was delirium.

Unless an acutely confused older patient is hit by a car or found with a heroin needle in a vein, they should be considered delirious until proven otherwise. Yet the doctors caring for bedbound ninety-four-year-old Mabel sent a toxicology screen. It may well be they did this out of habit or because they were following an (illogical, expensive) age-blind protocol. But those aren't the only possible explanations. I know because I had a "control" patient, also old and quite debilitated, who was seen in the same emergency department in the same month as Mabel.

For the better part of the last decade of his life, from his mid-seventies to his mid-eighties, my father became delirious every time he entered the hospital. He had delirium from a heart attack, a knee replacement, cardiac bypass surgery, pneumonia, an allergic reaction, a bladder infection, another orthopedic surgery, and two falls. On exactly zero of these occasions was a toxicology screen sent by the emergency department staff tending him. Since drug abuse is less common in females than males and less likely among the very old and homebound, it would have made far more sense to send a tox screen on my father than on Mabel. But that's not what happened, even though their presentations were similar. Medically, both were old and frail, with long lists of diagnoses. Socially, both were accompanied by supportive, educated families, and had me as their advocate. Really, aside from her negative risk factors of greater age and disability, the biggest difference between Mabel and my father was skin color. My father was white, while Mabel was African American. It seemed clear that the resident treating Mabel couldn't imagine her beautifully appointed single-family home filled with generations of family photographs and religious artifacts—not that any of that should have been relevant to the care she deserved or received.

I wouldn't send a tox screen on a bedbound ninety-four-year-old, but I might consider sending one for a younger person, and part of that choice might be based on skin color. If I did, I would note my prejudice, push it from my thoughts, and make an effort to see the patient with an open mind. That's progress, but according to the research on biases in medicine, it's probably not enough. And if people like me—or, worse, people who have such biases and don't see them as problems—are the ones shaping and running our health care system, is it any wonder so many types of people routinely receive lesser care? Almost all of us fall into one or more of the categories subject to health care biases, and even those few who don't today will one day, barring sudden death, by virtue of ill health or old age. When we reach elderhood in a world where a study of four- to seven-year-olds found that 66 percent wouldn't want to be old, no matter who we were beforehand, we all become part of a vast, vulnerable, and underserved population.

The handling of Mabel's and my father's delirium that month illustrates the importance of *intersectionality*, society's multiply interacting and historically ever-evolving systems of privilege and oppression, inclusion and exclusion. Intersectionality shows that it's never accurate to consider a person solely on the basis of just one of their defining categories. Mabel wasn't just black or female or old, she was all three, and also disabled, heterosexual, educated, Christian, well groomed, and so much more. All those factors are always relevant in human experience, playing out not only across individual lifetimes but through generations in ways both good and bad, depending on who you are and when and where you live.

Joan Didion had one explanation for Huey Newton's experience in the Kaiser emergency department until the facts shattered her understanding of him and his position in society. But what if her explanation remained true in some ways, just not in the way she expected it to? Wasn't he both a historical outsider *and* a Kaiser member? And what if all the other possible explanations on the differential diagnosis were also true? Indeed, what if her mistake was not in evoking the wrong theory or assumption so much as in believing any one explanation could be sufficient to account for human behavior?

At the risk of noting so many forms of bias that each loses its impact as list cedes to litany and the battle cry to which this writing aspires devolves into noise, I will merely itemize those for which I have seen scientifically sound and morally distressing data: racism, classism, sexism, ageism, homophobia, xenophobia, and prejudice based on religion, primary language, literacy, substance use, housing status, gender fluidity, behavior in the medical setting, and various diagnoses, both physical and mental. These medical biases lead to bad care and impaired trust and unnecessary suffering, as well as high costs, avoidable disease, and deaths. It's not that each of us manifests all prejudices or that we manifest one or more of them all the time, but—like all human beings—all health care professionals are some of these things at least some of the time, sometimes intentionally and sometimes not.

If two patients of the same age and grooming and class, one brown and one white, present with the exact same heart attack, the white one will receive heart- and lifesaving treatment sooner, especially if the white one is a he rather than a she. If two women arrive with abdominal pain eventually shown to be from the same cause, the white woman will get more pain medication than the brown woman, especially if the white one's primary language is English and the brown one's is not. Equally disturbing from the point of view of a well-intentioned doctor, it seems then that even if I mean well, make regular efforts to educate myself, and feel real and genuine connection with my patients whose background differs from mine, I may do them harm.

Perhaps even more concerning, systems themselves—the National Institutes of Health, my medical center, and that colossal enterprise called

American medicine—can reflect assumptions, norms, and values that perpetuate inequalities, endangering many of the same people those institutions want to serve. There are countless examples where a different norm is listed for older adults based on averages, not outcomes, from lab test results to thresholds for intervention. In most cases, we don't know for sure whether those different standards reflect age-specific norms or inadequately investigated age-based pathology. When I was in training, we were told old people's blood pressure ran high "normally" or "naturally." When the topic was studied a few years later, it turned out that when old people had "normal-old" blood pressures—numbers that would have been considered high in youth or middle age—they had more strokes, just like the young and middle-aged.

Medical norms often shape policy that in turn harms patients. Not only is hearing loss considered a "normal part of aging," allowing most insurance plans to refuse to pay for hearing aids, but American medicine and health policy call hearing "normal" in old people at levels that lead to early intervention in children in order to improve their ability to function, learn, and communicate. Meanwhile, we know older adults with hearing loss develop cognitive impairment 3.2 years sooner than those with normal hearing, and older people with mild, moderate, and severe hearing loss are two, three, and five times more likely to develop dementia. Although we don't know that hearing loss causes dementia (something else could be simultaneously leading to both), it's easier to treat the hearing part of that nefarious couple. Besides, hearing loss in old age is associated with functional loss, isolation, family discord, medical miscommunications, depression, anxiety, and paranoia. All that scientific data on harms, but we have higher thresholds for intervention in old age, and insurance doesn't pay for hearing aids.

Addressing biases and prejudices is complex. Doctors, it turns out, are people. Our behavior has all the variability, inconsistency, prejudices, and complexity that come with that categorization. The issue, then, is not whether "-isms" exist in medical practice but how they manifest, at what cost to patients, and what can be done to make medical care more just in the complex adaptive systems of medical culture, hospitals, clinics, and clinicians. This is where structural approaches are essential. Systems and policies can institution-alize or compensate for human biases and failings—the choice is ours.

Until 2014, kidney transplants in the United States were allocated using a "first referred, first served" system. That sounds like a fair, impartial proce-dure, and it was probably well intentioned. Yet practice data from across the country show that doctors are less likely to refer kidney failure patients of color for transplantation in a timely manner (or sometimes at all). Those later referrals meant African American and Latino patients had lower chances of getting a new kidney; substantially lengthened time on dialysis, a procedure that takes hours, often generates cycles of fatigue and nausea, and compro-mises a person's ability to work and live to their potential; and greater chances of dying. Since 2014, patients' places on the transplant list are decided by when they began dialysis, not referral. This has eliminated some of the struc-tural, race-based inequities in kidney transplantation. Others persist at the ever-moving, murky intersection of history, society, and medicine.

Sometimes systemic injustice is intentional. Other times it occurs because science prioritizes what's easy to measure rather than what matters. When a patient has a heart attack, we look at outcomes such as time from hospital arrival to catheter treatment, use of certain medications, and mortality. But the heart attack of an eighty-year-old with a seventeen-item problem list differs from the heart attack of an otherwise healthy fifty-five-year-old who collapses while jogging, even if the same heart vessel is clogged to the same degree at the same place. Standard medical measures leave out outcomes of critical importance to the older patient, such as return to prior cognitive function, loss of key abilities and independence, and risk of nursing home placement. Who a person is and where they are in their life always matters. Age blindness is another form of bias.

# 8. ADULT

In 2012 a group of doctors at Johns Hopkins made a video called *The Unknown Profession*. The setup was simple. One winter's afternoon, they walked around Baltimore with a video camera and asked people the question "What is a geriatrician?" They interviewed people of different ages, ethnic and racial backgrounds, and levels of education. Most had no idea and tried to guess. My favorite response was "a person who scoops ice cream at Ben and Jerry's." But the interview that sticks with me was of a middle-aged woman trying to find clues in the sound or root of the word *geriatrician*. She was shocked when she learned the real definition, telling the videographer that she had spent the last few years caring for her elderly parents and had never come across that word.

The specialty only emerged in the United States in 1978, and was just a decade old the year I started medical school. Geriatricians were a rare breed, and geriatrics was not on my or any of my classmates' horizon of possible specialties. I heard of just one in four years of med school. That geriatrician worked at one of the two small community hospitals outside Boston where students sometimes did rotations. Working in the emergency department there during my fourth year, I vaguely recall a sighting of her and a lack of clarity about exactly what it was she did. The doctors in the emergency department found her amusing, though they were relieved to summon her when they had an old patient they didn't know what to do with. From them I got the sense that because the geriatrician considered so-called social issues—Could the patient go home safely? Were there day-to-day activities with which he needed help? Why, really, had he come to the emergency department?—she was a lesser breed of doctor. True doctors, my supervisors made clear by their teaching topics and actions, dealt exclusively with biology and diseases and procedures.

San Francisco was no different than Boston in that regard. In our three years of internal medicine training, there was much talk about who would choose which subspecialty, but I don't recall anyone mentioning geriatrics. In my second year, as I began considering my postresidency career, I knew only that I wanted to be an expert in whole-person care and to serve people who really needed me. Many of us in the primary care track felt similarly. We debated whether to stay in academics or work in a community practice, whether to continue honing our skills as general internists or informally subspecialize in some way, maybe by working with AIDS patients. Although I enjoyed my older patients, I'd still encountered only that one geriatrician in Cambridge years earlier and had no idea what a geriatrician did or how it might differ from what a general internist or cardiologist or rheumatologist did when caring for an older patient. As a result, I didn't realize geriatrics was the one subspecialty that would give me everything I wanted, and more. I figured I'd be a general internist taking care of adults of all ages, mostly in a clinic and occasionally in the hospital.


In retrospect, I had gravitated toward older patients from the start but didn't take note until a medical student pointed it out. Our team had admitted a very old, very small Chinese woman who spoke little English and always had at least one, and usually several, members of her large family in her room to help her. She'd come into the hospital struggling to breathe, with no appetite or interest in anything going on around her. After treatment for pneumonia and heart failure, she was a different person. Her bright brown eyes tracked the people and conversations in the room, even when she couldn't understand them. When we told her through her translating relatives that she could go home soon, she put a hand in front of her mouth to hide the teeth missing from her giant smile.

Once my team had filed out of her room into the hall, I reviewed the day's plan with the intern and student in charge of her care. While walking to another floor to see our next patient, the fourth-year medical student grinned at me. She had been on my team at another hospital the year before, and we knew each other fairly well.

"You love old patients," she said.

I looked at her, surprised and a little defensive, as if affection for an older person qualified as a shameful secret and she'd just outed me. Although I didn't have the wherewithal to think it through in that instant, enough people made fun of older patients that I wasn't sure I wanted to be known for having a special interest in them. It took me a second to realize that my student had been grinning because I had been grinning, and I had been grinning because seeing our nonagenarian patient's smile and renewed hope had made me very happy. I'd also enjoyed working with her family, whose dedication filled me with respect and admiration.

But something else about my smiling patient appealed to me, something I'm now loath to admit, much less write: she was cute. Small things of all kinds have always attracted me, and our patient had started small and shrunken in old age. She had tiny, well-formed features and wore a maroon watch cap night and day over her short, salt-with-a-dash-of-pepper hair. In the large hospital bed, she tucked the sheets under her armpits so only her arms, neck, and head showed, a diminutive figure framed by the white pillow, white sheet, and pale blanket.

Calling an older person cute is considered infantilizing and insulting—largely because it is often one or both. As a social justice advocacy website based in San Diego notes, "'Cute,' said of an old woman, does not mean 'hot.' It means that she has said or done something that would not be at all remarkable coming from a normal person but does not fit the speaker's stereotypes about old . . ." Having seen its demeaning uses, I'm sensitive to people's distaste for its use about old people. At the same time, I wonder if the greater problem comes from the *old* than the *cute*.

*Cute* isn't the same as pretty or handsome; it implies an emotional attractiveness, not just a physical one. My family thinks I'm cute, and I love that. Since *cute* is also more likely to be invoked for something or someone small and we shrink with age, old people often earn that label. In old age, foot arches fall, spinal vertebrae and the spaces between them decrease in height, tendons and joints contract. I hope to be seen as cute once those things happen to me, though only if the word is used without condescension. The problem with much of today's use of *cute* is its relationship to mechanistic and commercial notions of human value. Those judgments lead younger people to make indiscriminate assumptions about old age and incompetence, and older people to bemoan and deny normal age-related changes, thereby contributing to their own devaluation. Yet most of the time being called *cute* is a good thing, and not just when applied to someone sexually attractive. It's positive when applied to kids, beloved animals, and winsome behaviors or objects. If used for old people to similarly express affection and appeal, it is not an insult but an acknowledgment that every life stage has unique charms.

Over the year after my insightful medical student's observation, I started paying more attention to when I was most intellectually engaged and emotionally fulfilled. She was right; I found old people, with their long personal histories and complex medical problems, a pleasure and a challenge in all the best ways. There was just one problem: we didn't have geriatrics at my medical center, and although I could have trained elsewhere, I wanted to stay in San Francisco.

Sorting out this situation would require one of the defining skill sets of a geriatrician: I needed to use a blend of scientific data, interpersonal skills, and pragmatic creativity to achieve my goal in a health system that wasn't set up with old people in mind.

LANGUAGE

Three of the most common expressions used to talk about old age are "silver tsunami," "exceptional senior," and "successful aging." One is a metaphor, the second emblematic, and the third a trope. Each is familiar and memorable. But on a deeper level what they are really saying is, respectively: our society's increasing numbers of old people will destroy life as we know it; old age is so instantly and universally incapacitating that ordinary activities become exceptional; and illness and death signify failure. This language is catchy, and seductive. Almost everyone uses it.

At a "reimagining aging" conference, a famous researcher lecturing on aging science and population trends used another popular expression, the aphorism "Seventy is the new fifty." The audience loved it, especially coming from him. While it would be great to help people maintain their health, comfort, and function in old age, his quip implied that younger is always better and seventy has nothing to recommend it. Perhaps most concerning was that this accomplished white-haired scientist couldn't see how some of the most popular sayings about old age do more harm than good.

There are sayings about aging that everyone likes, and others that people find reassuring when they are young or young-old, and preposterous as they grow older still. *You're only as old as you think you are* is one of them. Ursula K. Le Guin rebutted this popular falsehood and several others with her usual wit and brilliance: "If I'm ninety and believe I'm forty-five, I'm headed for a very bad time trying to get out of the bathtub." She goes on to note that when people say *You're only as old as you think you are* "to somebody who actually is old, they don't realize how stupid it is, and how cruel it may be."

Another expression I hear often, one my father invoked several times, is *Old age isn't for sissies*. Of that one, Le Guin had this to say: "Old age is for anybody who gets there. Warriors get old; sissies get old . . . Old age is for the healthy, the strong, the tough, the intrepid, the sick, the weak, the cowardly, the incompetent." She acknowledged that most people say such things with good intentions but equated telling her in her eighties that she wasn't *old* with telling the pope he's not Catholic. She concluded her thoughts on the subject with a most important and poignant insight: "To tell me my old age doesn't exist is to tell me I don't exist." In old age, as in so many other parts of life, when our self-delusions are indulged, our reality and true selves, along with all our needs and opportunities, are erased.

The language of death is telling too, although in different ways. Euphemisms abound, even among doctors. People rarely say someone died. Instead they say: *she passed away; we lost him; she's been gone five years now; he has joined his beloved wife/daughter/parents; she is no longer with us*. Read most obituaries and you will find people die in just one of several ways: *suddenly, after a long battle, surrounded by family, peacefully at home*, or *following a brave struggle*. More rarely these days we learn someone *shuffled off their mortal coil, succumbed*, or *finally gave up*. The religious sometimes *go home* or to *meet their maker, cross over, return to the Lord*, or *rest in peace*. The sacrilegious occasionally joke that someone *croaked, kicked the bucket*, or *bought the farm*.

We use the word *premature* to describe death before old age. The word signifies an occurrence prior to the point of full development, as if the person missed out on key parts of life. But when people do *not* die prematurely, they moan, "There's nothing good about this aging business." Both can't be true, so how does this happen and why does it persist?

Consider the panoply of popular insults for old people: *biddy, blue-hair, BOF* (*boring old fart*), *BOOF* (*burned-out old fart*), *buffer* (stupid but not unpleasant old man), *codger, cougar, crone, fogey, FOP* (*fucking old person*), *gaffer* (old man), *geezer, goat* (old man with sexual interest in women), *has-been, LOL, old bag, old bat, old crow, old fart, old fogey, old-timer, OP, over-the-hill, pop, rhino* (opposite of *cougar*), *sea hag* (ugly old woman), *witch*. These words denigrate, ridicule, and reduce old people, lifting up those who are not yet old and widening the gulf between age groups. They say old is "other," less than, unappealing, abnormal. In Susan Sontag's 1972 essay "The Double Standard of Aging," she explained that as the United States turned into an industrial, secular society, youth had become a metaphor for happiness by virtue of its association with energy and appetites. The economic and power structures required consumption for their continued flourishing, and what better way than to revere the new. By making novelty necessary for happiness, people aspiring to the American dream were compelled to throw away the old for the new.

Youth remains a dominant metaphor in American culture, but what it implies has changed in the digital era. As technology and science have replaced industry and religion as the fundamental belief structures, even among many people who disavow science and believe in God, happiness has ceded the stage to success. Youth's traits—speed and particular forms of beauty and productivity—have become the defining characteristics of achievement, fame, and prosperity. We don't just want faster, slicker devices; we want humans that way too. We prize youth, though doing so means that all of us will spend most of our lives in a state of failure.

Witness this *New York Times* review of Jay-Z's album 4:44: "'Old school' still has some currency in hip-hop. It nods to forebears, styles and history. 'Old' is a different story. 'Old' means you're past your prime. It means you have nothing new to say—and even if you did, who would want to listen? 'Old' means maybe you know what's new, but you want to do it the way you've always done it. So 'old' also means fixed, settled, stuck."

This passage also reveals a prevalent double standard. If a *Times* reviewer wrote comparable words about what *female* or *black* means, I doubt his review would have been published. He might not even have had a job the next day.

In 1978 Susan Sontag defined *illness metaphors* as "punitive or sentimental fantasies concocted about that [illness] situation: not real geography but stereotypes of national culture." While it may be too early to know for sure, I suspect that old age is the "illness" metaphor of this century. It invokes visions of the aged human body as broken-down machine or outdated software. And those are only the beginning. Other metaphors for old age and aging include a journey, a cycle, a season, our natural fate; a problem, burden, disease, or curse; a losing battle, or a clock winding down; the process of climbing a ladder or the state of being over-the-hill; a time that is golden or silver or gray. Punitive and sentimental indeed.

Words and metaphors can bring or strip distinction and status. We need to reclaim the unpopular words of old age to associate them with their original meanings. *Old* is the term for life's third act, just as *youth* is the word for its first. It refers to much more than the late-stage phase of loss and disenfranchisement. Better still, if we didn't deny people's humanity as they reached that late stage, there would be no need to lament the language and metaphors of old age.

## VOCATION

By my final year of residency, my outpatient clinic was full of old patients. When I didn't know something about their care, I asked for help. But even among our remarkable faculty, no one knew much about the particular needs of my oldest patients. I decided to give my third-year talk on dementia, a topic that had received little attention, even though we saw it all the time, especially in the hospital. The talk went well, and before I knew it, what had begun as fulfillment of a residency requirement turned into a presentation I gave for years.

The first and most daunting of these large group talks took place at the annual meeting of the American College of Physicians. I'd been invited because of my topic. Having read all the major and countless minor studies on dementia, I had formulated a coherent way to think about and manage this common and disturbing condition, thus qualifying me as an expert, at least within internal medicine circles. This would not have been the case with most common conditions treated by internists and other primary care clinicians for which there were already true experts with years of patient care and research on their résumés. I felt like a fraud until people started asking questions. This audience had recognized that they didn't know what they needed to know in order to take good care of dementia patients. Less was known about dementia then—many people still believed senility was a normal part of old age—but there was a widespread feeling that our training hadn't effectively prepared us to manage this common condition.

I hadn't even passed my medicine board exams at the time, but suddenly I was an expert. Clearly, there was a huge need for aging information and expertise.

After residency, I did an extra year of training at UCSF in the new general medicine fellowship aimed at preparing young doctors for faculty positions. My program director told me to pick a specialty in which to gain more knowledge, and suggested dermatology, gynecology, rheumatology, or orthopedics. I proposed focusing on geriatrics instead, and, to my surprise, he said yes. Better still, my chief sent me to the annual UCLA geriatrics conference, all expenses paid—a wonderful thing for a person earning thirty-three thousand dollars a year despite twelve years of higher education and training. But that wasn't why the conference changed my life. Until those five days I hadn't fully understood how geriatrics differed from all other medical specialties and why that difference mattered in people's lives as they aged. I say five days, but actually I had an "Aha!" moment.

Let me set the scene: a generic business hotel, a large room packed with tables and chairs, no windows, a conference with few breaks, little or no easily accessible water or food. By midmorning and midafternoon, my stomach growled and my brain felt as though it were floating. Many people skipped sessions to exercise, shop, or meet friends who lived nearby. Not me, not on my kindly boss's dime. Never mind that this particular hotel was on the ocean, or that the average daily temperature in Los Angeles that week was in the low seventies. I attended every talk. My only opportunities for fresh air came early in the morning, during the ten-minute breaks, and after dark. I had never learned so much in so few days that was interesting and relevant to patient care.

Midweek, during the middle of another long day, a bearded UCLA faculty member wearing white pants moved to the podium. Dr. Ken Brummel-Smith's topic was listed on the program as *Rehabilitation*. I'd learned close to nothing in medical school and residency about rehab medicine, and UCSF didn't even have a training program in that specialty. Dr. Brummel-Smith began by discussing the most common reasons older patients needed rehab: strokes, heart attacks, fractures, surgery, and so forth. I had a fairly good sense of that already, just as I also knew the pathological changes in the brain and in the nervous and musculoskeletal systems caused by those conditions. Those are the focus of most medical talks, but he blew through them. Then he blew my mind.

Instead of linking treatment to that pathology—the only approach I'd ever been taught by any teacher in any specialty in seven years—he focused on finding out what the person needed to be able to do to be happy and safe in their individual daily life. What a patient needed from rehab, he explained, and from medical care generally, depended in large part on their answers to that question. Equally counter to usual medical teaching, he told us that even when you couldn't fully restore the body, you could often fix a problem so the patient could do what they needed to do in spite of compromised abilities. Sometimes that required changing how they did things, moving furniture, using equipment, or using a different body part. When it came to function, which was what patients cared about, there were many ways of getting around the mismatch between what a body could do and what needed doing. Strengthening the body was essential, but it was just the beginning. To empower people in their lives and restore their independence to the greatest extent possible, you also had to work on their environment, social network, community, imagination, and adaptability. It sounds absurd to me now, but I remember sitting in that windowless, over-cool hotel ballroom and thinking: This is the most radical, sensible, paradigm-shifting lecture I've ever heard. I was giddy.

It was also the moment when I realized that medical training doesn't just erode doctors' empathy: it brainwashes the common sense right out of us.

The term *geriatrics* was coined in 1909 by the Austrian-born chief physician of New York City hospitals, Ignatz Nascher. In the most widely available photograph of him, the father of American geriatrics appears stocky, with a full face and broad shoulders. Close-cut graying hair hugs his mostly bald pate in an ear-to-ear semicircle above intense eyes, full lips, and a strong chin. He wears a dark suit coat, a striped tie, and a pressed white shirt. He looks like a businessman.

Choosing as his model that other age-specific realm of medicine, *pediatrics*, Nascher combined the Greek words for old age (*geras*) and relating to the physician (-*iatrikos*). By emulating another recently developed and already rapidly growing specialty, he hoped that the fields would develop together. As he later argued in *Longevity and Rejuvenescence*, he believed a word and field were needed "to emphasize the necessity of considering senility and its diseases apart from maturity—apart, that is, from adulthood. He used the word *senility* not as an indication of dementia but in its traditional Latin usage meaning the state of being old. Nascher also considered disease pathologies distinct from the "normally degenerating body" of the older patient, and he distinguished between diseases that might have complications in old age, those that didn't change with age, and diseases specific to old age.

The belief that older patients require specialized study and care has existed since classical times, although as Pat Thane, a historian of European old age, noted, its advocates "have never been numerous or powerful." In 1627 the French physician-professor François Ranchin wrote in *Opuscula medica* words that might emerge from geriatricians even today:

> The conservation of old people and the healing of their diseases . . . has been neglected by our forefathers and even by modern authors too. What has been written about the conservation of old people and the healing of the diseases of old age, is so bad and so unproductive that we get the impression not only that this noblest part of Medicine was not cultivated but even that, yes, it has been flatly suppressed and buried.

Like geriatricians today, Ranchin described the manifestations of general diseases in old people, the effects of aging itself, and disorders specific to older adults. And like old patients of today, those of his era had little or no knowledge of or contact with the small numbers of doctors focused on old age. "For most of recorded time," Thane reports, "neither philosophical nor medical comment on old age (a small proportion of the full range of medical discourse) touched the actual lives of most older people."

In mid-eighteenth century Europe, this began to change. With advances in pathology and microbiology, particularly in France and Italy, *gérocomie* became a well-defined area of medical specialization. By the mid-1800s, all medical teaching in Paris included dedicated sections on old patients. The impetus for this specialized geriatrics research and care came from *hospices*, residential facilities for the poor and mentally ill where older adults too frail to keep working often lived out the last years of their lives. Initially, visible age-related pathologies of specific organs garnered the most attention, while the pathological advances of the time contributed little to new therapeutics. Medicine could do little for conditions that regularly impaired and killed old people, such as pneumonia, cancer, and neurologic diseases, although the new attention to frail patients revealed the harms of long-standing practices, including bloodletting and induced vomiting. Treatment advances later in the nineteenth century introduced surgery for broken bones, cataract removal, and digitalis for heart conditions.

By the turn of the nineteenth century in France, its once exclusively custodial "hospices" were transformed into medical institutions for care, teaching, and research, much like public hospitals of today. Old people were not the only residents, but they were numerous, and physicians seeing large numbers of both adult and old patients began calling for the recognition of old age as a distinct life phase and for specialization in *médecine des vieillards*. Yet, despite the establishment of many other new specialties at that time, geriatrics did not become an official medical field in France for another century.

In most countries, even official status did not lead to recognition of geriatrics alongside pediatrics and adult medicine. In the United States of the early 1900s, Nascher lamented the lack of lectures about old patients in medical schools; in 2019, all schools have lectures, but only a small minority have required geriatrics rotations. At Harvard, long the nation's top medical school, the first geriatrics lecture was given in 1942, but when the school launched its latest curriculum in 2015, it included required clinical rotations in pediatrics, obstetrics, and surgery, even though most doctors will not take care of kids, manage pregnancy, or perform surgery once they finish their education. It did not include geriatrics, although most doctors will take care of old patients and many will do it often. The next year, UCSF's new curriculum increased geriatrics teaching more than sixfold. That sounds transformative, except we went from four to twenty-seven hours over four years while continuing to define *normal* and *pathological* by adult standards and keeping geriatrics an optional clinical experience. There are so many ways to communicate the relative unimportance of an entire category of human being.

In 1940, when Nascher listed geriatrics on a questionnaire, he was told it wasn't a recognized specialty. Today, when I go to the pull-down menus on websites asking for my specialty, geriatrics is often not one of the selections, a reality analogous to the one experienced by many older job seekers who try to enter their birth year only to find the options begin years or decades after they were born. Essentially, geriatrics is to medicine as old age is to society. This tends to bother geriatricians less than you'd imagine, perhaps because we know we are firmly planted on a moral high ground. As the British geriatrician Trevor Howell explained, geriatrics is "a reaction against the belief that after sixty a patient is too old to be medically interesting or therapeutically rewarding."

Nearly twenty-five years after my "Aha!" moment in Los Angeles, medical training and care include more of the lessons I learned at that conference—but not many more. This has set up a vicious cycle wherein geriatricians focus on the oldest, frailest, and most neglected old people, an approach that makes the specialty seem narrow compared to pediatrics or adult medicine, and that self-imposed restriction in turn makes geriatrics easier to dismiss. As a result, few doctors know much about aging, and it's likely that medical care harms and kills old people in ways and numbers far beyond what gets reported. After all, people are rarely surprised when a sick old person dies.

## DISTANCE

The urgent e-mail arrived at three P.M. on a Tuesday from a former high school classmate I hadn't heard from in decades. Allan's eighty-one-year-old mother had been hospitalized and his father was falling apart. His parents were still in San Francisco, though he had long since moved to L.A., where he had a full life that included a high-pressure career, a wife, and two kids. His younger sister lived across the country. Despite his Stanford education and professional success, Internet searches and a call to his parents' primary care physician, Allen had no idea how to contend with the fact that his parents' living situation made no sense, his mother's medical care appeared to be doing more harm than good, and there was clearly something very wrong with his father as well.

Regularly, e-mails like this one go out on our LISTSERV: "Anyone know a geriatrician in El Paso, Boise, Iowa City, Athens, Schenectady, Santa Rosa . . ." These queries come from friends, relatives, acquaintances met fleetingly, total strangers who find us on the Internet, and colleagues in other specialties. At parties, conferences, schools, and gyms, people say, "Can I ask you about my mother/father/husband/sister/self?" They come from everyone and everywhere, because most people grow old, and no one can easily and reliably get themselves the help and care needed for their aging parents, partners, spouses, or friends.

Allan's experience is the norm. After developing a relatively minor and treatable new problem, his mother had been given a dose of a drug suitable for a middle-aged woman. The side effects landed her in the hospital, where other adverse events soon followed: an infected IV site, a nighttime fall, and a broken arm. Meanwhile, with his mother hospitalized, his father's dementia, undiagnosed for years despite frequent medical care, was unmasked. Allan's mother had been compensating. Her husband did well enough if they kept to a routine, and she didn't want to bother or worry her busy children.

Allan had noticed that his father, Carl, was less sharp than before but figured it was a normal part of aging. He assumed that had there been a real problem, there would be a diagnosis, a variant of his mother's assumption that their doctor would have given her husband an official diagnosis if there was something to be done about it. Neither knew that many doctors count only drugs, surgery, procedures, and rehabilitative therapies as treatment. That overnarrow conception of care deprives people of useful, sometimes critical therapeutics—from food and physical therapy to symptom management and trained caregivers. Current dementia medications at best temporarily stall illness progression in some patients, while those other so-called less medical types of care help everyone. Not having a diagnosis meant Allan's parents had not accessed the many strategies and resources available to maximize Carl's independence, safety, and enjoyment of life. Carl also lost the chance to do certain things while he still could, from a much-anticipated Alaska trip with his grandchildren to reevaluating his financial and living situations to ensure his care didn't threaten his wife's health or leave her without resources for her own needs as she aged. It also meant their family didn't have the opportunity to plan ahead for crises like the one in which they now found themselves.

Over several days, Allan and I exchanged long e-mails. I told him what questions to ask the hospital staff about his mother and which assisted living facilities might meet his parents' needs, and sent him links to resources on dementia, falls, caregiving, and financial planning. We also squeezed his parents into our geriatrics practice. They moved a short while later, and their new community provided them with both the practical support they needed and a new version of the active social life they'd always enjoyed. Although they would have preferred to stay in their house, the entire family was relieved by the safer living situation and less harmful medical care. But most people don't know a geriatrician and can't afford high-end assisted living. Wealth and personal connections should not be required for older adults and their families to get needed care.

Yolanda had three daughters all with names that began with the letter C. I saw Cinnamon only once. I interacted with Charrdannay, the out-of-state daughter, regularly by phone, and never heard from Candy, the third, who lived a few hours away, though Charrdannay made clear that she and Candy were in close touch. After a while, I suspected the sisters might have been doing something that's incredibly helpful to a busy doctor: having one point person as liaison between the family and the medical team.

A week earlier, the visiting nurse who had referred Yolanda to our house-calls clinic called to ask if Yolanda could be moved up our waitlist. After her first visit, the nurse had reported Yolanda's case to Adult Protective Services (APS), but apparently, with "one daughter present," Yolanda had denied any problems. Since APS, unlike child protective services, cannot intervene against a patient's wishes in California, that was the end of that. "I know they're overworked," the nurse told me, "but you have to wonder how hard he really tried."

My GPS took me to a public housing complex I knew well from runs and dog walks. It was near a park in a neighborhood of Arts and Crafts, tract, and postmodern homes. I rang the bell and nothing happened. I rang again and didn't hear a chime, so I knocked. Cinnamon opened the door. She had smooth skin and dark depressions under her eyes. Cinnamon didn't say hello or introduce herself, just pointed down a narrow hallway and, with a twist of her wrist, around the corner.

On the doorstep, I already noticed the stench. Inside, it was worse. I didn't need to be told where my patient was; I followed my nose.

Cinnamon barely budged, and I had to turn sideways to pass her. There was a tiny kitchen on the right, a larger room ahead with a couch, TV, and purple cloths hanging over the windows.

I sensed Cinnamon watching as I made my way through the lavender darkness of what had to be the living room, trying to scan for any clinically useful information while pretending not to. Walking down a second, shorter hallway, I passed a bathroom. *Good*, I thought, *it's not far from the bedroom*.

Yolanda's room was square with white walls and very bright. I took in the absent shades, the two single beds, the boxes of medical supplies on the windowsills, and the older woman in the bed on the left, greeting me with a broad, denture-white smile.

We shook hands. She apologized for not getting up. I noticed her filthy, stained covers, her mussed, matted hair and the places she had obviously and unsuccessfully tried to tame it. I noticed, too, the wound supplies and the pill bottles and the fast-food wrappers and the smudged, empty water glass. There was no pillbox to organize her medications and no pink Advanced Directive sign on the wall, although the referral diagnosis was *widely meta-static cancer*, so knowing her preferences would be essential sometime soon and she'd be unlikely to be able to communicate them herself when her body shut down. Finally, I noticed Cinnamon leaning against the wall just outside the bedroom door.

I pretended not to see any of this. I explained that I was the visiting doctor, we had to fill out routine paperwork, and I needed to ask a few routine questions. I did not say most of what I usually say at the outset of a new patient visit in order to make clear that my care won't be restricted to diseases, but kept our conversation boring and standard until I heard the front door slam with Cinnamon's departure.

On the phone later that day, Charrdannay would tell me that Cinnamon took their mother's Social Security money and used it to buy cigarettes and drugs. Charrdannay said she was very worried about her mother, but she lived across the country, had a full-time job and three kids, and her husband was posted overseas. Candy was closer, but her husband was dying and she was overwhelmed. Neither of them could get away, and their sister could not be trusted.

Once I felt certain Cinnamon was gone, I asked Yolanda what bothered her most. "The diapers," she said.

I waited. From the smell in the apartment, I had a guess about why they posed a problem for her, but I had learned the hard way not to make assumptions. Different people are bothered in different ways by adult diapers, with complaints that range from the purely physical to the existential.

"They don't last the way they should," she said.

I asked to see one, looking over my right shoulder toward the boxes stacked on the windowsill. No diapers. Yolanda lifted her covers to reveal a deeply yellowed and fully soaked diaper. The sheets were also wet and stained. It appeared she'd been wearing the same diaper for at least two days.

"Cin might bring some new ones when she comes back," she said.

"Is that what she went out for?"

She shook her head. "I asked but usually she buy cigarettes instead."

I tried to keep my expression neutral while internally debating whether it was better to show my shock, horror, and sympathy or to act nonchalant in hopes of minimizing Yolanda's shame and allowing her to keep protecting her daughter. I felt confident that she would prioritize her motherly instincts over her own well-being.

Sometimes on a home visit, I move through a complete history and physical with relative ease. Other times, one issue takes precedence— shortness of breath, for example, or a stroke, a broken bone, an infected wound or high fever or a blood pressure that's too high or too low. And sometimes I think I've found one pressing issue only to realize there are several. Almost always in that latter circumstance, the problems are only partly "medical" in the narrow, traditional way my profession defines that term.

During the hour I spent with her that day, Yolanda often smiled and laughed, although she had multiple medical problems, including metastatic breast cancer, open chest wounds where the tumor had grown up through the skin, dangerously high blood pressure, pressure ulcers on her sacrum and hips from lying in bed, incontinence (she was too weak to walk to the bathroom), and significant weight loss. Such "medical" issues can rarely, if ever, be entirely separated from their social, political, economic, and cultural contexts.

Yolanda was what we call "dual eligible," a patient with both Medicaid and Medicare. She required those social supports because, despite working six or seven days a week for nearly fifty years, she remained poor. She had received a high school diploma but little education in her native Alabama, and the only sorts of jobs open to her as a black woman in the mid-twentieth century paid little, with no benefits. These new benefits didn't solve all her problems, but they did provide medical care, medications, and supplies. Because she had Medicaid, however, only some doctors would treat her. And because our insurance systems reimburse generously for chemotherapy, little for conversations of patient values and goals and wishes for end-of-life care, and nothing for the time a doctor spends figuring out how to get diapers and a commode for his patient with end-stage cancer and working to sort out her thorny family challenges, Yolanda had been getting regular, apparently useless chemo from a local doctor, but nothing that might have improved the weeks to months that remained of her life.

I told Yolanda Medicaid would pay for diapers and I could arrange to have them delivered. She looked at me as if I'd said something she didn't quite understand or that might be a joke. "Really?" she said in a soft voice. "Really," I answered, and she laughed with surprised pleasure.

We moved on to the rest of her physical exam and "complaints"—the official medical word for issues a patient wants to discuss with her or his doctor. The wounds were bad, and it seemed unlikely we could count on Cinnamon to care for them twice a day. Yolanda needed different treatment, something a visiting nurse could do a few times a week.

Before I left, I told Yolanda the home care nurse and I would be taking care of her together and that at first we would be checking in several times a week to get her medication and wounds sorted.

She wasn't actively dying, but she was at the stage where anything could happen. I needed to know whether she wanted to go to the hospital if she got sick or wanted to stay home, and whether she understood all that hospice offered and felt ready for it. Given her circumstances, there was also a question of whether she wanted to stay in her apartment as she got weaker and sicker or move somewhere else for skilled nursing or hospice care. I was reluctant to push her on the day we met and with her lying in a cold, wet diaper. In her place, that miserable reality might well influence my choices. I wanted Yolanda to have a chance to think through her options while physically comfortable.

She took my hand. "Thank you, baby," she said. "You come back anytime."

When I got back to the office that afternoon, our coordinator said Yolanda's daughter had called. That surprised me until I punched in the numbers and Charrdannay answered what was clearly her office line.

"It's worse than we thought," she said after I described my visit. Still, she had given thought to what her mother might want and not want as her death approached. Her take on things seemed just right, given the inevitable.

"Have you discussed it with her?" I asked. In my schoolgirl days, I would have crossed my fingers.

"Not a lot."

Darn. "Would you?" I was tempted to hold my breath.

"Yes. Of course. I'll try, anyway . . ."

We talked about my plans for her mother's care. "If you want to see her—" I began, toward what seemed like the end of our conversation.

Once again, our minds had gone the same direction. "I was just thinking . . . maybe I could ask a friend to take the kids, come out there for a day or two. I'll leave a message if I can make it work. Also, we have some savings here. It's not a lot, but I talked to my husband. If it would help my mother, I can send it. You just tell me where."

When asked the recipe for a good old age, I often give a list: good genes, good luck, enough money, and one good kid, usually a daughter.

At a Living Well, Dying Well meeting of the Hastings Center bioethics research institute, Joanne Lynn, a leading geriatrician, old age researcher, and aging-policy advocate, said something similar: "And in our current system . . . unless you've got three daughters or daughters-in-law, you should count on being an old person in a nursing home." In that same talk, she offered a reason for why we are collectively doing so poorly: we have a system that was built fifty years ago for a time when we "got sick and died—all in one sentence and all in a few days or weeks." Things have changed. Today, people die in old age from chronic illness after being disabled for an average of two to four years, and without any reliable caregiving system.

## VALUES

When I tell someone what I do for a living, they usually have one of two reactions. Either their face contorts as if they'd just smelled something foul, or they offer compliments about my selfless dedication to an important cause. Those in the former camp usually hurriedly change the subject; many in the latter group tell me, either outright or by implication via excessive praise and admiration, that I'm a saint. These apparently opposite responses are actually the same. Both imply that what I'm doing is something no one in her right mind would do.

Actually, in studies of physician career satisfaction, geriatricians come out on top. There are many reasons why doctors who specialize in the care of old patients are overall happier and more fulfilled. If you choose to do something that falls at the low end of the spectrum of prestige, power, respect, and income in a profession where all four are possible, chances are you are doing it for the reasons that give life meaning: it interests and inspires you, you believe in it, and it gives you pleasure. In other words, you are doing it for love.

People's reactions to my job choice (even to the word *geriatrics*) speak to our societal values. Medicine, calling itself a science while making choices based on those same values, almost universally prioritizes what is fixable and "worth fixing" over what is viewed as neither.

Many of the best geriatrics innovations—palliative care, transitions (home to hospital to nursing home, and all variations thereof), multimorbidity, home care, elder-friendly hospitals—have become part of general medical culture. To achieve that status, most have been divorced from their geriatrics origins. Not associating them with old age increases their appeal. Sometimes this is because they are useful to many types of patients; other times, the shift panders to ageism. But perhaps things are beginning to change. A recent article invoked Sheryl Sandberg's *Lean In*, advocating to move the conversation from what geriatricians (and old people) *are not* to what they *are*. This struck me not only as good marketing but the basis for every civil rights campaign that shifts focus from what certain people can't do to what they are already doing and all they could if they were allowed to.

For too long geriatrics has been like a small religion. We believers are fervent, and everyone else thinks we're fringe or unimportant. We believe that we know the truth, but others don't see it that way. When I teach communication to medical students, I tell them that when most people are not getting their message, chances are the problem is not with the audience but with the explainer and explanation. If as America ages—the baby boomers are entering legal old age at a rate of ten thousand people per day—the field of medicine devoted to the health of older adults remains small, there can be no question that geriatrics is doing something wrong. The better question is: How do we change our approach to ensure old people of all ages and backgrounds stay healthy as long as possible and get good health care when they need it?

In his introduction to Nascher's 1914 classic *Geriatrics*, the renowned pediatrician Abraham Jacobi asked, "Now why is it that the growing interests in many of the branches of medical science and practice has not equally been extended to the diseases of old age?" The minority of clinicians who paid attention to the special needs of older patients had been asking similar questions for centuries. Jacobi also provided an answer: "The cause of this neglect must be sought in the general mental attitude toward the aged."

Nascher was more specific: "Until it receives the attention its importance deserves, and we know more about the metabolic changes in the period of decline, we must fall back upon empiricism in the treatment of diseases in senility." In other words, because we didn't study old people, we didn't understand their unique physiology, and because we lacked that essential knowledge, we could not offer older patients the targeted treatments offered younger ones. As a result, treatment of older patients was based on coarse observations, not studies, and doctors didn't know why some strategies worked and others did not.

Nascher also addressed the presumed source of this "mental attitude," using language that perfectly captures the feelings of many people today, including doctors:

> We realize that for all practical purposes the lives of the aged are useless, that they are often a burden to themselves, their family and to the community at large. Their appearance is generally unesthetic, their actions objectionable, their very existence often an incubus to those who in the spirit of humanity or duty take upon themselves the care of the aged . . . There is . . . a natural reluctance to exert oneself for those who are economically worthless and must remain so, or to strive against the inevitable, though there be the possibility of momentary success, or to devote time and effort in so unfruitful a field when both can be used to greater material advantage in other fields of medicine.

As often happens today, Nascher conflates extreme old age with the entirety of that life phase and emphasizes the negative traits of a minority of old people while failing to mention any of the well-documented positives of the majority. His perspective also stems from a belief, equally prevalent now, that "the prolongation of life is after all the aim and goal of the physician's endeavors." One of the distinguishing features of modern geriatricians generally, and certainly this one, is that we believe the aim and goal of medicine is the optimization of health and well-being—whatever that means to a specific patient. Sometimes that includes prolonging life, and sometimes it does not.

People complain that older people complain too much. But we all speak of the stuff of our lives. Parents of babies talk about babies, parents of teenagers speak of teenagers. Those who work discuss work. Those who do and see more speak of doing and seeing more, and those who do and see less talk of the details and rhythms of their smaller world. Is smaller less or just smaller? Is a still life art, even if it's not a sprawling tableau of human life?

If older people talk more about their bodies, it's in part because of what the old body does or will not do, what it screams or insists on, has become more prominent in their lives. Comfort and abilities, facile to the point of unconsciousness in youth for most people, require attention, effort, or the recognition of impossibility. The relationship between person and body changes as we age.

The fading of certain activities from foreground to middle, then back across a human life, doesn't only occur because of biology. It's also because we live in a world designed for the young and middle-aged, one where an old person often needs a device or helping hand because no one considered them when planning that world. We all recognize the bodily transformation of age, and even if we can't fully explain it, we understand it as the product of genes and choices, luck and repeated use. But what of that shift of potentially competing interests from foreground to back? Do we examine, objectively and thoughtfully, its contributors? Do we consider, alongside debility and choice and character traits, that one reason bodily laments feature so frequently is that we have systematically and structurally stripped, for reasons both benevolent and nefarious in intention, old people from the larger world and the larger world from the lives of old people?

In contemplating what medicine is and should be, whether for old patients or younger ones, I prefer the famous words from the original Hippocratic oath: *to cure when possible, to heal sometimes, to care always.* But Nascher and I are agreed on some of the reasons that make caring for older adults so interesting and fulfilling. When a phase of life is considered difficult, and when, on top of that, the group currently living through that phase is neglected, disparaged, and vilified, opportunities to relieve distress and make a real difference are countless. Just as a dehydrated older patient may go from appearing to be at death's door to looking essentially back to normal after the infusion of a half bag of intravenous fluids, so can I make a meaningful difference in the life of most old people with a warm hello or a sincere interest in talking to them. It should take more than that.

Because old patients are near the chronological end of their lives, most medical decisions, and many in other arenas as well, invoke the grand issues, mysteries, and questions of life and death. In geriatrics, it is far harder to reduce medical care to a disease or organ. Most illnesses also raise existential issues. This may well be what some people dislike most. In a world where if infection = antibiotics and dying tissue = surgical removal, the grand unanswerable questions of existence may inspire passion and curiosity in some and feelings of distress or helplessness in others.

How doctors choose to spend their careers may depend in part on their tolerance for ambiguity and complexity, and their interest in questions that lend themselves as much to philosophy, psychology, and sociology as to science and statistics. In certain specialties, the most defining and time-consuming work takes place actually or essentially without the patient. Those doctors look at tissues and images of people who aren't present or provide most of their care when their patients are unconscious. That's great if they enjoy it, but it's not how I like to spend my time. I'd rather be talking to patients and working with them, their families, and caregivers. Many older patients have multiple medical problems with functional and social implications, which adds to the variety and richness of conversations that inevitably touch on questions of meaning, purpose, and identity. I see such discussions as interesting, unique to each patient, and a meaningful way to spend my time. Not everyone agrees. A recent study of medical student perspectives on older patients quoted a fourth-year student saying that doctors "assume that when an old person comes in there's going to be a ton of problems and it's going to be a pain to address all of those issues." The student did not mention that it's a pain to address those issues because the health care system is not set up to do so.

The most difficult part of patient care of any kind is dealing with the hardest parts of what it means to be human. But ask most people about their most significant, challenging, and worthwhile experiences in life, and most will name these same hard parts, from raising children to the death of a loved one. Hard isn't, of itself, a bad thing. What is bad is when, through avoidance, judgment, tradition, or neglect, we fail to do our best addressing problems that will affect almost all of us eventually, directly and indirectly. How much better and richer would life be for all of us in a society that cared for a ninety-two-year-old for the simple reason that the ninety-two-year-old is a human being, and we care about human beings.

Contrast the quoted medical student's view of old patients as "a pain" with those of the British surgeon Marjory Warren at the end of her training. Faced with an entire ward of bedbound old people, she neither despaired nor ran away. She saw a need and an injustice, and her response was to disrupt, to innovate, and to transform. The impact of her work remains visible everywhere in medicine today, yet the prejudices that inspired it remain.

For each of my patients, if knowing them and caring for them includes sadness and frustration, there is also, to the end, evidence of powerful humanity. Sometimes that takes the form of courage or humor, and other times it manifests as anger, even fury. Their rage can be long-standing, unrelated to current circumstances, or it can be just the opposite, a response to what their lives have become. It is there, in how we construct the circumstances of old age—from the sixty-eight-year-old who wants to work less but still work and maybe try something he didn't dare risk earlier in life to the centenarian who can't see, hear, or move as well as she'd like—that the world offers us so many opportunities to create an old age we need not dread.

For a long time, when people asked why I became a geriatrician, I answered in one of several ways:

"I didn't mean to" was the opening line of one story.

"I screwed up" began another.

"I just loved older patients" started the third.

Each reply was equally true, but even taken together they didn't tell the whole story. There are so many good reasons, it's hard to know where to begin. Since many people believe dealing with old patients is harder or less pleasant and fulfilling than dealing with younger ones, I often told the story about a Saturday night—or, rather, an early Sunday morning—when I was on call for the General Medicine practice. This was call from home—meaning I carried a pager overnight and on weekends, fielding calls that ranged from medication refills to grave illnesses requiring ambulances and handoffs to doctors in the emergency room.

I was sound asleep around two A.M. when my pager alarmed. I turned on my bedside light, rubbed my face to wake myself up, and called the page operator. She gave me the patient's details, the most salient of which was that he was an otherwise healthy twenty-two-year-old who had been out dancing and was complaining of shoulder pain. I dialed the number she gave me and identified myself as the on-call doctor.

"Oh, hey, Doc," he said. "How're you doing?"

"Fine, thanks," I replied, wondering whether the middle-of-the-night pleasantries meant his pain wasn't so bad after all or simply indicated stoicism and good manners. "I hear you've hurt your arm. Can you tell me what happened?"

"I don't know if I hurt it, but it definitely hurts."

I waited.

"I was out dancing—Saturday night, you know?"

I murmured affirmatively to suggest I might still be the sort of person who went out dancing, rather than a woman just ten years older than he was and thrilled to be in bed at ten P.M.

"The music was pretty wild, and whenever I did certain moves with my left arm, the shoulder seriously hurt."

I began asking questions to establish when the pain started in order to figure out how he'd injured himself, what the injury was, and what next steps were needed for diagnosis or treatment and to manage his pain. On call in the middle of the night, my main concern was whether he needed to go to the emergency department for a dislocated shoulder or fracture and, if neither of those seemed likely, to come up with a plan for damage control until Monday, when he could be seen in clinic.

"I didn't fall or anything like that," he said. "I'm not sure when it started. Maybe a month ago?"

I blinked. "Did something make it worse tonight?"

"Hmm. I don't think so. It's just that when you're dancing, you really notice it, you know?"

He woke me up to ask about a problem he'd had for a month that didn't interfere with his daily activities—didn't even stop him from going out dancing—and hadn't gotten worse. Did he think doctors sat up all night hoping someone would call?

I asked a few more questions to make sure I hadn't misunderstood.

"Well," he said at some point, "I told my buddy it was bugging me and he said I should get it checked out, so I called."

I told him that I couldn't make a diagnosis over the phone but that his friend was right, he should have it evaluated and treated so he didn't develop chronic problems. I added that the after-hours line was for emergencies and he needed to call back Monday morning for a clinic appointment but that I'd let his primary doctor know what was going on.

It took me a while to fall back asleep.

I'm an early riser, so I was up reading the Sunday paper when my pager went off again about two minutes past seven that morning. The caller was an octogenarian who had woken up in the early hours unable to use her left side. I called back immediately.

"Good morning, Doctor," she said with slightly slurred speech. "I hope I didn't wake you. I waited until seven but I know this is serious so I thought once it was morning I needed to call."

I confirmed her symptoms and safety, asked the 911 operator to send an ambulance to her house, telling the emergency department to expect a patient several hours into a major stroke. Then I sat with my cold cup of coffee mulling the obliviousness of the young caller and the thoughtfulness of the life-threatened older one. I considered that although I'd cared for wonderful adults of all ages, these two patients were in many ways representative of their age groups and generations. I knew without question which I preferred.

My older caller that night should have phoned sooner; her situation was precisely why doctors take calls. Yet I still remember her because even though she didn't know me and despite her crisis, she was thinking of me with concern and generosity. It's always a pleasure to deal with another person who sees you not simply as a means to an end but as a human being worthy of kindness and consideration. When people of varying ages are tested, older adults score higher on traits like emotional intelligence and wisdom.

Still, the doctor-patient relationship isn't a friendship; it's the doctor's job to care for the patient, not vice versa. At least, that's the ideal. In practice, doctors are human, even if we sometimes pretend otherwise. Since from the beginning one of the primary appeals of medicine for me was patient relationships, it seemed sensible to choose to work with a group of people who, on the whole, treated me well and cared about the quality of our professional relationship. On the patient side, there may be more to it than that, having to do with the gulf between what we all hope for from a doctor and what we must be prepared to accept. That gulf may be wider and deeper if you are in a category of person often unseen, discounted, or subject to disregard.

## TRUTH

In December 2011 just before Christmas, I locked my car and ran-walked the block and a half toward my destination, a dilapidated clinic down the hill from a recently renovated hospital. Every time my right foot hit the pavement, I was reminded why I needed the podiatry appointment for which I was about to be late. Nearing the entryway, I admired its worn grandeur: tapered semi-circular walls extended welcoming arms from either side of the sliding glass doors, and a half-moon of sidewalk stretched to the quiet side street.

That's when I noticed a woman standing at the curb. She had propped her cane on her walker and was squinting toward the nearby boulevard. It was about four thirty; I'd asked for the last appointment of the day for my pre-op so I could leave work as late as possible. The woman was well into her eighties, with a confident demeanor, and clothes and hair that revealed an attention to appearance and suggested a middle-class existence. She had a cell phone in one hand and seemed to be waiting for a ride.

When I came back out after five o'clock, night had fallen. But for her tan winter coat and bright scarf, I might have missed her standing in the shadows, leaning against the curved wall. She still held the mobile phone, but now her shoulders were slumped and her hair disheveled by an increasingly cold evening breeze.

I hesitated. On one side of San Francisco, my elderly mother needed computer help. On the other, our dog needed a walk, dinner had to be cooked, and several hours of patient notes and work e-mails required my attention.

I asked if she was okay. When she answered, "Yes," I waited. She looked at the sidewalk, lips pursed, and shook her head. "No," she said. "My ride didn't come, and I have this thing on my phone that calls a cab but it sends them to my apartment. I don't know how to get them here, and I can't reach my friend."

She showed me her phone. The battery was dead. I called for a taxi with my phone and helped her forward from the entryway wall to the curb. Tired and cold, she suddenly seemed frail.

We chatted while waiting. Eva owned a small business downtown—or she had. She was in the process of retiring, having been unable to do much work in recent months because of illnesses. She'd been hospitalized twice in the past year. Nothing catastrophic, yet somehow the second stay had dismantled her life. Since then, things had never quite gotten back to normal.

The doctor in me noted that Eva had some trouble hearing, even more difficulty seeing, arthritic fingers, and an antalgic gait that favored her right side. But her brain was sharp, and she had a terrific sense of humor.

Finally, the cab arrived. The driver watched as I helped Eva off the curb, an awkward, slow process because of her cold-stiffened joints, the walker, and our bags. As I turned to open the backseat door, he sped away without his passenger. I stared, dumbfounded, and pulled out my phone to call the company and complain. Eva was more sanguine.

"It happens all the time," she said. Just then, a taxi from another company turned the corner. He slowed down for my outstretched hand but saw Eva and screeched off into the night.

"Damn," she muttered.


It didn't take a rocket scientist—or even a geriatrician—to figure out why taxis didn't want to pick up Eva. Doctors and medical practices, community centers, restaurants, and employers of all stripes often invoke the same reasoning: Old people move too slowly, making efficiency impossible. And more often than not, things get complicated.

"I'll give you a ride," I said, having refrained from making the offer until then at least in part because of that uniquely American quandary: What if something happens to her and her relatives sue?

Her face lit up. "Oh, no. I couldn't let you do that."

It took almost as long to maneuver her into my front seat as it did to get across town. She directed me to an apartment complex on the steep slope of one of San Francisco's trademark hills. Twin rows of stacked apartments, separated by an expanse of shrubs and trees, rose up the incline like terraced fields, their landings connected by flights of steep, poorly lit steps. As it turned out, Eva lived toward the top. Before we started up, she handed me her keys and pointed, explaining that she needed to exchange her going-out walker and cane for her at-home cane, which was in the garage. Also, she added, it would be a big help if I'd carry her mail.

I phoned my mother to reschedule and called home to say I'd be late. Getting up the steps was slow going. Along the way, I learned that Eva had seen the podiatrist that afternoon as well, a visit she made every few months because she could no longer cut her own toenails. I told her what I did for a living.

She told me she had lots of doctors and, as often happens, wanted to know if I knew any of them. We discovered that she got all her medical care except podiatry at my institution, and I knew her primary care doctor and several of her specialists.

As I would write in an e-mail to my general internist colleague the next morning, getting Eva out of my car and up the forty-nine stairs to her apartment "took nearly an hour because of her grave debility. She is very weak, has audible bone-on-bone arthritis in all major joints, frequent spasms in her left hip, minimal clearance of her right foot and could not move her left foot; I basically had to hoist her." I had no idea how Eva ever made it up the steps unassisted.

On the way up the steps, we took frequent breaks so Eva could catch her breath and have a reprieve from the pain. During each rest stop, she told me more about her life. She'd had several romances but no children. Most of her friends were also old and ill, so she didn't see them as much as she'd like. She had lived in the same apartment since the early 1970s, loved it and would never live anywhere else. She had a blood cancer that she hoped was cured, asthma, some kind of heart problem, and both glaucoma and macular degeneration. After a recent hospitalization for pneumonia, she had been sent to a local nursing home and said she'd rather die than go there again, though she wasn't keen on dying. She hated that she could no longer work and couldn't understand why people looked forward to retirement.

Walking up the steps with Eva was interesting but also, intermittently, excruciating. Every few minutes, I felt a surge of that trapped, will-this-ever-end feeling. The sensation of slowness and less than optimally used time was familiar to me, as it would be familiar to any doctor or nurse—indeed, to most human beings. With each occurrence, I reminded myself that I was getting to know someone new and doing the right thing. But the truth is that for every time I thought, *I'm really enjoying this*, I would also think, *Poor Eva*, and then, *Poor me*.

Similar sentiments are common in patient care. Although older patients are by no means the only ones to elicit them, the very old do move slowly and often have more issues in need of attention. As a result, they require the one entity that constantly feels in short supply in modern life: time. The ticking clock creates tension, and the best way to relieve the tension is to get rid of whatever is slowing you down and move on, telling yourself the slowness isn't your problem and is hampering your ability to meet your responsibilities. That's the mind-set that leads doctors to cut patients of all ages off after just twelve to twenty-three seconds, cabbies to drive away from an old woman standing in the dark and cold, and people to roll their eyes as an older adult moves slowly down the street or unhurriedly produces their credit card at the grocery store. In all those situations, it's easy to forget that efficiency is a concept best applied to organizations and systems, not people and human interactions.

Forty-some minutes after starting our ascent, we arrived at her apartment. Inside, there was a living room crowded with stacks of books, magazines, and mail, and a small, cluttered kitchen. It also smelled musty, as if she hadn't opened a window in years.

"Shut the door!" she said suddenly, but not soon enough. A blur of dark fur grazed my leg, and her cat disappeared down the steps into the night.

We called him. No response. I walked down the steps, calling and looking. Nothing. After ten minutes of searching, there was still no sign of the cat, whose name, appropriately enough, was Heathcliff. Eva said this wasn't the first time he'd escaped, but, she informed me with a glare missing all the warmth of our exchanges just seconds earlier, when an indoor cat got out, you never knew whether he'd be back. As she steadied herself by leaning on the bulky handle to her front door, it was clear that, isolated by infirmities, her own and her friends', as well as by her building's topography, Heathcliff had become Eva's main companion.

I should have stayed longer to look for him, but I went home.

Before I left, Eva gave me permission to access her medical record, contact her primary care doctor, and make recommendations to help improve her function and well-being. What I found in her chart was a near-universal story of old age in America.

I learned that in the previous year Eva had made thirty visits to our medical center: nine ophthalmology appointments, five visits for radiology studies, four appointments with her lung doctor, four visits to the incontinence clinic, three appointments with her cancer doctor, two emergency department visits, and one appointment each with her cardiologist, a nurse in the oncology clinic, and her primary care doctor. This tally does not include the appointments she missed because, as is noted in at least two places in her chart, "the taxi never showed up." Eva also made frequent phone calls to her doctors' offices and was taking seventeen medications prescribed by at least five physicians. There are words for patients such as Eva and this pattern of care. On the patient side, the words are *complexity, multimorbidity,* and *geriatric.* On the system side, they include *fragmented, uncoordinated,* and *expensive.*

The notes in Eva's chart revealed clinicians providing thorough, evidence-based evaluation and treatment of the issue or organ system in which they specialized. Eva's doctors and nurses knew her, seemed to care about her, and were applying their considerable expertise on her behalf. Unfortunately, their expertise didn't include any of the skills that would have addressed Eva's most pressing needs.

Several notes hinted at what I saw as Eva and I made our slow trek up the steps to her apartment. They documented terrible arthritic pain, significant mobility issues, and ongoing transportation problems. Despite these important observations about Eva's most bothersome medical conditions and significant life challenges, none of the clinicians seeing her evaluated her joints and gait, did a functional assessment, treated her pain, or referred her to a social worker, physical therapist, geriatrician, or another clinician who might address these crucial needs.

Equally significant were the problems that no one mentioned. No physician commented on how many different doctors Eva had or the number of visits she made, both of which might reasonably raise questions about fragmented care and the need for care coordination. And they did not discuss her use of a long list of medications, a situation known as "polypharmacy" and associated with adverse drug reactions and bad outcomes, including falls, hospitalization, and death. Her clinicians did not address Eva's social isolation, living situation, or growing inability to take care of some of her most basic needs, from tending her feet to cooking dinner. Finally, and particularly remarkable for a woman in her eighties with multiple medical problems and no immediate family, no one documented her life priorities and goals of care, or discussed with her who she would want to make medical decisions on her behalf if—or, more likely, when—she was unable to do so herself.

The closest her record came to addressing those vital issues occurred during her hospital admissions when her inpatient doctors dutifully complied with federal guidelines and asked whether she wanted to be "DNR," or Do Not Resuscitate, if her heart stopped. Much has been written about the failures of such conversations, which too often take place in a hurried fashion among strangers and don't include the information patients need to make the right decision for themselves. In Eva's case, although she'd apparently elected to be "full code," such information would include her slim chances of being brought back from the dead given her age and numerous health conditions, as well as the high likelihood that if she survived, she would almost certainly have neurologic damage and worsened disability, and spend the rest of her days in a nursing home.

A second, equally important but infrequently discussed failure of such conversations is that they address only the last topic in a much larger conversation that should take place about a person's health and life priorities. Some people want to be alive in any state; others want hospitalization but not intensive care; and still others only want care they can get in their homes. The menu of what the health care system has on offer ranges from breathing tubes to hospitalization to antibiotics to human help. Eva had been asked only whether she wanted CPR if she no longer had a pulse, but no one had talked with her about how she wanted to live.

After exchanging e-mails with her primary care doctor, I called Eva to tell her what to expect. She wasn't nearly as concerned about her medical care as I was. She liked her doctors and, as is the case for many people, seemed to take for granted that each body part required its own specialist. It became clear that her medical visits served an important social purpose. When I mentioned that she could get her toenails trimmed by a home visit podiatrist rather than make bimonthly trips to the clinic where we had met, she exclaimed, "But I've been going there for years. And they're so nice to me!"

I tried to take a casual, conversational tone for my next question and asked whether she'd ever considered moving. A building on flatter terrain, without stairs, and closer to shops would offer her greater independence. Assisted living, if she could afford it, would provide those advantages plus cleaning services, meals, and a built-in social network.

"The only way I'm leaving here," she said, "is feet first."

Eva's choices made her life more difficult. Yet it was also true that the apartment had been her home for decades, and anywhere she moved would be many times the cost of her 1970s-era, rent-controlled, and long-personalized rooms. Like the vast majority of older adults, what Eva wanted most was help maximizing her abilities and environment so she could continue in the life and home she'd created for herself.

Before hanging up, I asked if I could put her on the waitlist for our geriatrics practice. I explained that if she agreed, she would get a new doctor who would take a different approach to her care. The geriatrician would manage her diseases as her previous doctors had, but would begin by establishing Eva's life and health priorities, address her function and transportation challenges, review her medications and appointments to see if all were truly necessary, and be available by phone or to make a home visit if she got sick to try to prevent hospitalizations.

Eva was silent for a moment. Then she said, "That sounds too good to be true!"

Each one of Eva's doctors was compassionate, smart, and dedicated. Indeed, her diseases were largely under good control. Yet Eva's health was declining, she was missing appointments, and she was increasingly unable to care for herself and her apartment. Several of her clinicians recognized this, but none took action. Their inaction was the inevitable result of their medical training and our health care system's sometimes myopic focus on diseases and medicine at the expense of health.

In a medical culture organized around organs and diseases, doctors will naturally attend to the area within their purview. This limited view may come at the expense of understanding how their organ or disease and its related medications and treatments interact with other parts, and the person overall. In our current health care system, we should not be surprised that clinicians struggle to personalize and coordinate patient care. It's far easier for people to see doctors than to get the social services that might improve their lives and decrease their need for medical care. In a profession that deems some skills and actions on behalf of patients doctorly, and equally health-promoting others not, it's inevitable that at times medicine will fail to provide care that is "necessary for the health, welfare, maintenance, and protection of someone."

Even if Eva's devoted, accomplished doctors had been inclined to address her rapidly declining health and quality of life, our health care system would have punished them for trying. Repercussions to clinicians for tackling this sort of patient complexity include diminished productivity scores, low quality-of-care ratings, longer work hours, and decreased clinical revenue. The game is rigged.

Here's how it works: Strokes and falls are both among the top five killers of older adults. When not fatal, as is often the case, both routinely lead to injury, debility, and lost quality of life and independence. We have stroke units and stroke specialists but neither of these for falls. Stroke occurs after a clot or a bleed deprives part of the brain of blood. Brains and blood and clotting cascades are things all doctors are trained to manage. But falls have innumerable causes: many diseases and also a person's physical environment, their fear of falling (which significantly increases risk), their balance, strength, coordination (issues for physical therapists, not doctors!), their medications, and much more. Additionally, whereas there are dozens of insurance billing codes for stroke, falls had merely an ancillary, non-revenue-generating code until just a few years ago. Similarly, electronic health records lack prominent, useful places to manage and document the care coordination essential for high-quality care of complex patients, including those who fall.

Eva mentioned her walking trouble to one doctor after another, but no one did anything about it, so she brought it up less and less. When nothing is done for a problem, people logically assume nothing can be done. When certain problems are defined as "nonmedical," patients often don't bring them up until they're so advanced that what might have helped now does little.

Old people also decide not to raise certain issues for fear of what the medical system will do to them. After the irreparable harm of her last hospital stay, Eva began avoiding some of her doctors in hopes of steering clear of the nursing home of her nightmares. This happens the world over. Struggling to breathe but certain the local hospital on sanctions by the British government would kill her, my mother-in-law refused to seek care without one of us present to protect her. In book 1 of *My Struggle* Karl Ove Knausgaard describes his Norwegian grandfather's last weeks:

> He must have known something was wrong, but had been reluctant to go to the doctor with it. Then he collapsed on the bathroom floor, close to death, and although they caught him in time at the hospital, and initially he was saved, he was so weakened that he gradually wasted away and, eventually, died.

The problem illustrated here is threefold: the limited scope of what counts as medical; the fact that the "medical" work of doctors counts more than the work of nutritionists, physical therapists, and social workers, even when those professionals might be necessary to ensure a patient's health; and nursing homes so fearsome that people don't admit to serious needs.

Across the planet, people say old age is different and costly to health systems, and then set up those systems tailored to the young and middle-aged.

Old age gets blamed for people's declining health when our strictly medical approach to care leaves out or limits services and treatments for many of the conditions that make old age most challenging.

Eleven months after I met her, Eva finally made it off our housecalls practice waitlist. During her first visit, the geriatrician elicited Eva's health and life priorities and documented the name and contact information of her health care proxy. Because she listed arthritis and pain as her biggest problems, she received steroid injections in her two most painful joints and a pain medication safe for older adults. As her specialists had noted on her recent visits, her blood pressure was quite high. It turned out Eva wasn't taking several medications because she hadn't been able to get to the pharmacy for them. She was taking a medication known to worsen incontinence, another shown to benefit middle-aged patients but not those older than age eighty, and a few that might no longer be necessary. The geriatrician adjusted the timing of her medications so the schedule was simpler and less burdensome and arranged for home delivery from the pharmacy.

Eva's geriatrician also learned that on days when Eva couldn't manage her stairs at all, getting to the medical center was outrageously costly. She had to pay three dollars per step to be carried down and later back up the steps to her apartment. Since there were forty-nine steps, that meant a total of three hundred dollars per appointment, not including the fare for the cab ride. Fortunately, she didn't need to visit the medical center nearly as often as she had been. The geriatrician could treat her incontinence, stable lung disease, and other chronic conditions, as well as monitor her for cancer recurrence, during home visits. Other members of the team—in this case a nurse, physical therapist, and social worker—helped align Eva's self-management skills, activities, and home environment with her goals. The only specialist Eva still needed was the eye doctor. And with the money she saved on transportation, Eva could hire more help at home.

Helping an older adult find a caregiver, delineating the caregiver's tasks, monitoring the caregiver's work with the older adult, and ensuring the caregiver's own well-being are not traditional medical tasks, nor do they need to be done by a physician. They can be, however, among the most important interventions to ensure the well-being and safety of frail older adults. Eva's geriatrician could speak accurately to those needs and was willing to do such uncompensated, "nonmedical" work for the sake of her patient's health and well-being. Once in place, Eva's caregiver picked up medications (so she didn't have to pay for home delivery), assisted with cooking and exercise, and cleaned the apartment. She also provided Eva with social interaction and foot care.

Nearly three years later, Eva was looking forward to her ninetieth birthday. She was frailer than when I first met her, and turned out to be a "difficult patient" who would fire her caregivers, not do her exercises, and sometimes even refuse the care she'd been so enthusiastic about when her health was better. Still, she remained out of the hospital, out of a nursing home, and in her beloved apartment with Heathcliff, who, thankfully, did eventually come home.

BIOLOGY

In the sixteenth century, when Shakespeare wrote *As You Like It*, he divided life into seven stages. By middle age, he said, "all the men and women" develop wisdom but also a "fair round belly," which in older age turns into "spectacles on nose" and a "shrunk shank," and finally, in "the last scene of all, that ends this strange eventful history," the oldest old end up "sans teeth, sans eyes, sans taste, sans everything." It's this final fate that gives aging such a bad rap.

With advancing age, our cells and molecular building blocks change and break down, losing the ability to self-regulate and repair damage. This has anatomical and physiological consequences for organ function. Some changes are unique to a particular part or system; the immune system's dendritic cells, for example, are less and less able to effectively respond to threats. Others affect multiple systems; as enzymes form cross-links in skin, cartilage, and bones, those tissues become less elastic and resilient. All body parts are eventually affected, although different parts age at different rates, and some changes are more apparent than others. We can easily see wrinkles as our skin thins and loses elasticity, or gray hair as the pigment cells called melanocytes disappear from the bases of our hair cells. Less obvious until something goes wrong are changes such as the hardening of arteries from thickened blood vessel membranes and calcification, or thinning of bones as they lose essential minerals. In many places, the deterioration manifests as decreases: shrunken brains, less muscle mass, thinner intervertebral disks, sunken eyes, smaller kidneys. In others, it's about increases: the heart gets bigger and heavier, ears continue to grow, the lens of the eye thickens.

Most people think of these changes as exclusively negative. Also, ugly. Angela Morales offers another perspective. In "Nine Days of Ruth," she describes her grandmother's dying: "Her skin feels like the surface of a mushroom (amphibious perhaps), and I wonder if decomposition has already begun . . . Autolysis means 'self-digestion' . . . thus, the body begins the recycling process. Such beauty, even in reverse!" I have had similar thoughts watching an old person die. It's nature at work, and nature is beautiful. It's a different beauty than a young body in motion, quieter and more understated, and also less pleasurable to witness, even if the person is ancient and ready. Still, being with such a body, all the senses are involved and the feeling is one of symmetry and completion. We call our excursion from birth to death a life *cycle* for a reason.

Not all species age, and those that do don't all age in the same ways. There is no indication that prokaryotes, organisms such as bacteria or blue-green algae that lack chromosomes, a nucleus, and other membrane-bound organelles, undergo senescence. Among eukaryotes, there is good evidence that single-celled populations are immortal and that senescence occurs in all multicellular organisms—plants and animals—that undergo somatic, that is, non-germ-cell, differentiation. Organisms age at wildly different rates. Flies die suddenly right after maturation. Pacific salmon reproduce and die soon thereafter. Humans and other placental mammals gradually deteriorate from maturation onward, while trees and reptiles don't appear to experience post-maturational increases in mortality.

Although scientists have made progress in documenting what happens to the human body as it ages, determining why and how those changes occur has proved more challenging. Of the dozens of circulating theories, not one is universally accepted. Because evolutionary, psychosocial, and physiological theories tackle the same questions in different ways, it may be that some combination of them offers the most accurate and comprehensive explanation for why we grow old.

Evolutionary theories come in two basic types. One posits that natural selection doesn't affect genes that act primarily once we've reproduced. The second suggests a package deal with harmful aging traits bundled with highly prioritized others needed for successful reproduction. Psychosocial theories explain aging in relation to behavior. They view old age in three primary ways: as a process of natural maturation; as a coping strategy for adjusting to biological changes; or as the progressive confirmation or rejection of past perspectives, relationships, and activities. These processes aren't mutually exclusive with each other or with physiological theories that explore what's going on at the cellular level. Physiologists offer sometimes competing ideas of aging as genetic damage from radiation and chemicals, accumulating errors in genes and proteins, or depletion of necessary cells or cell parts. Here, too, it seems likely that several types of changes might be happening at once. Physiologically, senescence could be a state of declining immunity and chronic inflammation and also the result of wear and tear after longer use and exposure to disease risk factors, as well as time enough for even slow-moving pathologies to do damage. Genetic factors clearly play a role too.

The speed and degree of aging vary widely not only between people but also within the same individual. The biology of aging mirrors its lived experience: cellular changes depend on a multitude of factors both inside and outside the individual. Like diseases, aging disorders bodily structures and functions. It also increases a person's vulnerability to injury and illness. Perhaps the most accurate understanding of aging, then, is as the biological manifestation of living.


One cool October day a few years ago, my colorist, who is only somewhat younger than I am but whose smooth skin and black hair expand the gap between us, met me with a bemused grin. I had reached the three-month mark in my effort to grow in my gray hair. That past summer, I had come to the conclusion that I should be doing a better job of embracing my own aging. What kind of hypocrite, I asked myself, champions old age while masking at least part of her own aging? I resolved to see what my head would look like *au natural*.

I went gray in my early thirties, an event unheard-of on either side of my family and one that I attributed to the stress of medical training. At thirty-four, still single, I asked the man who cut my hair to return it to its original dark brown. For the next nearly two decades, I steadfastly refused high-lights and other embellishments, insisting that I wasn't going for glamour, I just wanted to look my age. Once in my early fifties, that argument no longer worked. Almost all fifty-year-olds have gray hair, whether you see it or not.

"So?" My colorist stood behind my chair as we stared at my head in the long mirror in front of us. In honor of our appointment, I had not used my trusty color wand to hide the gray and white hair at my hairline and along my part.

I admitted to relief each time the magic wand obscured the gray demarcation line.

"You're not into it, then," she said, again looking amused.

I explained that I was fairly sure—if not entirely certain—that my objection was to the telling transition between dyed and native hair, rather than to the white-gray hairs themselves. It looked sloppy and ugly to me. In a context in which most women dye their hair, I also worried that I would appear older than I was or somehow less professional. And more than anything, I felt horrible about feeling that way.

My colorist suggested she add highlights to blur the demarcation line, and I said yes.

Biology is only part of the story of aging. Call it the nature portion of a complex process in which "nurture" plays an equally critical role. How and when we age, and how we experience that aging, also depends on our environment, coping mechanisms, health, behavior, wealth, gender, geography, and luck. All humans belong to the same species and have the same biological life span, but these "nurture" factors greatly influence aging. In wealthy Monaco, the average life expectancy is nearly ninety years, which means people are counted as among the aging for nearly a half century and among the old for decades. By contrast, in impoverished Chad the average life expectancy is below fifty years, aging begins earlier, and old age is shorter. Even within the United States, discrepancies are marked: Asian Americans in

Massachusetts live, on average, to age eighty-nine, while South Dakota's Native Americans die on average a generation earlier, before their seventieth birthday. Biology matters, but it's not everything.

In the early 2010s, a colleague and I did geriatrics consultations at a local prison. We saw every inmate aged fifty or older. When a fifty- or sixty-something prisoner was on his first incarceration and less than a few years into his sentence, we could speed through the evaluation; the man was middle-aged and had no geriatric issues. But if an inmate in the same age range had lived his entire life in poverty, been in and out of prison repeatedly or incarcerated for decades, or if he had serious mental or physical illness, his body resembled that of a seventy- or eighty-year-old.

Anyone born healthy begins life with organs working far better than they need to. Biologically, this phenomenon is called redundancy, and it's present in all organs. Our eyes, ears, lungs, kidneys, ovaries, or testes are redundant because most of us have two of them, although we can manage well enough with just one, even one that's less than perfect. Our single organs also have enough excess capacity that they can decline yet continue to function adequately under normal conditions. That caveat, "normal conditions," is key. Above all, aging is a loss of homeostasis, a decline in our ability to self-regulate and maintain equilibrium under duress. So thinner bones seem not to matter until you fall, resulting in a fracture you wouldn't have sustained in younger years when you had stronger bones. And the heart pumps less effectively as it thickens and stiffens with age, although you probably can't tell while sitting in a chair or walking on the flat. But ask it to work harder, by climbing stairs or getting sick, and the presence and degree of compromise may become apparent.

The Berkeley professor Guy Micco's napkin drawing of a relentlessly downward trajectory with age appears to accurately capture the biology of aging. Choose any anatomical or physiological component of a human body at the level of a tissue or organ: numbers of sensory nerves or fast-twitch muscle fibers, blood flow through the kidneys, amount of circulating sex hormone, saliva production, or lung capacity. Across the life span, each of these steadily decline: fewer neurons and fibers, less blood flow and saliva, lower hormone levels and lung capacity. It's enough to make a person agree with Philip Roth that "old age isn't a battle; it's a massacre."

This is precisely where medicalization does us a disservice. Looking through that single lens, we see only part of the larger picture. Most of us are far more interested in what we can do at the level of the whole human than in what's going on with our parts. Notably, a person's ability to perform a task—as opposed to a cell's or an organ's—depends on more than biology. This plays out in a variety of ways.

Some functions decline but not to a point that is noticeable. Others can be slowed with choices and behaviors—actions that are easier for some people than others. As with most things in life, the fortunate have more health-related resources, access, and education, and this helps them make better choices. Some communities also support healthy options more effectively than others.

Perhaps most important from a policy perspective, how well a person functions often depends on factors that have nothing to do with biology. For example, if we chart the hearing of an average twenty-year-old, fifty-year-old, and eighty-year-old, the image is one of decline. But whether the decreased hearing matters in their lives depends not just on their auditory function but on where they are. All three of our hypothetical people may have little trouble at home or work, but put them in a busy restaurant or conference hall and the eighty-year-old may struggle to hear above the background noise. In that situation, it's not the person's function that's changed—certainly they didn't lose more cochlear neurons, hair cells, and hearing on their way to dinner—but the threshold itself. If there's enough noise, even the fifty-year-old, who under normal conditions can't tell any difference between their current hearing and their hearing thirty years earlier, may have trouble. And if it's louder still, the twenty-year-old will also struggle, even though their ears function optimally. Worse, those healthy ears may be getting injured, increasing the person's chances of later deafness. Thus, the impact of biological changes on our lives at all ages can be made worse—or better—by our environment.

Despite the highlights added by my colorist, as my gray hair grew in I found it was a disappointingly nondescript shade, without enough silver or white to make a fashionable salt-and-pepper mix or luxurious-looking new age-appropriate look. This posed a problem, and not just aesthetically.

Discrimination against workers over forty is well documented across employment sectors. To many people, gray hair signals old, and old means out-of-date, used up, on the way out. I wanted to look "normal," and normal in the segments of society I inhabit generally does not include gray hair on women until old age, and for a good many not even then, unless it's beautiful. We are supposed to pretend we're not aging, and many of us comply, not wanting to stand out as Other, especially when that Other comes with so many prejudices and assumptions about one's appearance, competence, and relevance.

Gloria Steinem summed up the situation well in 1974, describing an exchange at her fortieth birthday party: "And a reporter said to me, kindly, 'Oh, you don't look 40.' And I said, just off the top of my head, 'This is what 40 looks like—we've been lying for so long, who would know?'"

Just after Thanksgiving, I called the salon and told them I could come in anytime. When I arrived, my colorist smiled sympathetically. She knew I'd be back. Although the Bible states that "gray hairs are a crown of honor," times have changed.

Two years later, I'm trying again, and I'm not the only one. To many of us, hair suddenly seems an important form of political and social action. Biology means fifty-five looks different than forty. I'd rather live in a world where I could spend less time, money, and effort on delusion and put all those precious resources toward showing what each of life's decades actually look like and how they can be enjoyed. And every day I wonder whether I'm being brave or foolish.

## ADVOCACY

Four weeks after his quadruple bypass and valve repair, three weeks after the bladder infection, pharyngeal trauma, heart failure, nightly agitated confusion, and pacemaker and feeding-tube insertions, and two weeks after his return home, I was helping my seventy-five-year-old father off the toilet when his blood pressure dropped out from under him. As did his legs.

I held him up. I shouted for my mother. As any doctor would, I kept a hand on my father's pulse, which was regular: no pauses, no accelerations or decelerations.

My mother was seventy-one years old and, fortunately, quite fit. She had been making dinner and said she dropped the salad bowl when I yelled. She took the stairs two at time. Something about my tone, she said.

We lowered my father to the bathroom floor. I told her to keep him talking and to call me if he stopped, then I dialed 911.

In the emergency department, after some fluids, my father felt better. My mother held his hand. We compared this new hospital with the last one where we'd spent so many weeks. The doctor came in and reported no ECG changes and no significant laboratory abnormalities, except that the test measuring the effect of his blood thinner was above the target range. The doctor guessed the trouble was dehydration. He would watch for a while, just to be safe.

My mother waited with my father. The rest of us filed in and out, not wanting to crowd the tiny room. Then my father's blood pressure dropped again. I told the nurse and stayed out of the way. She silenced the alarm, upped the fluids, and rechecked the blood pressure. It was better. But less than half an hour later, we listened as the machine scanned for a reading, dropping from triple to double digits before it found its mark. The numbers flashed, but the silenced alarm remained quiet. I pressed the call button, and when the nurse arrived, I asked her to call for the doctor. When no one came, I went to the nursing station and made my case to the assembled doctors and nurses. They were polite, but their unspoken message was that they were working hard, my father wasn't their only patient, and they had appropriately prioritized their tasks. I wondered how many times I had made similar assumptions and offered the same assurances to patients or families.

After weeks of illness and caregiving, it can be a relief to be a daughter and leave the doctoring to others. But I had been holding a thought just beyond consciousness, and not just because I hoped to remain in my assigned role as patient's offspring. I didn't want to be the sort of family member that medical teams complain about. Now that I'd apparently taken on that persona, there was no longer any point in suppressing the thought. His medical history and overly thin blood suggested internal bleeding to me.

I rested my hand on my father's arm to get his attention and said, "Dad, how much would you mind if I did a rectal?"

We doctors do many things that are otherwise unacceptable. We are trained not only in how to do such things but in how to do them almost without noticing, almost without caring, at least in the ways we might care in different circumstances or settings. A rectal exam on one's father is exactly the same as other rectal exams—and also completely different. Luckily for me, my father was a doctor too. When I asked my crazy question, he smiled.

"Kid," he replied, "do what you have to do."

I found gloves and lube. I had him roll on his side. Afterward, I took my bloody gloved finger out into the hallway to prove my point.

I realize that walking to the nurses' station holding aloft one's bloody, gloved hand is not an optimal tactic from a professionalism standpoint—but it worked. A nurse followed me back into my father's room, saw my panicked mother holding a bedpan overflowing with blood and clots, and called for help. Within seconds, the room filled, and minutes later, when the ICU team showed up, I stood back, a daughter again.

In retrospect, what is most interesting is how much more comfortable I felt performing an intimate procedure on my father than demanding the attention of the professionals assigned to care for him. Abiding by the unspoken rules of medical etiquette, I had quieted my internal alarms for more than two hours. Instead, I had considered how doctors and nurses feel about so-called difficult families. I had prioritized wanting us to be seen as a "good family" over being a good doctor-daughter.

Although many physicians would have made different choices than I did, the impetus for my decisions lay in a trait of our medical culture. When we call patients or families "good," or at least spare them the "difficult" label, we are rewarding acquiescence. Too often, this "good" means you agree with me and don't bother me and let me be in charge of what happens and when. This definition runs counter to what we know about truly good care as a collaborative process. From the history that so often generates the diagnosis to the treatment that is the basis of care or cure, active participation of patients and families is essential to optimal outcomes.

Most patients and families who are considered high-maintenance, challenging, or both are simply trying their best to manage their own or their loved ones' illness. That we sometimes feel besieged or irritated by these advocates speaks to opportunities for improvement in medical culture. The physician and nurse representatives of that culture would benefit from a lens shift, seeing more vocal patients and families as actively engaged, presenting new, potentially important information, and expressing unmet needs. That won't happen unless the health care system begins valuing and rewarding the time that clinicians spend talking to patients and families.

Many years later, the most vivid image I have of that night is not my father wobbling in the bathroom surrounded by cold, hard tile or a mustard-yellow bedpan filling with bright red blood. The image is this, a worst-case might-have-been scenario had I not been there: my parents, sleepy, snuggled together at the top of the gurney, my mother resting her head against my father's chest, their eyes closed, faces relaxed. His systolic blood pressure, usually 130, dropping to 80, then 70. The monitors turned off or ignored. The lights dim. A short nap and they'd feel better. A little rest and maybe it would be time to go home.

## OUTSOURCED

By the time I got back, it was too late.

When I had left two weeks earlier, Neeta was in the hospital after a fall and hip fracture surgery. A few days later she'd been discharged to a skilled nursing facility—one I wouldn't have chosen. There they'd managed her delirium with sedating drugs, and she'd barely eaten or begun physical therapy. Now she was bedbound with a huge pressure sore, malnutrition, and a wound infection. Her only option became hospice care.

Already I missed how before the fracture, over the course of home visits, Neeta would age: telling me when I arrived she was ninety-two, then ninety-five, and ninety-seven, and so on, until she was over one hundred years old by the time I would leave. I loved the way she had called me "my love" or "darling." She remembered she liked me if not my name. I had looked forward to her jokes.

"Why did the police arrest the belt?" she asked with a grin as I set up for a blood draw. "Because it held up some pants!"

Her son and daughters—who lived on the same block as her, who had continued working after they might have retired in order to provide her with years of in-home care twenty-four hours a day—were heartbroken that she was dying. "How could this happen?" her son asked when I called. "I thought the hospital and surgery were the dangerous parts."

There were so many ways to answer his question. At nearly every step in her illness, Neeta had received care that was typical but not what she needed—nor was it optimal for a frail older adult.

Increasing numbers of hospitals offer orthopedic and geriatric co-management of elderly hip fracture patients. The surgeons repair the hip; the geriatric medicine specialists take care of everything else, from co-morbid conditions to care and life priorities. With this approach, patients get to the operating room sooner, have fewer unnecessary tests, are less likely to experience delirium, leave the hospital sooner, and are more likely to be walking and living meaningful lives a year after their fractures.

But what happened at the hospital was just one part of what went wrong. I had to keep myself from reminding her son that I'd warned him. Before leaving for vacation, Neeta's son had said they were thinking about the facility where she ended up because it was located near their neighborhood.

"That way we can see her before and after work," he had said.

Rather than repeating the bad rumors about the place he mentioned, I had lauded two better places. I should have been more emphatic about the consequences of choosing the wrong nursing home and stressed that no matter where Neeta ended up, they should not just hand over her care to the facility, assuming everything possible would be done as well as it could be, or even well enough. I should have explained that even when I fought to get my own father into one of the better places in the city after his surgeries, we remained with him, taking turns to ensure one of us was there 24/7 initially and then hiring someone to help overnight once the worst was over. I had spent enough time in hospitals and nursing homes to know that if we didn't, bad things were likely to happen.

Neeta's family also assumed the hospital doctors and discharge planners were equipped to offer the needed guidance. Speak human-to-human to most health professionals, and they seem well aware that most nursing homes make a casket look inviting. But with quality of hospital care and optimal resource utilization linked to patient discharge, hospitals put steady pressure on staff to discharge patients after a set diagnosis-dependent period of time. Since those doctors get little training in outpatient medicine, geriatrics, medical transportation, and home care, nursing homes are often the best and easiest way for them to discharge people who aren't ready to go home. The trouble is, doctors don't know much about nursing homes either.

A 2017 medical journal article looked at how hospital-based doctors handle transfers to nursing homes. They described pressure to speed up discharges, a tendency to use skilled nursing facilities as "safety nets," the absence of a decision-making system or framework for matching patients and places, and little knowledge about the quality or patient outcomes of local facilities. This common reality explains how Neeta ended up at a low-quality nursing facility despite my warnings and her family's best intentions.

In *A Woman's Story*, the French writer Annie Ernaux described a key transition in her mother's life, a series of events that happen every day to older people. On a warm day, her mother fainted and was taken to "the medical service of the old people's home," an option not available in the United States. Rehydration, food, and a few days later, feeling back to normal (and not realizing that her normal had become less than what it had been), Ernaux writes that her mother insisted on leaving: "'Otherwise,' she said, 'I'll jump out the window.' According to the doctor, she could no longer be left on her own. He advised me to put her into an old people's home." The author takes her mother home. The subsequent events culminate in this comment: "And here her story stops for there was no longer a place for her in society."

But it didn't stop. The pages that follow detail confusion (mother), traffic accidents (daughter), fury (both), forgetting, hallucinations, strange eating habits, and a hospitalization where "the nurses had to tie her to her chair because she kept trying to escape from the ward." From there her mother moved to the nursing home unit, a modern building behind the hospital that sounded lovely and smartly organized. There, her daughter found her one evening, "already asleep at half past six, lying across the rumpled sheets in her slip. Her knees were up, showing her private parts. It was very warm in the room . . . Within a few weeks, she lost her self-respect."

She may also have been drugged. Likely, she was bored. Those who can often refer to themselves not as "residents" or "patients" but as *inmates*. Walk the halls of most nursing homes, and you will see people "parked" in the hallways, sleeping or staring or screaming. The odor tends to be anything but homelike. Ditto the food. The people working there wear uniforms, not clothes. They are paid very little. Some are there because they enjoy working with older people; many more because they need a paycheck and this is their best option. Much of the time, neither those who live at the "home" nor the staff want to be there. Old people abandoned by society to such places often earn labels such as "noncompliant" or "difficult," as if resisting unwanted care or trying to leave lockup in a regimented nonhome represents something other than rational self-preservation.

Neeta ended up in that sort of place, a place that essentially killed her. It looked and smelled like a subpar hospital and bore no resemblance to a home. People were tied down, vocalizing, ignored—not always, but often enough, and how often is too often? If you love a person, or believe human beings in need should be treated well, it's hard not to answer *Never*.

People often assume that, until recently, advanced old age was different: old people remained at home cared for by their families. In fact, institutions providing basic care to older adults have existed for thousands of years. In some ways, they were needed more in the past than they are today, since, for most of human history, living into old age often meant outliving one's children. Notably, while approaches have varied over time, old-age institutions have almost always come in one of two flavors: sympathy and antipathy.

Prior to the advent of retirement and pensions in the late nineteenth century in Europe and the twentieth century in the United States, anyone who wasn't rich—most people—and who didn't have family or friends to support them had to keep working. When illness or advanced age made that impossible, they became impoverished and homeless. In some eras, they suffered and died in that state. In others, they were thrown into workhouses or poorhouses with criminals and the mentally ill. The inability to work was seen as a sign of poor character, no matter a person's age. Often, institutions got people off the streets but housed them in cold, dirty, crowded facilities with a small amount of food so living there wouldn't appeal to "vagrants." At other times, religious organizations or governments built facilities in an attempt to respond with compassion to the needs of their oldest citizens. These patterns recurred across time and countries.

During the Roman Empire—a period renowned for its efficiency—a system of homes called *gerocomeia* was established, beginning in Constantinople. Rather than being tucked out of sight as inconsequential, residents were visited annually by the emperor in recognition of the potential political power of older adults. In the early days of Christianity, monasteries often provided food, shelter, and care for the old and infirm. This practice of offering hospitality led to the name and institutions we know as hospitals, though initially they were more custodial than medical, more like modern-day nursing homes. From these initial local acts, the Byzantine emperors, church, and benefactors began building nursing homes alongside or near monasteries throughout the empire. This assured that no matter where a person lived when they became ill or old or disabled, they could get help.

Although old age always eventually brought the need for assistance, when religion dominated, it had spiritual value. Old people were closer to God. When the state took over from the church, advanced old age transitioned from a spiritually valued life stage to a social problem. Separation of frail older people from the rest of society was used as a means of control or a form of punishment, and it was often an act of expediency. Putting many people with similar needs in one place focused resources even as it facilitated systematic segregated dehumanization. The state managed people to civilize them, preserve the social order for everyone else, and demonstrate its capacity to handle all classes of citizens. Having the streets full of poor or old people, dirty and hungry, implied a failure of governance.

Comparing England with France over centuries illustrates how governments can affect the quality of older lives for better or worse. In England, the church-based system worked well until a new administration changed everything for reasons that had nothing to do with old people. During the Reformation, King Henry VIII abolished the monasteries in an effort to ensure the domination of Protestantism over Catholicism. With the monasteries went the nursing homes. Not until the Poor Laws centuries later did the British state again support local parishes in taking responsibility for their impoverished and elderly citizens.

The French didn't set up their hospitality institutions, or "hospices," until after a royal edict in the mid-1600s, when conditions in England were already in decline. The hospices were not initially hospitals in the sense of the word today—that didn't happen until after the French Revolution in 1789—but institutions that simultaneously served as prisons, insane asylums, and residential homes for the disabled of all ages and the elderly. The grouping of older adults with criminals, the mentally ill, and the chronically disabled was telling. While people in those different categories are now separately housed (not that those various conditions are mutually exclusive), our general attitudes toward them are largely unchanged. Each is seen as costly, burdensome, and of little social value. From the start, their treatment has raised questions about whether their sequestration enabled the focus, help, and care they needed or served other purposes. While many have argued for the segregation of criminals to protect the public, the segregation of those with mental illness or debility helped families by transferring custodial and care responsibilities to the state. But if they offered protection, it was of the sort that allowed people *without* those conditions to live lives in which those *with* those conditions did not exist. People could go about their days without the "lesser" and "burdensome" others visibly present and pretend that they, too, might not end up in similar straits. In country after country, more and more families abdicated their responsibilities.

Sometimes, too, the so-called afflicted refused familial shelter and care, ending up on the streets. Again, we see how little changes. In the 1970s, in the wake of revelations of abuse and neglect in mental institutions, deinstitutionalization became the standard in the United States. Walk down the streets of San Francisco or any other American city today, and you will see people huddled in doorways, under overpasses, in sidewalk tents, and on traffic islands. We still haven't found a satisfactory solution to a situation that transcends centuries and cultures. It's hard not to suspect that our approach is fatally flawed.

In the twentieth century, with the huge progress in medical diagnosis and treatment, old age became medicalized, offering new ways to see old people as "problems." Suddenly it wasn't just the poor who ended up in nursing homes but anyone whose body was seen as requiring ongoing management. Those institutions, designed for societal undesirables, retained much of the workhouse era's attitude toward residents in their structures and systems. No one saw much point in investing in or truly attending to the lives of people who were, as a nonagenarian once said to me, "past their use-by dates."

And then, once again, the options changed for reasons ranging from good intentions to profiteering. Recent decades have brought a shift from public to private institutions and a flourishing of alternative facilities, from small mom-and-pop board-and-care homes to high-end assisted living centers that somewhat resemble a college dorm or cruise ship. This has made nursing homes even more repellent. It has also created new challenges. Ancient, frail people with resources and options increasingly spend the last months or years of their lives in assisted living, places generally not set up with them in mind. The less moneyed end up in unsafe living conditions without adequate food, help, or human contact, or spend down until they become eligible for Medicaid, and then only certain sorts of places will have them. Once there, they are subject to the very "deprivatization of experience" for which old age is reviled.

Although facilities are often the stuff of horror stories, the same is true of some old people's lives with their families. In both situations, vulnerable people are behind closed doors with more able and powerful people. As much as the bodily changes of old age, that fate has made the final years of old age fearsome. The worst could happen to anyone. And it does: elder neglect and abuse occur in people of every social class, background, and geography. Today, there are more choices than ever for where to spend one's old age but still relatively few that hold much appeal. Meanwhile, we close our eyes, individually and collectively, avoiding our friends and loved ones once they are debilitated, until one day we find "they" are us and it's too late to do anything about it.


A photo I sometimes use in teaching shows a hallway in a nursing home with a line of older women in wheelchairs. Heads hang down, are held in hands, eyes are closed. Is this old age, or a way to cope with a certain brand of old age, one no more appealing to old, frail people than to the rest of us?

Nascher noted that "in institutions where the aged have light tasks assigned to them, they do not break down mentally, either as soon or as completely as whenever the aged have nothing to do but sit on a bench and brood." Marjory Warren, confronted with so many delirious and defeated old patients in West Middlesex, similarly insisted any life could be improved by more stimulation and pleasant surroundings, and it was worth determining recovery potential in people with *any* disability. A notable percentage of her patients returned home, and even those whose improvement was limited led more comfortable and meaningful lives.

In 1950, fifteen years after Warren transformed her patients and unit, the UK Ministry of Health announced: "The workhouse is doomed. Instead local authorities are busy planning and opening small comfortable Homes where old people . . . can live pleasantly and with dignity. The old 'master and inmate' relationship is being replaced by one more nearly approaching that of a hotel manager and his guests." But the tides of history wax and wane. Governments choose their weapons from a limited arsenal. Ahead of the 2016 Super Bowl hosted in the Bay Area, San Francisco's mayor had the homeless population moved and removed, housed and given tents in out-of-the-way places. That same year, our local newspapers featured articles about our aging homeless population.

"Nursing homes are charged with an incredible endeavor—taking care of the failing," Robin Young commented in *Here and Now*. Yet we keep using them. We put "loved ones" in them, underfund them as a society, and hope never to need one ourselves. It sounds better to say *We're sending her back to the home*, or *He lives in a home now* than to say *We're sending her back to the institution where she will spend the rest of her life bored and unhappy until she dies*, or *He lives in an institution now because we couldn't fit his care into our lives*. But it's too easy to blame individuals for something that is complex, multifactorial, and at least partly structural. That last quote should finish with these words: *given how little our society supports such efforts*.

ZEALOT

Sometimes I hate my colleagues.

When he developed cancer, Juan was eighty-six years old. Already, he had heart disease, arthritis, and diabetes, as well as one-sided weakness and mild dementia from a stroke. The oncologists put him through ten months of permanently debilitating chemotherapy and radiation and then said the disease wasn't curable and there was nothing more they could do.

Another day, Deborah, a patient who'd just signed up for hospice, was sent to the emergency department by someone at her assisted living facility who had neglected to check her file before calling for an ambulance. Her distraught and disappointed family called her primary doctor, who called the emergency department, explained the situation, and asked them to send her home. The hospice and primary care teams would take it from there. The emergency doctor said they needed to do a CT scan because Deborah might be having a stroke and need a potent blood thinner. He could not understand that he didn't have to do those things, that they wouldn't change the fundamentals of Deborah's life at that point, or that it was not only legal but ethical and kind to respect the patient's wishes at the end of her life. He said, "We can't just not provide care." For him, only certain sorts of activities (scans and certain drugs) and places (hospitals and emergency departments) counted as medicine and health care.

Then there was Albert, my ninety-four-year-old patient who was cut off from friends by his deafness, unable to hear much despite his hearing aids. He increasingly struggled to walk, spent most days alone, and was getting sick more and more often, when he fell outside his building and hit his head. A passerby called the paramedics, who wanted to take him to the hospital. Albert refused, since he didn't have a cut that needed sutures. The paramedics argued that he might be bleeding into his head. A doctor himself, Albert said, "So what?" Given where his life was and where it was headed, lapsing into a coma and dying in his bed would be a better end than anything the hospital had to offer for a brain bleed. He microwaved a frozen dinner, watched some television, and finally went to bed, where, to his disappointment, he didn't die.

Albert was unusual. As the end of life nears, most people don't know what they want or can expect. They do as they are told, deferring to the knowledge and assuming the benevolence and objectivity of their physicians. But doctors are flawed and fallible, the products of their culture and time like everyone else. As the Canadian physician Balford Mount, who coined the term *palliative care*, wrote years ago: "We [in medicine] emerge deserving of little credit; we who are capable of ignoring the conditions which make muted people suffer. The dissatisfied dead cannot noise abroad the negligence they have experienced . . . We don't imagine that we, who strive to be and view ourselves as well-meaning and competent, might be neither . . . And patients are afraid of insulting or upsetting those responsible for their care."

Since the twentieth-century medicalization of aging and dying, medicine has mainly seen itself as a means to wage battle against death, not as one of many tools with which to ease that inevitable transition. Education about how to conduct so-called difficult conversations, give bad news, assess patient priorities, and manage symptoms at the end of life only became standard in medical schools in the 2010s, and remain ignored or underutilized by many specialists. Geriatrics and palliative care, the two fields in which those tasks are elemental, are called in—or worse, they're not. Indeed, ongoing efforts at reform notwithstanding, medical culture and financial rewards for dialysis, chemotherapy, and procedures persist, even when they are unlikely to benefit a patient.

Meanwhile, death is outsourced to palliative care, as if it were something uncommon.

# 9. MIDDLE-AGED

Throughout ancient and medieval times, old age was defined as a distinct life stage. Though the number of stages varied, most commonly including three, four, six, or twelve, each stage was thought to have unique behavioral and health attributes but unclear transition phases. Aristotle identified three stages: growth, stasis, and decline, the last two correlating roughly with later notions of fit and frail elders, respectively. Perhaps in part because of mystical notions of the number seven, the Ninetieth Psalm fixed the life span at seventy years with seven age groups. This view of the human life span as made up of distinct stages persisted in the West until the eighteenth century.

The industrial age called for specialization of social and work functions for adults and a more distinct phase of childhood, and it deemed old age a brief period defined by the mixed messages of well-earned retirement and uselessness. "Middle age" came later, propelled initially by efforts to distinguish increasingly powerful midlife adults from older ones, and as a catchall for the decades between young and old as lives lengthened. New institutions and terminology developed in response to each new life phase. Here is the social historian Tamara Hareven:

> The "discovery" of a new stage of life is itself a complex process. First, individuals become aware of the specific characteristics of a given stage of life as a distinct condition. This discovery is then passed on to society in popularized versions. If it appears to be associated with a major social problem, it attracts the attention of agencies of welfare and social control. Finally, it is institutionalized: legislation is passed and agencies are created to deal with its special needs and problems.

Through this mechanism, society both supports its citizens and reduces them.

In the modern era, a variety of substage names have been proposed for old age. The psychologist G. Stanley Hall proposed *senescence* as a late-life analogue of adolescence: "There is a certain maturity of judgment about men, things, causes and life generally, that nothing in the world but years can bring, a real wisdom that only age can teach." In 1974 it was the psychologist and aging scholar Bernice Neugarten who divided old people into *young-old*, meaning those between the ages of fifty-five and seventy-five, and *old-old* for those ages seventy-five and above. Ten years later, to capture the distinct characteristics of the increasing numbers of people over age eighty-five, Richard Suzman and Matilda White Riley added *oldest old* to Neugarten's model. In the public arena, three stage divisions are also common, particularly the catchy and somewhat irreverent *go-go*, *go-slow*, and *no-go*.

Geriatricians also divide old people into stages, most commonly identifying four based on disease and function: healthy, chronically ill, frail, and dying. A more relational five-stage approach has been proposed by Dr. Mark Frankel as independence or self-sufficiency, interdependence (when occasional help is needed), dependence (when a person needs regular, daily life help), crisis (when professional care may be required), and death.

The stages of old age are complicated by the fact that people can move forward and sometimes backward among them, something that never happens in earlier phases of life. After an accident, or heart surgery, or chemotherapy, a person might appear "aged," looking years older than they did just months earlier. They might even skip forward a stage or two of development, requiring a walker or wheelchair and help bathing. But months later, after time for healing and physical therapy, they might get "younger" again. Similarly, if an older adult decides to start exercising or begins an exciting new job or falls in love, they can suddenly seem years younger or as if they "had a new lease on life." The stages of old age are more fluid than those of childhood and adulthood. They can be skipped and returned to, though overall, in old age as in its predecessor stages, there is a typical progression.

\*  \*  \*

Trajectory matters. Like babies and children, very old people are often small and dependent. But while our landscapes at life's start and end share some attributes, they are fundamentally different, and not just because in youth we know little but are headed toward most of life and in old age we have already traversed that territory and are closer to death. Ignatz Nascher used biology to refute the notion of advanced age as second childhood:

> A comparison of the organism in childhood with the organism in old age will show that there is not an organ or tissue, not a function, mental or physical, identical at the two periods of life. Vitality, metabolism, even instinct differ. The process of senescence is progressive, not retrogressive, there is no reversal in the order of development and not a single tissue reverts to an earlier type.

Physiologically as well as developmentally, then, the Victorians were right: life is a journey, not a cycle.

Nascher also recognized that medicine's approach to childhood health offered an ideal model for approaching health in old age. We don't think of childhood as an immature perversion of adulthood, characterized by an underdeveloped psyche, intellect, organs, and tissues. Anatomical struc- tures (an infant's big head, a child's smaller body and parts), physiological functions (what counts as normal in muscle strength or pulse rate), appear- ance, and behaviors that would be deemed pathological in adulthood are considered normal and natural in childhood. "We must," Nascher advised, "take a similar view of senility."

A little over a decade later, in her 1930 book *Salvaging Old Age*, the American psychologist Lillien J. Martin suggested the problem of old age in America was conceptual, not biological: "When we have arrived at the place of looking at old age as a period of life rather than as a bodily condition, we shall give it the intelligent and careful study that we have applied to other such periods, infancy, childhood, adolescence . . . as a period with its own struggles, its aspirations and its accomplishments."

I have begun to think of life this way: it's as if child, adult, and elder are life's three primary colors and all its substages are derived from those three fundamentals, just as all other colors are made by combining red, yellow, and blue.

HELP

The frantic call came from Frank Cavaglieri's assisted living facility just after two in the afternoon. I was in my office catching up on paperwork.

"Oh, God," I said after taking the call, pushing back my chair and reaching for my visit bag. "Tell them twenty minutes."

When I arrived at the handsomely restored building with its English manor house landscaping and City Landmark status, the knife had been removed from the table next to Frank's lift recliner. He'd set it beside the jar of sour lemon candies his daughter, Susan, kept continuously stocked because he loved sweets and his mouth was always dry, and because she loved him.

The cut was on the back of his hand an inch down from the knuckles. It bled, though not much, and not nearly enough for his purposes. Shallow as it was, it wouldn't even require stitches. He'd used the only instrument he could find, a butter knife lacking a true blade, worn nearly smooth from years of institutional use.

Seeing me, Frank tried to smile. Well dressed as always, he wore a soft gray sweater over a patterned maroon shirt, and his white hair was neatly combed.

"I can't even do this," he said. "I can't even kill myself."

I squeezed his hand but didn't speak right away. I didn't want to insult his intelligence by pretending this was a problem I could fix.

With Frank's soft, warm skin against mine, I struggled to show I cared without actually crying in front of my patient, this lovely ninety-two-year-old man who desperately wanted to be dead, and found himself, day after meaningless day, still alive.

Three years earlier, I had pulled up to a pale green house with rows of flowering geraniums below each front window in rectangular planters painted to match the white trim. On the passenger seat of my car sat two folders of new patient paperwork. The couple, both in their late eighties, had lived in the same modest home for sixty years. It stood on a short street overlooking a freeway in a rapidly gentrifying once working-class neighborhood.

My visit was supposed to be a consultation. They already had a primary care internist they liked, as well as a bevy of specialists: a cardiologist, neurologist, podiatrist, and pulmonologist for him, and a neurologist and dermatologist for her. But their daughter was convinced they weren't getting what they most needed, though she couldn't say exactly what that might be. She hoped someone with expertise in the care of the very old might help her figure out what to do to improve her parents' lives. All she knew for sure was that they were neither happy nor thriving. That wasn't like them at all, even if it was how most people think of advanced old age.

When Frank tried to kill himself, he was widowed and lived in a studio apartment in the assisted living facility. His room was large and the place fairly nice, but it was an institution. Even with some of his own furniture and photographs, it wasn't home. There were group meals and activities, but by his second year living there, he couldn't taste much or hear very well, despite expensive hearing aids. He stopped participating in card games when he began regularly making mistakes, and he no longer went to performances by visiting musicians. He couldn't walk either, and although he received regular visits from his attentive and loving family, they had jobs and school and travel, so mostly there he was, alone in his room.

The staff came in to help him dress, wash, and get to meals. They cut the meat on his plate, gave him his medications, and told him what time to eat, get up, dress, bathe, and go to bed. He regularly fell while trying to transfer himself from chair to wheelchair or wheelchair to toilet, in part because he wanted to do such basic things himself and in part because even when he did call for help with these tasks, the wait often was longer than he could tolerate. Eventually, the facility's caregivers insisted on diapers, and he conceded.

Frank told me he wished he were dead. We tried antidepressants, which didn't help. Though worth a try in case they might mitigate his distress, it seemed unlikely to both of us that they could address his fundamental problems.

Frank had three of the six conditions participants in a recent study identified as worse than death: *bowel and bladder incontinence*, the *inability to get out of bed* (he could still get up, but at least one person and a mechanical lift device were required to transfer him from his bed into a wheelchair), and *needing around-the-clock care*.

He would never develop two of the other three unacceptable states, *needing a feeding* or *needing a breathing tube*, but in the slow lead-up to his death he would have more and more of the sixth, *being confused all the time*. There was nothing he or I or anyone could do about it.

That helplessness, of course, is part of what people dread about old age. It's not just the lost functions and roles, from the fundamental to the just plain fun, but the loss of control over one's body, situation, and life. Given sufficient longevity and a certain balance of luck, both good and bad, that outcome seems biologically determined. At some point the good luck of not dying early and of developing conditions that medicine can at least partially treat begins to look like all loss and no gain, an inexorable accrual of negatives with no potential upside. The fortunate live this way for days to weeks; for the less fortunate, it can go on for years.

While not rich, Frank had more advantages and resources than many people, including a family who loved him, who regularly showed up to visit and always when called, and who never stopped trying to find ways to make life better for him. Yet he clearly suffered. But the changes that eventually became his advanced old age actually started earlier—for him, as for the rest of us, in our forties or fifties, though at that stage they don't dominate, presenting instead as small flares on the larger background of our functionality and engagement.

We joke about worn-out knees and receding hairlines and find workarounds for nouns or facts we can't quite locate at the exact moment we'd like to use them. Those are serious and real changes, and only the beginning of a process that becomes advanced old age decades later.

There is old and there is ancient. Live long enough and eventually the body fails. It betrays us. Our flesh wrinkles, sags, and sinks. Strength wanes. We lose speed, agility, and balance. Abilities once taken for granted are accessed only verbally, using the past tense. Sometimes the mind follows the body's descent, words, logic, insight, and memories dropping away. We fall ill more often and more gravely. We become frail. The smallest, most ordinary tasks—eating, showering, walking—become time-consuming, difficult, dangerous, or impossible. Absent purpose or agency, frustration, boredom, and discomfort provide the landscape of our days. In the end, we are defined more by what we are no longer than by what we are. We fight and flirt with death.

The day I first met Frank, I followed his daughter, Susan, up a long set of steps into a cheerful living room where her parents sat waiting. Frank used the arms of his chair to push himself to standing and, once upright, extended his hand. He was a slight man with a full white mustache, a large, flat nose, and a strong grip. Despite his good manners, I could tell my visit was his daughter's idea.

His wife also rose, though more slowly and with a boost from Susan. Her hair stuck out from her skull, dense white and fluffy, reminding me of a dandelion, and her words emerged in the quiet, mumbled way of people with middle-stage Parkinson's disease. I had to concentrate to catch what she was saying. Although her name was Carol, she told me to call her Cookie.

She, too, had a winning smile, though her tiny, tremulous hand felt fragile in mine.

Despite his small stature, Frank had been a skilled worker who rose to foreman and provided his children with the college education he didn't have. He fixed everything around the house, from the dishwasher and radio to the deck and roof. Until he couldn't. That was shortly after his stroke and several years into Cookie's decline. A year before I met him, he'd first tried to kill himself. The subject came up when I asked about past hospitalizations. He had been so sincere during our conversation up until that point, his answers punctuated with amused and sometimes resigned smiles, that I remember being shocked when they told me about the suicide attempt and his subsequent stay on a locked psychiatric ward. There was nothing about Frank that said mental illness: he was a sane man who didn't want to live dependent and disabled, and who had decided to take control of his situation in the best way he could, as he was accustomed to doing.

None of the family members wanted to talk about it. Susan rested her hand on his arm, her eyes bright. Frank spoke softly, alternately looking at me and staring at his lap. He hadn't liked the unit where they'd kept him after the stroke, he said, or how they had treated him, and he really hadn't liked the psychiatric unit. I couldn't tell which of the identity insults of illness bothered him most, only that he had felt powerless, sad, and ashamed. That day at their house, Frank admitted to often feeling down and hopeless, although he denied suicidality. As he said he wasn't thinking of trying to kill himself again, he looked first at Susan and then over at Cookie, glances that suggested a different truth than the one he'd put into words.

From the start, Cookie had been Frank's perfect match, as compulsive about cleaning, cooking, and tending their home and family as he had been about providing for them. Even smaller than he, she was also more nervous and timid. Or maybe she had become that way by the time I began taking care of them. I suspect those qualities, always present, had risen to prominence as others receded. That sort of change can happen in old age, people becoming "more so" in ways both good and bad. It's a process that resembles what happens to ears and noses over decades; not only does the cartilage in those structures keep growing throughout life, long after bones, muscles, and fat have stopped, but the skin and parts around them diminish, accentuating their enlargement. Still, as the Cavaglieri family stories would make clear in subsequent visits, in her kitchen and at her dinner table, Cookie called the shots.

Frank and Cookie had been married for sixty-five years. Once, a decade or so before I met them, their son had taken his father on a "boys'" trip with his own sons, a one-off family adventure that required a plane trip to another state. They were already in the wilderness a thousand miles from home, with the sun setting and the tent up, when Frank said, "I wonder if I'll sleep. Except during World War II, I've never spent a night away from your mother."

Their son laughed when he told me that story, his amusement equal parts incredulity and wonder.

Frank managed those few nights of the camping trip. But later, after Cookie's death, he'd find it much harder to be the sole representative of a successful pair—not just because his marital other half was missing, but because so much of him was too.

*   *   *

Shortly before Frank and Cookie joined our housecalls practice, their "kids" had begun making arrangements for them to move to assisted living. Parkinson's rendered Cookie stiff and slow, and a stroke had slowed and weakened Frank. Their house had stairs outside and inside, and they struggled to accomplish even the most basic of household tasks, from showers to meal preparation. For a while, Susan said, it had worked to have household help and for her or their daughter-in-law to keep them stocked with prepared meals, but eventually even that wasn't enough. Sometimes Cookie couldn't get out of bed. Or they couldn't manage getting the ready-made meals warmed and onto the table. Although the key rooms of their house were on a single level, a flight of stairs separated them from the street. They were trapped, and they couldn't afford twenty-four-hour care at home. Shortly after my first visit, they moved.

I adjusted their medications so he'd stop fainting or nearly fainting and so they'd both be able to move around better with less pain. I also arranged for physical and occupational therapy—the former to work on strength and walking, the latter to devise strategies to keep them independent in at least some tasks of daily living. Each of these geriatric interventions helped, but not nearly as much as they would have a year or several earlier, and not enough to markedly improve what bothered them most. This was partly because the facility looked nice but, as with most such places, still operated like an assembly line where the product was frail, elderly humans. But also, it seemed neither Frank and Cookie nor the therapists working with them believed that old and frail people could make significant physical gains. None of them tried as hard as they might have had they known about, or believed, the studies showing how much change is possible even in advanced old age with the correct doses of the right exercises. But it was also because my own geriatrics approach, though far broader than that of most other branches of medicine, was too narrowly focused on illness and disability. As their doctor, my role was management of their diseases and geriatric syndromes, but that wasn't what they needed most. Even, or perhaps especially, once good health was no longer attainable, they needed well-being in the form of purpose, meaning, and relevant options. Getting those health essentials would require both a society that didn't reduce old people to their bodies and ailments and a health care system that valued health and wellness as much as it did diseases.

When people think of old age as depressing, they are likely imagining scenarios like Frank and Cookie's. Ditto when medical students, doctors, and other health professionals think about geriatrics.

Missing from those apprehensions are the distinctions between fixing and helping, between depressing and sad, and between the easy, comfortable moments most people prefer and those that define and give meaning to our lives. Equally absent is acknowledgment of the interplay between biological destiny and the consequences of our social constructions of old age, which include houses built with the assumption that no one lives past sixty or seventy to institutional warehouses with the thinnest veneer of hominess over the trappings of a prison or hospital.

I am telling just one side of this story here, the side that highlights the worst of old age; it's also possible to construct analogous horror stories of childhood or adulthood. What most of us see when looking at very old people in institutions seems entirely sensible, until that person who is isolated, ignored, and warehoused is our mother or father, friend or self. Only then, too late, do we consider that our individual and societal decisions, often based on such reasonable considerations as convenience, economics, or well-intentioned efforts to keep aged people safe, have in fact created an advanced old age nobody wants.

But there is also this: in telling Frank's story, I have done what we often do when we talk about old age, devoting thousands of words to the bad part of his long life and just a few lines to the good. In reality, over nine decades of living and three of those in old age, the proportions were just the opposite. Frank had over eighty good years, a few years that were not so good, and one to two years that were bad. The bad matters, and we need to make it better, but to say all of life, even all of old age, is bad is to tell a story that isn't true.

Frank and Cookie were in their sunny one-bedroom apartment in assisted living for less than a year when she got pneumonia. We treated the infection, but she never fully recovered. Cookie became bedbound, barely ate, and developed pressure sores. We held a family meeting and decided on hospice.

In the weeks leading up to her death, Frank lay nearby, trying to keep awake at night to listen for sounds of distress. Their marital bed had disappeared. Now Cookie was in a hospital bed across from Frank's new, single bed in their apartment's small bedroom. He had fought this furniture arrangement, this separation of the two of them, and—like most battles at that stage of his life—he'd lost. According to medical conventions and the government's rules for such facilities, the hospital bed was considered necessary for the safety of both Cookie and her caregivers.

When she moaned, he'd rise and try to tend her. Several times, he fell crossing the small divide between their beds. Sometimes he got himself back up. Other times he crawled to the call button and waited for an aide. "They sure don't come running," he told me.

In those days, the bags under his eyes nearly reached his mustache. He looked shattered. Seventy years, I kept thinking. They'd been married nearly seventy years. I hadn't even been breathing for fifty at the time.

Cookie died, and at first, to everyone's pleased surprise, Frank did okay. Worried about her, he hadn't participated in many facility activities. Now he went on trips to the coast and to musicals in the beautifully appointed "great room." He played cards twice a week, made new friends, and sat with "the boys" for meals. He enjoyed watching the children who came to perform and going to his son's house for dinner. It wasn't the best year of his life, but it was acceptable.

But when his hearing got worse, neither the ear doctor nor hearing aid specialists could help. He began having more heart symptoms. He had another small stroke. His thinking slowed and faltered. From that point on, things went steadily downhill. At each visit, when we were alone together, he talked about how much he wished his life would end.

Several times, I asked Susan or another family member to meet me in his room. In the presence of his family, Frank would backtrack from our conversations and deny wanting to be dead. He would tell them he loved them and that he would try harder. He would tell them it wasn't so bad.

Even at this moment when he could no longer do so much of what had defined him, he couldn't help but continue to be a good father, prioritizing his children's welfare over his own. As his life became more of what he didn't want it to be, he remained patient with all of us who were supposedly helping him, even when it was clear we couldn't give him what he wanted most.

Frank's fate often tops people's list of the problems with old age. For many, it's more terrifying than death, the version of "old" they fear and dread. In gerontology, that final stage of life before death is known as "the Fourth Age," the phase when we pass "beyond any possibility of agency, human intimacy, or social exchange . . . [into] a hyper-reality from which there is no . . . return."

A year and a half after Cookie's death, Frank's suffering became undeniable. By then, it was clear that nothing could be done to improve his hearing, walking, or continence, and, related but perhaps even more important, his sense of purpose. When he asked what could be done, I explained to him, as I have to so many others, that I could not kill him but we could make some changes that would at least lessen the medicalization of his life and might allow death to arrive sooner than it would if we continued with a disease-focused rather than a more person-focused approach to his care. That day, we stopped his heart medications, a step his family couldn't imagine taking even a few months earlier. We also agreed that if he got sick, we would start hospice and morphine rather than move him to the hospital.

And still he didn't die. For weeks, then months, nothing changed. It seemed he hadn't needed all those medications, something I often see. But he remained chronically dying, increasingly confused and thoroughly, miserably still alive.

How universal are the factors that give life meaning? How do we decide the meaningfulness of another person's life? What can or should we do when that meaning seems irretrievably lost? People offer a wide range of answers to those questions, from leaving it in God's hands to passing assisted dying laws. But faith doesn't preclude human efforts to improve the station of others, and many assistance-in-dying laws have little or no applications in the lives of the people most likely to die: the oldest among us, people like Frank. Aid-in-dying laws require a terminal disease with a six-month prognosis, good mental capacity, and the physical ability to take the lethal medication unassisted. Frank could not self-administer drugs and was increasingly confused, and his form of dying didn't have either a single cause or a clear end point.

For his family, and for me, Frank's life had meaning and importance right up until the end—he did eventually die, of course. But to look at it that way is to do to Frank in death what we did to him throughout his last years, which is to make it about us—the young and middle-aged and young-old—and not about him. Shouldn't he, like the rest of us, have been able to articulate and get what he wanted? His last few years didn't feel meaningful to him, and there was no chance he'd get back what mattered to him most.

Speak to almost anyone in their fifties, sixties, and seventies, and they can tell you about a loved one who ended up in a situation like Frank's. It's a tragedy and a travesty that our "modern, developed" society can't have an honest conversation about advanced old age when a majority of us will experience it. If our beliefs and institutions gave Frank the ending we fear, it's time to change those beliefs and institutions. We need to look at old age with compassion and creativity, to reimagine and improve it, from its early fit, functional stages to its less appealing final years. That won't do Frank any good but it will help the rest of us—and it would have made Frank happy to know those years he felt so useless were actually changing the world.

## PRESTIGE

In medicine, as in society, biases shape what and who counts. People who take care of kids, the mentally ill, the poor, or the very old are paid less—and sometimes respected less—than those who care for adults more generally. Always at the top of the power ladder are those whose focus is surgery, parts, procedures, technology, and machines. Always at the bottom are the doctors who deal with psyches, holism, complex physiological systems, so-called social issues, and long-term doctor-patient relationships. Basically, the narrower the focus, the shorter the interaction with the patient, and the more high-tech and procedural, the higher the status on the totem pole of medical specialties.

If you use physicians' annual income by specialty as a marker of perceived professional status, entrenched systemic priorities emerge. To wit:

- Exhibit A—All top-ranked health systems on the planet rely on primary care to keep people healthy. In the United States, ranked thirty-seventh among nations by the World Health Organization, we have trouble recruiting doctors to primary care, in part, perhaps, because in addition to having a broader purview, they are paid on average over one hundred thousand dollars less per year than specialists.
- Exhibit B—Internists (adult doctors) are paid more than pediatricians. Orthopedists are paid more than rheumatologists. Neurosurgeons are paid more than psychiatrists.
- Exhibit C—In internal medicine and pediatrics, primary care doctors complete the same residencies as hospitalists, yet the latter are paid an average of thirty thousand to fifty thousand dollars more per year. Yet ask most hospitalists if they would do primary care, and they'll say, *No way; it's too many hours, too frustrating, too stressful, too hard.*
- Exhibit D—Most of the specialties at the top are procedural and majority male, and the more relational ones at the bottom are mostly female. Also, urologists make more than gynecologists.
- Finally, Exhibit E—geriatrics and palliative care, despite their advanced training and certification procedures, decades-old professional societies, and presence throughout the country, don't even appear on most specialty ranking lists.

The messages embedded in the rankings are clear: High-tech care is best. Inpatient is better than outpatient. Adults matter more than kids. Stereotypically male skills are worth more than ones commonly considered stronger in females. Curing beats caring. The powerful and able-bodied matter more than the vulnerable.

These hierarchies of relative value work counter to society's needs. They also harm patients—some of us all the time, and all of us some of the time.

By preferentially directing resources and clinicians, it restricts options and access, often away from what patients need most.

Among the justifications for power, compensation, and prestige differences among medical specialties are training time and perceived difficulty—arguments with some merit. Should there be cause for someone to do some cutting and rearranging of my brain, I want that person to be highly trained and exceptionally skilled. But that would be no less true if I developed schizophrenia. Neurosurgical training is longer than psychiatry, so maybe the surgeon should have a higher salary, but I'm not convinced that brain clot or epilepsy focus removal skills are worthy of more respect than help with debilitating depression or psychosis. Similarly, can it possibly be true that it takes two to three times as much skill to read an X-ray or MRI of a two-year-old child as to figure out the cause, explain to the parents, and initiate tests and treatments of illness in the same two-year-old child? One might think so, given that the radiologist is paid two to three times more than the pediatrician, even though it is the latter who not only must put the X-ray findings in context but also do a physical exam and take a history and negotiate what will and will not be done with the worried parents and their insurance company—and, long after the billable, productivity counted visit, field their concerned calls while seeing other patients or tucking in their own two-year-olds.

These figures suggest modern medicine is an anti-intellectual profession: those whose work is based on interaction and negotiation and analysis, on looking at the big picture, and on deciphering the cognitive puzzles presented by patients with particular bodies and lives, social circumstances and complaints, symptoms and health insurance-related options, are paid significantly less than those whose patients are absent or who can focus on one part of the body and ignore everything else.

One could argue that our health system's perverse priorities are a natural outgrowth of medical history. The interview and physical exam have been around for millennia. Many of the greatest innovations of the last century involved technology and procedures, and, as is the case for most new things, the newer skills were seen as sexier and priced at a higher level.

But this, too, is true: when studies examine differences between men and women, they find that men more often value the left-brain skills associated with technology and procedures and women the right-brain ones associated with communication skills and relationship building. But here, as most everywhere, culture interacts with biology. When women first became doctors, they were strongly encouraged to go into psychiatry and pediatrics. Now they are going into surgery and radiology and emergency medicine in large numbers, and reports from the field suggest their patients have the same—or better—outcomes. And still, look at a list of the highest-paid medical specialties, and you find that all but dermatology are left-brain specialties where men predominate. On the list of the lowest-paid specialties you find the specialties are more relational, cognitive, and right-brain, the specialties where women are in the majority.

A randomized controlled trial published in 2016 sent identical applications for a lab manager position to science faculty, half with a man's name, half with a woman's. The male applicant was rated as more competent and hirable and offered a higher salary by both male and female science faculty. We are all part of the same culture and we are all biased, even when we think we're not, even when we try not to be, and certainly when we think talking about bias is a form of bias against those who routinely benefit from our most entrenched and beloved biases.

People who earn more money have more money, as do companies that make a fortune off drugs and devices and technologies. And people with more money have more power and greater capacity to lobby for their self-interest. Radiologists, who fall to the top of the specialty pay heap, lobby hard for mammograms in age groups where they have been shown to do more harm than good and in situations where other technologies and approaches appear more effective. More mammograms mean more money for them. Pediatricians, by contrast, do not lobby for themselves but for kids to have better schools and food and opportunities. And so they remain, decade after decade, in the bottom rungs of the pay scale; after all, children don't vote or have power, and taking care of children is women's work and so worth little on the marketplace.

Rarely in salary discussions do doctors or fee-setting committees mention the needs of the populace. In fact, it's only recently that people in medicine have begun to consider what is now called "Population Health." In many ways, a focus on social needs is un-American. In a culture where self-determination is paramount, individual doctors are entitled to go into radiology and orthopedics and dermatology and anesthesia rather than into primary care (where they are desperately needed, where care more efficiently and effectively prevents disease and decreases costs). But they don't make those decisions in a vacuum.

Like many humans, many medical students gravitate toward respect, prestige, money, and power. They see who counts in the culture of medicine and in our larger society, and (surprise!) they feel far more competent in the hospital-based, interventional, organ- and disease-specific specialties where they do most of their training. Also, at most medical schools, the vast majority of students incur vast amounts of debt. They graduate owing hundreds of thousands of dollars, a figure that has grown dramatically over the last two decades. Lucrative specialties make debt repayment easier at a time of life when people want to buy homes and start families. Students from traditionally underrepresented backgrounds are more likely to need financial aid and graduate with greater debt loads. Unlike their peers, however, those students are more likely to work in poorer neighborhoods trying to help those who need it most.

In our current system, then, we provide incentives to enter fields without shortages and disincentives to enter those where our national need is greatest. And in a profound rebuttal to arguments for background-blind admissions policies, the people from traditionally underrepresented groups, whose backgrounds often mean they take the greatest risks and incur the greatest debt burdens, are the ones most likely to do the right thing for Population Health. They improve our society, and we punish them for it.

## COMPLEXITY

Laila Said lived in her daughter's house on a sloped street midway between a public housing complex and a quickly gentrifying shopping area. On my first housecall, a caregiver showed me into the bright front room, where a pack of small terriers and spaniels encircled my feet and doctor bag, sniffing with enthusiastic curiosity. Ten years after being diagnosed with dementia, Laila sat primly on her couch. When I said hello, she glanced at me, then looked away. I explained who I was and told her I needed to ask her some questions. She stared out the window. Over the next hour, she never smiled or offered more than one-word replies. Fortunately, her daughter had left notes, I had recent hospital records—lots of them—and when it became clear Laila couldn't or wouldn't answer my questions, the caregiver led me into the kitchen to show me her charge's medications. Shutting the door behind her, she said her job was very difficult. Laila could be really mean. The caregiver pulled up a shirtsleeve to show me fingernail scratches on her arm. "Be careful," she said.

When I returned to the living room, Laila hadn't moved. She had perfect posture in her tiny, emaciated body and the same hard-sad-vague expression on her face. I wanted to do a physical exam, but not without giving her warning. I held my stethoscope where I knew she could see it, trying to communicate to her that my stranger's touch meant help, not harm. The instant I placed my hand on her shoulder, her primal screeching began.

This is what many people dread most—for their future selves, for their families. For anyone. Even for doctors and nurses who experience it regularly and must do things that worsen the distress of the dementia patient they are trying to help. The situation can be made morally tolerable when the patient can still express their wishes for treatment or has provided clear guidance to a legally designated proxy decision-maker, and when the treatment is clearly helpful, resulting in the patient feeling better and returning to a more familiar environment. All too often, none of these mitigating factors exist. Afraid of old age, incapacity, and death, people don't designate a proxy and discuss with that person what they value most and want to avoid, a reality that drastically reduces their chances of receiving the care they want later. Absent any direction, the default position of the American health care system is to "do everything." More often than not, this approach does not actually include "everything," since it so rarely includes essential conversations about a person's future, care designed to minimize distress and maximize comfort, information about likely life expectancy, and options for treatment in a familiar environment. Each of those approaches is well studied, proven effective and cost-effective, preferred by many patients and families, and generally not provided in today's technology-obsessed and profit-driven health systems.

When Laila began screeching, the dogs fled the room and the caregiver and I stood back. Then I made a show of putting down my stethoscope and began speaking in what I hoped was a soothing, matter-of-fact tone. That didn't help. As I was debating what to do next, the screeching stopped as suddenly as it had begun. Laila was again perched on the couch with her hard-sad-vague expression.

Dementia doesn't invariably make people angry, sad, aggressive, or unreachable, but it makes many people those things on occasion in the disease's long course, and it makes some people one or more of those things for years. Sometimes the issue is the disease itself, early-stage grief of what will be lost to Alzheimer's, anger at what's been taken by a stroke in vascular dementia, frustration of fluctuating alertness, confusion, hallucinations, and physical control in Lewy body dementia, or the personality changes of frontotemporal dementia.

Other times, the triggers are situational. Imagine your reaction if a stranger started taking off your clothes. If you felt cold but couldn't find or ask for a sweater, or you had to pee but couldn't undo your clothes or were in a new place and couldn't find the bathroom. And what if you looked in the mirror and didn't recognize yourself, or sat in your home minding your own business when a stranger appeared claiming to be a doctor, asking you questions you couldn't answer, then wanting to touch intimate parts of your body?

In Laila's case, it was also possible stethoscopes and doctors signaled pain, confusion, and further loss of control to her. Before we took her into our housecalls practice, she had been back and forth from hospitals. Because of her diabetes and dementia, she had little sensation in her feet and usually forgot her walker. She frequently fell and developed infections or acted out in ways her family didn't know how to handle. For each problem, they called 911, and the paramedics arrived to find an ill or upset old woman with multiple serious medical problems. It was a no-brainer for them to take her to a hospital and a no-brainer for hospitals to admit her. She was old and sick. Wasn't the hospital where she needed to be?

After the housecalls began, her family started calling us first. In person or by phone, we helped them care for her without the added trauma of a hospital, with its chaos of strangers, unfamiliar rooms, bodily assaults, and invasions. We didn't cure Laila's dementia or other problems, but gradually figured out the interpersonal and medical reasons for her screaming. By tackling those problems with family education and medication and by working with our center's exceptional home health nurses, we improved her quality of life, as well as the lives of those around her. There was less screaming (by everyone), and they all felt less anxious, spent more pleasant time together, and slept better.

Because we cared for Laila in the early 2010s, we were not paid for the phone portion of the time spent doing this cost-saving, life-enhancing work. If you think of billing as a barometer of what matters in medicine, this becomes information relevant to most people. It was not until 2015 that our health system created care coordination billing codes and recognized patients and caregivers as part of the health care team. And there remains a second, equally important way that care of patients like Laila shows up critical blind spots in our health care system. Although Laila's home care saved tens to hundreds of thousands of health care dollars, it did so in a way that still doesn't appear on federal or local medical center ledgers.

Success for most hospitals is primarily measured by how full they are: how many bodies fill how many beds. This, despite our national focus on cost cutting in our high-price, low-value health care system, and federal penalties on hospitals for readmissions since the enactment of the 2012 Hospital Readmissions Reduction Program. Indeed, since that program covers just six common conditions (heart attacks, heart failure, pneumonia, chronic lung disease, hip and knee replacements, and coronary artery bypass graft surgery), there is little incentive for medical centers to strive for true, universal quality care by anticipating and solving problems before they reach the crisis proportions that warrant hospitalization. Good health is bad for business.

For several years until Laila's death, our home health team, my colleagues, and I rushed to her house as needed: to diagnose and treat pneumonia, an intestinal bleed, multiple episodes of worsened confusion, and, finally, a stroke. We talked her daughter and son-in-law through late-night crises and collaborated with home health nurses and social workers to help provide Laila the care she needed at home. It was still hard on everyone, and it was also much better.

Around this same time, our medical center moved to an accountable care organization approach—one linking organizations and providers across care sites to (in theory) provide collaborative, coordinated care for patients or populations. This didn't mean the hospital recognized the savings from keeping Laila out of the hospital, however. The inpatient and outpatient parts of health care still aren't connected in most systems. But the medical center did start supporting our housecalls program, eventually providing a social worker, nurse coordinator, and administrative help. For almost twenty years before that, "Care at Home" had been viable only by virtue of grateful patient and family donations.

Those giant institutional leaps forward explain our confusion when our medical center decided to shutter its home health program—a unit of nurses, physical and occupational therapists, social workers, and dietitians who provided care to patients temporarily homebound while recovering from hospitalization, illness, or surgery, or permanently homebound because of serious physical or mental disease. Home health care helps people leave the hospital sooner than they once did, continuing their care and serving as eyes and ears for physicians and nurse practitioners. The reason for the closure was the same as for many other academic medical centers: they were losing money. In a fragmented system, it's easier to close a program providing essential patient services than to recognize its uncounted gains and fight to restructure the system so they count.

Two of my colleagues, among the best and most passionate geriatricians I know, got wind of the potential closure a few weeks before it happened. They sent detailed letters to the administration that explained why home health agencies, just like medical centers (ours is rightly proud of itself), are not created equal. We all worked there for a reason: to provide the best, most up-to-date care in a system that neither rewarded (as fee-for-service does) nor penalized (as managed care sometimes does) clinicians for doing what was right for patients. One letter explained why we needed our own agency, how it differed from others in our city and region, and how its approach helped bridge the chasms of our divided health care system for patients of all ages with the greatest needs. The letter also says a lot about its physician-author. He's the sort of doctor who, when one of his patients dies, writes the story of their life and death and sends it to everyone who cared for that person as an inpatient or outpatient over the years. Residents and students describe him with awe. I wasn't surprised that he stayed late after a long day of work to write a polite, detailed letter on his patients' behalf, but since he's that very best version of a doctor-employee a medical center is likely to encounter, our institution's nonresponse did surprise me.

Of course, the second letter came from a similarly stalwart character. Among her many points:

> I have been told that [home health] accrued a . . . deficit in its last operating year. I may be wrong, but I would be interested in knowing what was assessed as the "ins" and "outs"—because knowing how hard it is to find analyst time and assignments to help evaluate program outcomes . . . I would want to be sure that consideration is given to the downstream savings [home health] can provide a health system (which I suspect was not factored into the $ . . . loss) and not just costs of running the program vs insurance reimbursements. I certainly agree that there is room to improve the operations . . .
>
> . . . there are MANY programs and areas of [our institution's] operations that "cost" money but are supported with the focused intention of supporting patients and their outpatient clinicians, and reducing avoidable downstream high-cost health systems utilization. [Home health] is no different . . .

A creative thinker, she offered four synergistic, system-savvy approaches to cutting costs and increasing efficiency without losing the unique services offered by our home health agency.

The person at the top of the institutional food chain to whom these letters were addressed did not respond. One of his henchmen thanked my two colleagues for their thoughtful comments, acknowledged the difficult situation, and assured them that the powers were looking at all options with our complex, older patients in mind. The next month, the medical center's CEO sent an e-mail to all staff announcing the closure.

No community discussion. No recalculation using all relevant metrics. No evidence of "other options."

The e-mail noted the financial challenges and the many other local home care programs. It argued—contradicting evidence, patient stories, and testimonies of my colleagues and the nurses who protested outside the hospital a few weeks later—that because our patients still had access to home care, they were not being deprived of essential services.

The announcement came as a done deal. To most of us, it felt like yet another nontransparent, noncollaborative, top-down decision inflicting harm on both patients and clinicians. They appeared to be checking boxes rather than ensuring optimal care. It felt as if they didn't care about either their hardworking primary care clinicians or the largely voiceless patients the home health program served. It's hard to work as well as you might at a medical center and in a health system where decisions are based on flawed evidence and partial data, where certain types of care and patients and clinicians are favored over others, and where leadership makes decisions that harm patients from behind closed doors, actual and digital.

## COMBUSTION

I had always imagined that when a straw broke a camel's back, the animal would buckle, her legs folding beneath her, her defeated body landing on the ground with a resounding thud.

But when it happened to me, it wasn't like that at all. It was actually very quiet.

I stood alone in a sixth-floor conference room after a meeting, checking e-mail on my cell phone. I was having a good day in a great month and terrific year as a doctor and medical school professor. That afternoon, none of my patients was seriously sick or actively dying, I had recently been awarded a major national grant and acquired two prestigious new job titles, and the meeting, the first with one of my grant teams, had gone very well.

When my phone rang, I almost didn't answer. But the person on the other end of the phone was the sort of person whose call you should answer if you possibly can, and so I did.

After I gave progress reports on my pending tasks and received responses of pleasure and gratitude, the person said something that was something fairly normal in our world, something small, something light. Something very much like a straw.

That was when I felt the snap. When my metaphorical back, or perhaps the doctor part of me, broke.

I remember looking at my watch. I remember thinking: Oh, and Oh shit. I remember finishing the call in a friendly, businesslike manner.

After hanging up, I noted the sounds from surrounding offices: clicking keyboards, voices from behind a closed door, a copier's whir and swish. Nothing was out of the ordinary for a workday midafternoon, yet for me, everything had just changed. Reality as I had lived it for over twenty-five years had shattered. The breakage seemed to me less like a dropped ceramic flower pot, obviously fractured but in large shards that might be glued back together, and more like a car's windshield after a collision: a still-intact surface in hundreds of tiny, irreparable pieces.

I'm mixing metaphors. But when a person is broken, she becomes a jumble of seemingly incompatible thoughts and emotions. What I didn't realize in the aftermath of that fateful phone call was that a broken person is also given the opportunity to see her life, and the world, differently. What I did realize was that I was experiencing what over 50 percent of American physicians are also currently experiencing: burnout. These levels of distress are unprecedented, and as bad for patients as for their doctors.

The person at the other end of the telephone that fateful day had been well intentioned and supportive. The words leading up to my snap were about looking forward to the good work we both expected me to do. Suddenly, I knew I couldn't, and that terrified me. I had known I was unhappy, unhealthy, and exhausted, that I was spending most of my clinic time on the computer, not with patients, and most of my academic time on projects that were good for my career and bad for me, but I hadn't realized that I was in such rough shape that words like *Keep up the great work* could break me. The standard in medicine is to ignore discomfort and distress of all kinds—physical, mental, emotional, and spiritual—and to carry on. That's what I'd been doing for months, or maybe years.

Burnout has three criteria. The first is emotional exhaustion. In that state, a person is tapped out at the end of the day and unable to recover with time off. This was certainly the case for me. By early 2015, I had stopped reading at night and begun sitting in front of the TV, unable to do anything more constructive or restorative unless shepherded by someone else. I wasn't depressed; I still enjoyed my patients, my family and friends, good food, and much more. But I jumped at the slightest unexpected sound and found myself suddenly, aggressively pulling our good-natured dog across the street at the tiniest hint of danger. During my ten- to twelve-hour workdays I ate little, letting my cells do the screaming I could not. Their demands became the background music to my days, giving them an extra edge and urgency, a metaphor writ imperceptibly on my body. At night and on weekends, after working and starving, I ate and ate, filling the void and sedating my distress. Because I came out even on body weight, I thought I'd invented a creative new version of work-life balance.

This is not the story my spouse would tell. That story would go like this: I had become scary. The slightest thing would transform me from the calm, cheerful person I mostly was with patients and colleagues into a whirling dervish of wrath. I behaved as if everyone and everything was out to get me: the idiot in the car ahead of me who stopped at the newly yellow light when I had no time to spare; the godforsaken computer that wouldn't let me format a document the way I needed to; the woman in our neighborhood with her rambunctious off-leash dog; all the people everywhere who didn't seem to do their jobs as well as I thought they should. (Luckily, getting help made a big difference, and we're still happily married.)

My internist didn't believe me about the depression. As she checked boxes in the electronic medical record, she had me complete a depression screening test. I sped through it.

"Oh," she said when she saw the confirming results. "Well, you said you weren't depressed." We smiled at each other and moved on to my vision and arthritis, fatigue and cough.

Just before I left, she said, "Wait. Let's do this one too." It was the anxiety scale.

I sped through that one too.

We counted the boxes I'd checked. The scoring options went from no anxiety to mild, moderate, severe, and very severe. It seemed I belonged in the last category.


In medicine, we use the word *erosion* to describe places where surface tissue—tooth enamel, say, or skin, those essential outer parts that protect the whole—has been gradually destroyed by chemical or physical action causing a wound. If you are too sick to turn yourself over, the constant pressure of your own weight can wear away skin and produce ulcers at your tailbone or hip, heel, or ankle. In teeth, cavities form when normal mouth bacteria convert food sugars to enamel-destroying acid plaque. Notably, erosion in medicine is evoked exclusively for physical processes and parts and not for a person's more abstract components, such as their agency, hope, psyche, soul, and self.

For every hour they spend face-to-face with patients, doctors now spend two to three hours on the electronic medical record, or EMR. They also spend "pajama time" at home at night finishing electronic notes they can't finish during their long workdays. Many of us lament this. Much less discussed is how technology that has undermined efficiency and the doctor-patient relationship became the national standard. Or why medicine bought electronic record systems from businesses with vastly different priorities from those of clinicians and patients, or why, having seen the harm to clinicians in systems that already adopted that technology, more and more health care organizations followed suit. Instead, we discuss the alarming, increasing rates that doctors get sick, take drugs, get divorced, and leave medicine, and how they commit suicide at rates higher than the general population. We institute programs on wellness and resilience, but don't change anything fundamental about the priorities and systems that make such programs necessary. We blame the victims.

As a doctor, I use the particular electronic medical record that holds the health information of a majority of Americans. It's a system designed to facilitate billing, not care. Its greatest asset is that the accounting department can quickly find the information needed to plug into formulas that link activities to charges. To make their jobs easier, we clinicians must provide required data in specific places in interconnected windows that resemble nothing so much as a fun house where doors lead to doors, and mirrors lead to confusion. We are also strongly encouraged to use standardized text, as if my visual disability or cancer surgery or inflammatory arthritis were identical to yours. Or as if one doctor's take on a particular patient were always identical to another's. This need to input copious information in particular language and places incentivizes cutting and pasting old notes to make new ones, and erring on the side of leaving things in rather than highlighting what may matter most. Medical notes are now so full of noise and jargon that it's often impossible to figure out what actually happened during a specific encounter. One night on call, the lab paged me about a dangerously abnormal test result in a cancer patient I don't know. I read and reread her notes, unable to tell which of the three cancer diagnoses on her chart was active. This is typical. Meanwhile, patients' illness stories and their doctors' analyses of those particular experiences, neither of which aid billing, are often altogether absent.

Electronic medical records are not the only contributors to physician burnout, but they are the technological embodiment of the nefarious values driving our health care system. The biggest EMR company apparently dismisses complaints from patients, doctors, and nurses. Our concerns don't matter, I've been told by multiple sources, because we're not their customers. Medical centers and health systems are, and they just keep on buying the product. In defending their actions, health leaders tout the EMR's reliability, its accessibility from anywhere, and its usefulness for research and quality improvement. Those are significant benefits. Unmentioned is its often redundant, recycled, and outdated information or its frequent, significant, systematic information gaps with real potential to harm or kill patients. Such flaws would not be tolerated by most businesses or consumers. As anyone who works with data knows: garbage in equals garbage out.

I do not feel sentimental about the days of handwritten patient notes and the illegible, sometimes unsafe, hard-to-find, and practically impossible-to-share records they produced. But I do feel nostalgic for something essential that was lost when they were replaced by electronic record platforms. Heedlessly and unnecessarily, this particular approach to cyberdata collection has desecrated the most precious, meaningful elements of the patient-doctor relationship: the human connection, direct and intimate, laden with subtleties, significance, and respect for each person's unique feelings and needs. In our brave new world, very little worth is accorded to activities such as spending a clinic visit talking through the impact of a patient's new diagnosis on her health and life or building the sort of relationship that enables discussion of the real reasons why another patient can't lose the excess weight causing his diabetes and high blood pressure. The things I most want from my doctors and try hardest to give my patients—things like attentive listening, shared decision-making, and individualized treatment—don't much matter. In such a system, I am penalized if my patient doesn't get a colonoscopy, something the EMR and my health center track, but struggle to find a place to document the half hour I spent with her and her daughter discussing why her multiple advanced illnesses and short life expectancy mean that she would likely incur all the risks and inconveniences of that screening test but none of its benefits.

The screen-focused physician is one reason patients complain doctors don't listen or know them. It's one reason 81 percent of physicians now say their workload is at capacity or overextended; half would not recommend medicine as a career. It's not that electronic records are the sole cause of the historically unprecedented disillusionment of doctors today, but they are paradigmatic.

Erosion results in a wound, the worn-away part present like the negative space in a sculpture. When I tried to learn how best to use our new electronic record system, my institution sent me to trainings with a young man who informed my large group of doctors that he hadn't been trained on what he called "the clinician interface."

Months later, when I went to the lead doctor in our practice to ask for help because the system-generated notes seemed so worthless that I found myself creating both those required checkbox, robotext records and also narrative notes that captured the important elements of my patient visits, her unspoken words and actions made me feel that she thought my concerns were the time-sucking ramblings of a technologically inept person with an irreparable cognitive deficit and an annoyingly flawed character.

The second criterion of burnout is depersonalization, which shows up as cynicism or a negative response to job duties. Here's where, when the snap occurred, I lit up the burnout scale. My situation felt hopeless. Our health system had ads and billboards all over town and radio spots I heard count-less times a day, yet adult patients of all ages waited over an hour on the phone only to be told there were no new primary care appointments. When I contacted the call center manager, I was told the administration was aware of the situation but providing more people to answer phones, and showing respect for potential patients' time and health needs, was low on the list of priorities. With no marketing at all, the wait list for our geriatric housecalls practice was at nine months, and people routinely died before we could get to them.

The human brain constructs stories from available information even when that information is partial. When a medical center CEO's multimillion-dollar salary is reported in the local paper the same month that center's janitors' barely livable salaries are cut in half, a story emerges. When a medical school teaches that black lives matter while providing copious training in medical science but token teaching about the structural and social determi-nants of health, a story is being told. When health care organizations proclaim value-based patient care is their top priority but institute productivity metrics that prioritize numbers of patients seen over whether those patients' needs are met, when they adopt electronic record systems that undermine the doctor-patient relationship, when their clinicians experience record levels of burnout and work dissatisfaction and they do nothing to alter the fundamental mechanics of daily life in their hospitals and clinics, an Orwellian story unfolds in the imaginations of patients and doctors alike.

One contributor to my burnout unspecified in the criteria but now getting some press was the feeling that the institutions I worked for did not share my values and goals. Our leaders used words like *health*, *primary care*, and *patient-centered* at the same time as they systematically undermined those pillars of good medicine by focusing their deeds, attention, and money elsewhere. With the people framing medicine this way holding most of the power and resources locally and nationally, setting the policies and agendas that shape our health and health care, and controlling the facts of your job, you cannot help but conclude that you may never again get to do the work that drew you to medicine in the first place. Doctors across the country are suffering this sort of moral distress. It affects their work, lives, and health, and it's the reason they stop practicing.

The third burnout criterion is reduced accomplishment, as the doctor wonders whether what she does really matters at all. After the final straw, it became clear to me that there was no point in seeing patients, helping with our new medical school curriculum, or leading the innovative programs for which I'd won grant support. Each of those activities suddenly seemed to me about as useful as moving chairs to an upper deck of the *Titanic*.

SEXY

Television serves as a rose-tinted mirror held up to our societal obsessions, conceits, and fantasies. Increasingly, it is weighing in on the topic of old age.

In the show *Grace and Frankie*, Jane Fonda (age seventy-nine in the third season) and Lily Tomlin (age seventy-seven) played scenes that often included jokes about one's hearing and the other's memory loss. Meanwhile, their now romantically partnered gay ex-husbands, Martin Sheen (age seventy-six) and Sam Waterston (also age seventy-six), after years of secrecy, at last let themselves come out to family and friends. Age liberated them from the conventions to which they submitted for decades, and the men finally claimed their true sexuality and identities.

In contrast to most casting, the male leads are younger than the females. Not by much, but Hollywood usually pairs men with women ten to thirty years their junior. Apparently, the rules of the game change in old age. This is Hollywood's traditional approach to heterosexuality across the life span: For the most part, teens fall for teens and young adults for young adults. In middle age, things change. Men fall for younger women, and women become mommies and bosses—roles commonly presented as mutually exclusive with sexuality and romance. In old age, the playing field evens up again, or maybe women gain a slight advantage. But it's not just women who are misrepresented. The association of manhood with virility is so strong that older men are put in a lose-lose situation, either portrayed as impotent in all senses of that word or described in language that suggests their sexuality is surprising, inappropriate, unbecoming, or repulsive. Jokes along the lines of "Grampa got game!" (said of Robert De Niro in the movie *The Intern*) commend thoughts and behaviors considered normal from age twelve through adulthood.

Despite its charms, *Grace and Frankie* sends mixed messages. The leads are all attractive, even if Fonda and Tomlin would not have been considered aesthetic peers in decades past. (Old is old is old . . .) None of the characters have completely gray or white hair, and given the commonness of hair loss in male old age, it's hard to believe that the selection of two still follicularly endowed male actors isn't meant to signal ongoing vitality. We are not the first generations to link sexuality with youth or to downgrade women years or decades before men.

A widowed friend in her seventies is often assumed to be much younger than she is. She has a great brain, a good sense of humor, flawless grooming, and a full life, but men don't look at her much anymore, and she hates that. When I last saw her, she regaled me with stories about her recent adventures in online dating. Her conclusion: "I don't want to be a nurse or mommy and only men looking for one of those look at me." The ones who might have interested her were looking downward chronologically, not across.

Other straight women find relief in the sexual invisibility of their old age. This has less to do with a loss of interest in sex than with the pleasure of shedding the need they once felt to groom, preen, perform, and perpetu-ally prove their worth by asserting their attractiveness to the male gaze. Those women still make an effort to look good but are happy to worry less about attractiveness, to have more time for other pursuits, to feel safer out in the world, and to celebrate a more honest and accurate alignment of their inner and outer selves.

Some have argued that because of gay male culture's focus on a young, buff, and beautiful version of sexual attractiveness, aging may be particularly difficult for gay men, especially those who are estranged from family or lost many peers in the early years of AIDS. Some of this is supposition, as little research has been done on sexual attractiveness and activity of LGBTQ elders. A search of the literature on the topic yielded primarily articles about sexual identity and health-related sexual challenges in old age. We know even less about lesbian, trans, or gender-fluid old people, though we do know that as groups they are more marginalized and have poorer health, two situations not generally correlated with sexual appeal.

Regardless of sexual identity, men are often said to have more options, and while that appears to be true, their romantic old age has its own disap-pointments. Men report surprise when their once effective charms aren't even noticed or, worse, are considered cute or absurd. All they want is what they've always wanted. The sportswriter and essayist Roger Angell, in his nineties, put it this way:

> More venery. More love; more closeness; more sex and romance. Bring it back, no matter what, no matter how old we are. This fervent cry of ours has been certified by Simone de Beauvoir and Alice Munro and Laurence Olivier and any number of remarried or recoupled ancient classmates of ours. Laurence Olivier? I'm thinking of what he says somewhere in an interview: "Inside, we're all seventeen, with red lips."

Not all men feel that way. Some are done. They let their beards grow and change their clothes less often, joking that this is how they always would have lived but for social norms and the need to be appealing. Others struggle to unify their identity and appearance. A nurse twice told me the story of a gay men's musical theater group he's been going to since the 1970s. He said he loved it but always joked how, himself and a few others aside, the audience was full of old farts. Nearing seventy, it only recently occurred to him that he now fits right in.

The psychological literature of old age attests that all these reactions are common. A person's response to being demoted from sexual being to "old person," a state commonly if mistakenly assumed to be asexual, depends a good deal on how much they still care about sex, their romantic aspirations and prospects, and the role of sexuality in their life to that point. As with everything old-age-related, responses vary, and the reactions of the not-old are telling. The wedding of a couple in their nineties or hundreds makes the national news, as if at that age people should no longer want romance or companionship, affection and communion. Donald Hall found he could no longer write poetry once his testosterone levels reached their nadir. Diana Athill notes that "about halfway through my seventies I stopped thinking of myself as a sexual being, and after a short period of shock at the fact, found it very restful. To be able to like, even to love, a man without wanting to go to bed with him turned out to be a new sort of freedom."

Once, when I took care of two sisters, one in her late eighties, the other in her early nineties, the younger one told me the older one was still having sex with her husband and insisted that I speak to her about it. When the older sister arrived, I could tell from her averted eyes that she, too, had received the propriety lecture. A few questions established that she and her husband both enjoyed their couplings. I told her there was no medical or other reason I knew of for stopping, and she beamed.

The opposite of sexy isn't so much unattractive as invisible. The first time I noticed I could no longer be seen, I was at a park near my house. My dog sniffed a shrub's damp leaves near a young woman's feet. She spoke into her cell phone. "No," she said as I stood a few feet away. "There's totally no one here."

"Talk to me, not my daughter!" demanded an octogenarian after salespeople repeatedly directed their questions to her fifty-something-year-old daughter, even when her daughter repeatedly turned to her mother for the answers.

In a trendy new restaurant before a famous author event in a large auditorium nearby, my mother began talking about the couples closely seated on either side of us. "Mom," I said pointedly, giving her a look that was meant to signal that not everyone has hearing loss and the people whose dress and behavior she was commenting on were right beside us. "Don't worry," she answered. "I'm invisible."

It has been said that for straight white males, being seen and treated as old can be their first real experience of being on the downside of social assumptions and discrimination. In old age, they lose the sexiness of their former social power and stature. They describe becoming invisible, invoking experiences long familiar to people of color and women. Roger Angell tells of a dinner out with younger friends:

> There's a pause, and I chime in with a couple of sentences. The others look at me politely, then resume the talk exactly at the point where they've just left it. What? Hello? Didn't I just say something? Have I left the room? . . . (Women I know say that this began to happen to them when they passed fifty.) When I mention the phenomenon to anyone around my age, I get back nods and smiles. Yes, we're invisible. Honored, respected, even loved, but not quite worth listening to anymore.

Angell's friends were not so young that one might imagine they didn't know better. They were in their sixties. It's often the almost or newly old who go to the greatest lengths to distance themselves from old age. Both tragic and ironic, they distinguish themselves from even older people by mimicking the way many younger people treat them.

Donald Hall describes a similar experience: "A grandchild's college roommate, encountered for the first time, pulls a chair to sit with her back directly in front of me, cutting me off from the family circle: I don't exist." Both Hall and Angell told these anecdotes to the world in high-circulation magazine essays that were sufficiently popular that they grew up to be parts of notable books. Putting aside the obvious rudeness and cruelty these men faced, their books provide evidence that both were not only compos mentis but witty and insightful (two traits I find quite sexy) at the time these incidents took place. In old age, even the brilliant, famous, and fairly unimpaired are ignored. The implications for the truly unsexy and invisible, those who can't quite follow a conversation for reasons from hearing loss to dementia, are terrifying.

Sexiness also matters in the world of health care, where the unofficial label for higher-caste diseases, patients, problems, and solutions is *sexy*. Heart disease is sexy. Cancer is sexy. All things procedural are sexy. Aging is not sexy. Since hearts and tumors are neither attractive nor desirable, the problem isn't one of aesthetics. It's one of value, both medical and social.

Lots of "not sexy" ailments can accompany old age. People with incontinence, falls, arthritis, constipation, insomnia, and vision and hearing loss often give up jobs and treasured activities. They lose confidence, comfort, and eventually friends. Some fall prey to profiteers promoting unproven therapies. This downward spiral doesn't affect just the afflicted individual; it affects us all, socially and economically, directly and indirectly. Fear and shame lead to inactivity and shrunken social circles, two of the strongest predictors of poor health and the need for expensive services.

Imagine being incontinent. Your underpants are wet, cold, and itchy against your skin. You worry that you smell. You live in constant fear of accidents, the wetness showing through your clothes. You avoid events that last too long or without easy bathroom access. At some point, there's an episode that leaves you so embarrassed and ashamed that you stop going out. Thirteen million Americans are incontinent, and half of noninstitutionalized people over age sixty-five report urinary leakage. Incontinence is among the top medical reasons preventing people from going out and leading to institutionalization—outcomes that adversely affect health and quality of life. Traditionally, doctors and nurses haven't asked about incontinence the way they ask about other common symptoms, and patients haven't brought it up. Many assume little can be done. In fact, often little is done because, like the general public, doctors and nurses receive inadequate education about how to manage it.

All geriatric problems have multiple effective treatments. But only some offer cures with the clean-cut outcome of cataract surgery, one of the sexier treatment options for an age-related disease. Yet the "less sexy" treatments often make life worth living. Imagine what might be possible if these conditions and management strategies were given the same respect as high blood pressure or athletic injuries and their treatments. Just as caste systems keep lower castes in a relentless cycle of poverty and drudgery, so does medicine's sexiness hierarchy deprive millions of Americans of healthier, fully engaged lives.

One year, I decide it's time to stop wearing a bikini. The next year, I give up exercise shorts.

I notice for the first time that most women my age and older do the same. A year or two later, I decide tank tops, too, have become unbecoming. I donate mine to a charity. Some friends tell me the problem is in my head; I'm fit and reasonably trim. I think of a colleague who, in her middle sixties and older, dressed in trendy clothes that would have looked cute on one of our medical students but on her often struck me as incongruous, maybe embarrassing. I reason that I didn't wear at thirty-three what I wore at thirteen, so it makes sense that different clothing suits me better now as well.

Since clothing is an expression of self, it's only logical that a person's clothes change over time, just as bodies and people do. At fifty, even the most gorgeous men acquire a certain jowliness. After menopause, even slim women develop at least a hint of "menopot." By the eighth decade and beyond, most bodies shrink, hunch, bend. A flattering outfit from a few years earlier suddenly doesn't fit or seem attractive. The Puritans had strict rules for old-age attire: "For old men to be gay and youthful in their apparel, or if aged women dress themselves like young girls, it exposeth them to reproach and contempt." Translation: what looks trendy on a twenty-year-old body might differ from what looks fashionable on a sixty- or eighty-year-old body.

But even here, at this juncture of sexiness and invisibility, fashion and function, there's an interplay of culture and biology. In *Women and Power*, the classicist Mary Beard makes a convincing case for the origins of our present notions of male and female speech and power having originated in ancient Greece. Similarly, when it comes to old age and appropriateness, it seems my own beliefs, which previously struck me as pragmatic and thoughtful, have their origins in American Puritanism. Recognizing that raises an important question: Since bodily changes with age are natural and universal, couldn't clothes differently manifest style and sex appeal across all age groups? Presumably, they can and, certainly, they should. It's not only fair and kind, but a considerable business opportunity languishing unclaimed in the marketplaces of clothing and fashion.

Over coffee, a young man who works at a large, familiar tech company tells me they are moving into the "aging space." There's money there, he says, and opportunity—in other words, it's becoming sexy, at least to the higher-ups with their eyes on changing demographics and the corporate bottom line. Farther down the company food chain, however, the staff isn't feeling the passion. Being assigned to the aging project is considered the worst assignment: Sad. Lame. A drag. A bummer. A punishment.

My acquaintance confides that he only agreed to lead this project to get his foot in the door, but as he's spoken to actual old people (something he'd never previously done), he realized two things. First, spouse-partner-friend caregivers are shocked that he's using the words *older adult* to refer to them, not just the person they care for, though to his eyes they are "no question, old." Second, he can't get even his middle-aged colleagues to approach the aging project in the same way they approach all other projects: objectively. Instead, they tell him about their father or grandmother, going straight to stories of disaster and decline. In company brainstorming groups where discussions are usually based on facts, they ignore the research reports he has provided and instead exchange loss and debility anecdotes. He can't get them to see that the experiences they are emphasizing may not be representative and that old age can be approached with the same open mind and intellectual rigor as every other topic.

Geriatrics frequently elicits the same reaction. One of the most well-known and influential physicians in America has described my specialty as "difficult and unappealingly limited." I'm biased, obviously, but how can a field devoted to caring for all medical conditions of all people in one of life's three decades-long age groups be described as limited? It's similarly worth considering why we hear a lot about surgical difficulty, but never that it lacks glamour. To me, all that cutting and rearranging is repetitive and dull—I cannot imagine spending my days that way—but I'm able to appreciate its value to patients and the world.

In medicine, some specialties are tops, while others are bottoms. But here's the rub: when we treat entire categories of people as less interesting and worthy, we devalue part of their humanity, and forfeit some of our own.

## DISILLUSIONMENT

In the months leading up to my burnout, I experienced two types of problems, one physical, one psychological, and, in retrospect, intimately interrelated. Physically, I struggled to do basic things like see well enough to work on a computer or drive my car. I couldn't walk without pain or exercise to relieve the stress of my lost functions and frustrations. Responses to these developments—mine and those of my supervisors—didn't help. Like a good doctor, I soldiered on. Like a typical doctor, I didn't consult a clinician other than the one in the mirror.

When, pre-snap, I mentioned challenges at work, I was offered a large monitor and other workstation modifications that took over fifty hours and several months to find, understand, and manage, time I could ill afford to lose. Luckily, our proactive administrators, with understated kindness, helped me place orders for adaptive equipment. My doctor-bosses, by contrast, made mild noises of sympathy but, busy and overworked themselves, failed to make any of the changes that would have helped me work around my physical challenges. In medical culture, one doctor's struggles are another's inconvenience. Knowing that, I should have been more emphatic and explicit about my needs, and more empathetic and forgiving about theirs.

But this was not my finest moment; I had no reserves from which to draw such a sensible and generous approach. Instead, I tuned out or quietly rebelled. If, for example, having mentioned again that I couldn't see the tiny screen on which we were being shown the new charting task we clinic providers were required to do in the electronic medical record, and again having been ignored, I felt entirely justified in simply not doing it.

This is not the wisest strategy for a person who wants to be a good doctor and decent colleague.

We know the origins of the common usage of the term *burnout*. In the early 1970s the German American psychologist Herbert J. Freudenberger used it to describe work-related stress he saw in physicians. Freudenberger observed that medical practice changed some doctors from passionate idealists to depressive cynics who treated their patients with cold indifference. Investigating further, he found the disillusioned doctors all shared certain traits: a strong work ethic, high achievement, and a tendency to see their work as essential to their identity. Once burned out, they also shared symptoms including disturbed sleep, mood fluctuations, and difficulty concentrating. Long-term stress adversely affected their bodies and minds, keeping them on high alert, as if they continuously faced a lethal threat. Their combination of high work engagement and incessant strain led to a vicious cycle of self-neglect, value revision, changed behavior, challenged relationships, withdrawal, and inner emptiness.

Increasingly, I had found myself easily startled and unable to recall simple words and statistics. I lay awake most nights between two and four in the morning, thoughts racing and heart percussing. I worried about my patients: Would S's daughter show up? Had I done the right thing for H? Would M fall again? I also ran through long lists of all the things I hadn't yet done and all the people who were making my life so unpleasant, then conjured up things I might have said or done and, finally, plausible escape routes: a broken hand that precluded typing, the sort of cancer that would get me off work for a good long time but wouldn't kill me, a family crisis that required my particular presence. I'd drift into an exhausted sleep just before my alarm went off to a new day with a full inbox, a schedule that allowed no time for meaningful note writing, countless other competing tasks and responsibilities, and wholly inadequate time for actually doing those things that could legitimately earn the label *patient care* or felt meaningful.

What I was seeing was happening everywhere and doctors were beginning to speak and write about it. In Omaha, Byers "Bud" Shaw, a transplant surgeon, stopped practicing when he found himself too anxious to leave his office, much less pick up a scalpel. In Boston, the internist Diane Shannon left medicine because of the constant tension between the sort of medicine she wanted to practice, "compassionate, safe, dependable, connected, and humane," and a health delivery system that seemed to value and prioritize everything but those elements. An unnamed hospital-based doctor quoted on NPR said, "If I took the time to actually talk with my patients, which is what drew me to medicine in the first place, it meant I fell behind and then spent hours and hours at home in the evening doing the required data entry." An outpatient-clinic doctor colleague of mine noted different but related pressures in his setting. Even if he finished his notes before heading home, he spent "2–3 hours every day/night on in-box stuff (e-mails and phone calls from patients, nurses, and pharmacists)—this is uncompensated, underappreciated work that we do on a daily basis and bleeds into our evenings and weekends. This work happens whether it is a clinic day or a non-clinic day. There is no escape and no relief." A doctor's interests and inclinations push one way, toward patients and care, and the system pushes the other, toward computers and tasks that are essential but not factored into our work schedules.

A 2015 study conducted by the American Medical Association and Mayo Clinic found that over half the doctors in America are experiencing burnout. The rates have increased yearly in recent years, and are far higher than for the general population, even among people with similar education and work hours. They also are, by far, the highest rates recorded among physicians since Freudenberger identified the phenomenon. The study's authors explain that this epidemic should be of grave concern to all Americans because, in addition to the personal toll on doctors and our rising suicide rates, "burnout appears to impact the quality of care physicians provide, and physician turnover, which [has] profound implications for the quality of the health care delivery system." That's bad news for patients, and we are all patients or potential patients. It's also bad news for American health care, which is seeing more and more doctors reducing their work hours, giving up clinical practice, or taking early retirement at a moment when the Department of Health and Human Services predicts a shortage of forty-five thousand to ninety thousand physicians by 2025.

As a doctor, if one of my patients has a serious, undesirable side effect to a medication or treatment, I change that medication or treatment. I continue it only if there are no alternatives and the patient and I believe the outcome will be worth the attendant agonies. But those in charge of American health care seem unfazed by our current system's many destructive side effects, including burnout and its harms to patients and clinicians. Much like our senators and representatives who deprive their constituents of health care coverage while continuing their own extra-special congressional health benefits, they behave as if they believe that people get what they deserve. Words such as *resilience* and *self-care*—the trait and skill, respectively, that we are encouraged to develop to combat burnout—suggest the failure is within America's clinicians, that we have unwisely used up our precious fuel, that we are weak and don't know how to take care of ourselves. The ubiquity of burnout across specialties and geographic regions suggests our distress is but a symptom alerting the health system to a potentially lethal underlying problem. In the same way a person can have arm pain during a heart attack when a critical artery is blocked, burnout is physician distress signaling that the health care system needs critical care.

Read any of the growing numbers of poignant essays about burnout, and you will find most doctors report what I, too, felt, even at my lowest point: that I still wanted to be a doctor, that the work for me has always been more vocation than job, but that the structures and demands of the health care system had begun preventing me from providing the sorts of care and healing I believed my patients needed, and that was something I couldn't abide.

### PRIORITIES

In the months after the snap, I had many doctor's appointments. One week, I had two just days apart, one in general medicine and the other in orthopedics, both at the same highly ranked medical institution. Occurring so close together, these visits quickly morphed in my mind from personal experiences with individual doctors into metaphors for the current state of U.S. medicine.

I saw my internist first. Her practice is in an older part of town where I can sometimes find street parking and avoid the astronomical fees at the patient parking garage—fees not covered by health insurance, though of course I can afford them better than most. The offices are clean but drab, and the clinic runs relatively efficiently. It has separate lines at the front desk for checking in and out, and shortly after my arrival, a friendly medical assistant called me in to take my vital signs and review my medication list.

Ten minutes later, I was in a narrow exam room and thirteen minutes after that, my internist appeared, looking tired yet radiating her usual warmth and concern. She apologized for running late, and I told her it was no problem. I didn't tell her that I always block out ninety minutes for my twenty-minute appointment and come prepared to work. As I answered her questions, we studied each other. I noted the subtle tension in her torso while we discussed my multiple concerns, each of which required decisions, tests, and referrals, and each of which she had to attend to given her broad skill set and primary care purview. Because of me, we both knew, she would end up running further behind.

At first, I had her full attention, but soon her fingers moved along her keyboard while we talked, and her eyes strayed from me to her screen. I knew she was working to fit my problems into the electronic record's template with its dozens of menus, billing-required but often clinically irrelevant checkboxes, and subsections not sequenced in the way our conversation was proceeding. Meanwhile, as I knew all too well from my own geriatrics practice, her clinical inbox was filling with an ever-growing list of tasks, all amounting to hours of work for which no time was allotted in her clinic day.

Of course, many of the challenges my internist faced that day aren't unique to primary care. That's why some practices have adopted two workarounds that increase efficiency—midlevel providers and scribes—strategies I got to see in action later that week at my orthopedist's office.

Although part of the same institution, my orthopedist works in a new, glass-walled building in a rapidly revitalizing part of town. There's no street parking, but a café on the ground floor serves farm-fresh salads and organic drip coffee. I went to see her not because I needed an appointment but because I'd been unable to get answers to a simple follow-up question via the patient portal. The problem wasn't that I couldn't get a response, just that I couldn't get one from her. I sent versions of the same query a few times, and each time it was handled without resolution by a different nurse practitioner who didn't know me and either couldn't, for reasons that might range from not having read my chart to not having the necessary knowledge, or wouldn't—since I wasn't their patient—answer my question.

After I checked in, the front desk person told me someone would call me shortly for an X-ray so I should sit by the X-ray room door.

I said I didn't need an X-ray.

He said everyone got an X-ray.

"Before they even see the doctor and whether they need one or not?" I asked in as even and polite and cheerful a tone as I could muster.

I told him I'd already had an X-ray at this same clinic for this same doctor about this same problem, and nothing had changed. He called his supervisor and asked her whether a patient could be seen if she refused the X-ray.

Fortunately, the supervisor said yes. I sat down, and a short while later a medical assistant called my name and took me back into a large, sunny exam room, entered my chief complaint in the computer, and told me where to sit and what clothing to remove.

I had only just begun working when my doctor came in followed by a young woman carrying a laptop. We exchanged pleasantries and then I was introduced to the scribe, who sat discreetly to one side, saying nothing during the visit while her fingers moved quietly on the keyboard.

For the entirety of the appointment, I had my doctor's full attention: eye contact, smiles, a targeted physical exam, and answers to my questions— the original one and some others I came up with to make the visit more worthwhile, though all related to the single body part that is her focus. She didn't seem to miss the X-ray I hadn't had and showed no interest in my other medical issues, or the parts of me that, while not orthopedic, might influence my treatment preferences and recovery. With some prodding—I used words like *physical therapy* and *exercise*—I was able to get her recommendations for approaches other than medications or the sort of high-tech surgery the medical center touted daily on local radio, television, and billboards but that was unlikely to address my primary concerns.

Once we'd made a plan, she left the room, telling me to wait there for her physician assistant, who would review with me my discharge instructions.

Miraculously, she walked out the door, her note written, having done nothing but attend to me during our encounter. We were both pleased and relaxed as a result.

My internist and orthopedist are both highly trained, highly skilled, and hardworking doctors. While I don't know their specific salaries, annual surveys by the American Medical Group Management Association (AMGA) between 2013 and 2017 cite median compensation figures ranging from $193,776 to $259,765 for internists and from $525,000 to $759,086 for ortho-pedists, a two- to threefold difference that grossly exceeds their training time differential and belies my internist's greater experience.

And, of course, that's only part of a larger and more complex financial system that incentivizes procedural and hospital-based care and specialties over relational and outpatient ones.

It would be hard, even morally suspect, to suggest that the salary dispar-ities among medical specialties in American medicine are the most pressing inequities of our health care system. Yet they are representative of the biases underpinning health care's often inefficient, always expensive, and some-times nonsensical care—biases that harm patients and undermine medi-cine's ability to achieve its primary mission.

Usually when we discuss disparities in medicine, we are speaking of patient populations. But there are disparities, or "differences in access to or availability of facilities and services," between my internist and orthopedist, too, ones that reflect systematic nationwide biases in how we value and reward different medical conditions and types of care. This favoritism toward certain sorts of doctors, medical conditions, and treatment approaches devel-oped as side effects of medicine's greatest twentieth-century successes. As scientific progress brought unprecedented gains in health and longevity, we assumed newer, more invasive, higher tech, and more specialized care was always better, and set up a system that prioritizes and generously rewards that sort of care. We confused the occasionally miraculous with the everyday essential, ignored the mounting evidence of economic and health harms of our faulty assumptions, and, in taking an increasingly business-based approach to health care, failed to recognize the ways in which human beings will always differ from other "commodities."

Our health care system's biases affect not just physician salaries but institutional, educational, and research priorities, and indeed, the very culture of medicine. At a recent meeting of the Harvard Medical School Alumni Council, a first-year student was asked about his debt. "Huge," he answered, shaking his head and adding that he also had college debt. "What will you do?" asked the council president. The student grinned. "Oh, I'm not worried. I'm going into Ortho."

In study after study, primary care has been shown to prevent illness, decrease mortality, and lower costs, all with higher patient satisfaction. A growing literature also demonstrates system-wide high rates of overuse and waste, as well as serious harms as a result of higher-tech, more aggressive, specialty-driven care. Internationally, the countries and regions with the most robust primary care systems have the best health outcomes. Yet primary care remains American medicine's second-class citizen.

In most clinics, appointments are scheduled in a one-size-fits-all manner that distinguishes only between new and returning patients and not between mostly healthy patients and those with complex conditions. Every aspect of those appointments assumes that the doctor's most important activities are diagnosis, prescriptions, and procedures. This discounts the entire range of critical activities that help clinicians match care to patients' realities and preferences, increasing the chances that they can and will follow their treatment plan and that the plan will help them. Such activities include skilled listening to what the patient is saying, all that isn't being said, and body language. It includes giving the patient time to absorb complex information or terrifying new diagnoses, express their concerns, and formulate questions relevant to their specific lives. It includes checking for alignment between what was said and what was heard, reading the medical record if you don't know the patient or if they have been hospitalized or seen another clinician since their last visit, establishing truly informed consent, negotiating language and literacy and health literacy barriers, and doing values elucidation, medication review and reconciliation, motivational interviewing, patient education, and counseling.

The terms *structural violence* and *structural inequality* pertain here. As the physician-anthropologist Paul Farmer explained, these concepts offer "one way of describing social arrangements that put individuals and populations in harm's way. The arrangements are *structural* because they are embedded in the political and economic organization of our social world"— in this case, the political and economic organization of American health care. A study of health care spending in eleven wealthy countries found costs in the United States from 2013 to 2016 far exceeded those of the other countries, all of which had better health outcomes, including lower infant mortality, less obesity, and longer life expectancy. The culprits? Prices, which reflect values and the structure of a health care system, particularly: administrative costs (all the paperwork and negotiation necessitated by a system-less system as well as, as one editorialist notes, the essential monopoly of some producers), "goods" including (especially brand-name) medications, and labor (some salaries more than others, clearly, but all driven up by the outliers' excesses). A commentary added high-cost procedures such as joint replacements and unnecessary imaging (CT, MRI) to the list.

Follow the money and hype in medicine and you will find that in the United States we prefer treatment to prevention. Bones matter more to us than children or old people, and patient benefit is not a prerequisite for treatments or procedures. We seem to believe that drugs work better than exercise; that doctors treat computers, not people; that death is avoidable with the right care; that hospitals are the best place to be sick. We value not having wrinkles or warts more than hearing, chewing, or walking.

This situation brings the words of Charles Dickens to mind. Ours are the best of times in American health care, and ours are the worst of times in American health care. Ours is the age of tech and the age of inequality, the epoch of innovation and the epoch of burnout, the season of #blacklivesmatter and the season of colossal health center marketing budgets. In the twenty-first century, we can do so much for people, from quickly curing infections to replacing damaged joints and organs, but we fail to prioritize care that most helps patients, making it far harder for clinicians providing those types of care to succeed.

SYMPATHY

The first week after the fateful phone call that inadvertently shifted my burnout from suppressed to florid, I didn't go to work. It was partly that I felt like I couldn't and partly that I knew I shouldn't. By the second Monday, I had returned, but only long enough to hand off, delegate, and delay before a fortuitously timed, long-planned vacation. By the end of those two weeks, I knew I needed to go on leave. I needed to do for myself what I would have counseled a patient to do: I put my health and well-being before my work.

Did I say as much to my colleagues as I should or could have about what was happening to me? I did not. I avoided some people, mentioned only the physical problems to others, smiled, and tried to look as normal and healthy and well as possible in public.

In a recent, deeply personal, and beautifully written essay in the *New England Journal of Medicine*, a trauma surgeon named Michael S. Weinstein, writing of his own burnout, noted that colleagues had tried to reach out and found him wholly unreceptive. His practice in operating rooms and the hospital was visible to others in ways that mine, making housecalls to patients in their homes and working on grants and projects in an office with a door, was not. Still, I can think of a couple of instances where I deflected queries. Much more common were unspoken questions leaking from kind eyes— those two administrators again, our clinic support staff, and two young doctors, very much my juniors, who helped me disentangle from all I could no longer do. There were also many lovely, supportive e-mails from colleagues, all of which I ignored. By definition, I was impaired.

I wished I could stop feeling so angry and hopeless. I had a meaningful career, a steady job, a good salary, and a happy home life. I was the one who had ignored my body, health, and well-being, so there could be no question of who was to blame for my situation. And yet I hadn't changed too much over my years as a physician, while health care itself and the daily tasks and demands of doctoring had.

For weeks after I went on leave, the worst part of each day was the time devoted to health care—procuring it, not providing it. I had terrific health insurance, the best plan my huge institution offered. I called my primary care doctor's office, and they told me she could see me in six weeks or I could see someone else who didn't know me or my history. I got around that by sending my doctor an e-mail, something that's easier to do if you, too, are a doctor—an unfair advantage, since all patients deserve care when they need it. She helped with most of my problems, but we agreed I needed a specialist to help with my psycho-existential crisis. My costly insurance said it covered mental health. The primary website sent me to a secondary one and then to a third. The journey was long and slow, full of digital roadblocks, distractions, and dead ends. They seemed to be fulfilling the letter of the contract but not its spirit.

The list of potential providers was many hundreds long. Each required a separate secondary search to determine where the office was (since I couldn't drive), what services were provided, and the doctor's ability to take new patients. Very quickly I learned to start with whether they had openings, since most practices had none.

When a person is in crisis, even the smallest tasks are hard. Encountering this labyrinth of hindrances, I cursed and raged. If a doctor who understands the system, speaks fluent English, and has optimal insurance can't get help, how on earth could anyone else?

Neurologists speak of localizing the lesion, finding the anatomical change that explains a patient's signs and symptoms. What lesion was responsible for my burnout, I wondered, and if there were many, did one in particular predominate? This was among the several questions I considered with the psychologist I paid out of pocket to see. Others included: Do I still want to be a doctor? And, if I don't, what else can I do that would provide not just income but health insurance to two middle-aged people with "preexisting conditions"?

My physical ailments were more easily treated than my psychological ones. Although I began to function again, I sensed my mental improvement was not because anything significant had changed but because I'd built up my reserves enough to again feign being fine.

A few months after going on leave, back at work but still steering clear of many activities that had contributed to my crisis, I had an epiphany. The system is created by people, and I was furious at some of them. Could they not see how much of our health care is unnecessarily costly, inefficient, prejudicial, and malevolent? Or did they see and not care? Maybe, I thought, burnout wasn't fundamentally about any of the things that appear in all the studies and articles about it. Maybe it was really about sympathy.

More precisely, maybe burnout was a by-product of a *lack* of sympathy in our health care system and its leaders. I felt no compassion in the official responses to the burnout epidemic generally or to my particular distress. In its place, I was left to feel that I had failed, that I was weak and defective, that I was disposable, and that my concerns and needs were unseemly.

Underappreciated in discussions of burnout is the impact of other people's responses to those who are struggling. There are simple things that too often don't happen. Sincere—not automatized, not institutional— acknowledgment of moral distress. Avoiding obvious, facile solutions that any intelligent, struggling person would have already tried and either found unhelpful or in violation of their core values and interests. Taking action toward changes that might simultaneously mitigate the damage and show kindness. Allowing for flexibility and differences in people, whether they are doctors or patients, nurses or families.

With the right support, burned-out physicians might continue to practice; without it, they go on leave, stop seeing patients, commit suicide. Most weeks of 2017 and 2018 have brought new articles about burnout and new lists of nonclinical jobs doctors can do. Those efforts are steps in the right direction, but we also must address how our bosses and system have responded to the burnout crisis. It's hurtful and disappointing to be kicked when you're down, to be offered not sympathy and succor but insults and disrespect, to have colleagues you trusted and admired smile at you while rubbing salt into the wounds you showed them after gathering up what remained of your small courage. Trust is like Dresden in World War II or New Orleans after Hurricane Katrina; you can rebuild after the devastation, but it will never be the same.

# 10. SENIOR

AGES

In 1960, the bespectacled, royalist-anarchist director of France's Institute of Applied Research for Colonial Fruits in Paris made a radical claim that had nothing to do with bananas, papayas, or jackfruit. "In medieval society," Philippe Ariès wrote in his classic, *Centuries of Childhood: A Social History of Family Life*, "the idea of childhood did not exist."

As is often the case, the French took this news with more equanimity than the Americans. When the book appeared in the United States two years after its French release, the "discovery of childhood" inspired considerable excitement and equally impassioned criticism. Language was partly to blame: where Ariès used the French word *sentiment*, implying both a concept and a sense of feeling, *idea* appears in the English version of the book, losing the fuller meaning of his text. He wasn't arguing that children hadn't existed before the seventeenth century but that social, political, and economic changes ushered in an era in which childhood was newly recognized as a distinct and valued life phase. That he did not approve of this change was also lost in translation.

Ariès's claims and methods remain controversial. Yet his work helped make the institution of family a topic worthy of scholarly attention. He popularized the use of more varied sorts of historical evidence, and his work led to greater awareness that human experience of different life stages varies depending on where and when people live. In history, as in science, what is looked at determines what is seen and known. More traditional historical data—birth, death, and tax records, inventories, property transactions, and the like—tell one story, while letters, newspapers, art, literature, and textbooks tell another. Ariès's biased presentation of such data notwithstanding, it seems likely that the truth includes both those stories.

Take a person's age. These days, we all know how old we are, but the practice of knowing for certain one's birth date and age didn't become universal in Western societies until the eighteenth century. Before that, some people knew their exact ages—Greek and Roman writers were precise, and presumably accurate, about how old they were—and most did not. A person was referred to as "a youth" or "an old person" based on how they looked and acted, not on how many years had elapsed since their birth. A forty-year-old might earn either label.

We don't need to span centuries to find transformed ideas about life phases. In the early 1950s, when my mother was in her early twenties, my grandfather worried that she was becoming an old maid. As her friends married, my grandparents watched with growing alarm as my mother dated and broke up with a variety of perfectly acceptable suitors. They were relieved when, at the ripe old age of twenty-four, she and my father became engaged. One generation later, I can count only a small handful of friends who got married in their twenties. For most of us, it happened in our thirties. My family's social circumstances didn't change over those decades; what was considered normal did.

Widen the lens further, and the changes are even more dramatic. If my mother and I had been born in Europe in the latter Middle Ages or early Renaissance, we might have married at twelve. In those days, menarche equaled maturity, and the notion of adolescence, much less a female young adulthood of higher education, career advancement, and intimate relationships not leading to marriage, did not exist. By our early thirties, had we lived that long, we would have been grandmothers, not the parent of two small children, as my mother was, or a still-unmarried doctor, as I was. What's normal depends not only on when you live but where and who you are in that place and time.

The human brain naturally makes categories. Chinese, Iranian, and Greek authors write of boys, men, and old men. Since the age distribution of our species changed so quickly in recent years, our language and institutions for the years after fifty or sixty haven't caught up. Nor have they accurately captured the variety of who we are or maximized the individual and social potential of people across a newly enlarged canvas of human potential.

The French seem to have an aptitude for naming life stages. In the 1970s they began educational and engagement programs for retired people that were called Les Universités du Troisième Age, or Universities of the Third Age. Both concept and phrase jumped the pond to England before the term *Third Age* was generalized by the historian Peter Laslett, who felt it helped fill "the perennial need for a term to describe older people, a term not already tarnished." Laslett also advanced what he himself termed a radical notion: that the Third Age is the apogee of personal life. He added that the stages, while usually sequential, are not divided by birthdays and supposed that a person could be in the First or Second and Third Ages simultaneously, if that person reached their apogee in youth (as female gymnasts do, for example) or while also working and raising a family. But the Third Age "emphatically" could not overlap with the Fourth. Here, then, is where Laslett's schema falls apart: he defined the first two categories by customary age-related activities, the third by personal realization and a particular set of behaviors that transcend age, and the fourth by biology. There can be no clarity, and no justice and equity, among age groups when they are identified using different metrics.

The Third Age and the Fourth Age can differ in chronological age—young-old and old-old—but are primarily distinguished by their differences in health, activities, and consumer roles. People in the Third Age are "aging successfully," while those in the Fourth are frail and dependent. Laslett called the postwork, postchildren life phase the "crown of life" and the "time of personal self-realization and fulfillment." The Third Age, he argues, is made up of the years and decades recently added to the human life span. It should be used for the "founding, shaping, sustaining, and extending" of duties and institutions. He defines five challenges addressed by the Third Age: recognition of our changed demographics; supporting large numbers of people no longer required to work; cultivating attitudes and morale in the face of inaccurate stereotypes; developing an outlook, institutions, and organizations to give purpose to all those added years; and coping with the problem of the Fourth Age. Although he doesn't fully explore the influences of a person's economic and social situation on their ability to enjoy a Third Age, he does acknowledge the risk of foisting on the Fourth Age all the prejudices that now universally attach to anyone over sixty. He asserts the goal of delineating the two ages was instead to make the most and best of each.

Some have argued that more attention has been paid to the Third Age than the Fourth, but this discounts geriatric medicine: to its credit and detriment, my specialty has traditionally paid much more attention to the Fourth than the Third.

Third Agers are active participants in our mass consumer society. Although many are partly or completely retired, they retain agency—in fact, that ability to act for oneself is one of its two defining features. The most fortunate Third Agers buy anti-aging products and join gyms and social clubs. They travel and volunteer. The Third Age, then, is more a set of behaviors and attitudes, a lifestyle particular to middle-class and wealthy members of our consumerist culture and sociohistorical time. It's the grown-up version of the 1960s emphasis on youth, beauty, choice, and self-expression. It's also a continued effort to define oneself and one's peers as something other than "old."

Not everyone past middle age is part of the Third Age, and many such people have agency but use it in ways that don't fall under the Third Age concept. The Third Age can seem universal because it comprises the people who are most likely to write, speak, and create the art and marketing that have defined it.

Laslett saw the Fourth Age as biologically determined and timeless. Live long enough at any time in our species' history, and you would enter it and be subjected to its inevitable decline and "ignominy." Chris Gilleard and Paul Higgs argue that the Fourth Age is the product of "the combination of a public failure of self-management and the securing of this failure by institutional forms of care." The result is "a location stripped of the social and cultural capital that is most valued" in society. They assert that "the appearance of a fourth age . . . has been contingent upon developments in health and social policy during the course of the twentieth century." It has also been the "bitter fruit" of Third Age efforts to create an image of older people as attractive, useful, and relevant.

Laslett's goal was to counter the "hostile and demeaning descriptions of the elderly which have denied them their status and their self-respect."

That is a worthy goal, though only insofar as it helps *all* older people achieve status and self-respect. If instead it allows the younger and fitter old to gain those essentials at the expense of those who are neither, then such efforts are counterproductive. In Matthew 12:25 Jesus says, "Every kingdom divided against itself is brought to desolation," words echoed by Abraham Lincoln on June 16, 1858, in his "A house divided against itself cannot stand" speech. Similarly, old age divided between Third Agers and Fourth Agers is unsustainable; indeed, it has been of little benefit over its half century as a concept, except to offer false succor to those in the Third Age, followed by worsened degradation when they reach the Fourth. Prejudicial segregation breeds degradation, and we value some lives or parts of lives over others to our own peril. The most fundamental consideration must be the moral one: Will we treat all human beings as human beings regardless of differences, or treat some as lesser beings? The unattainability of absolute equality is no excuse for the ruthless devaluation of individuals or social groups.

Advanced old age invokes negative associations: repugnance at bodily aging, fear of loss of function, a position of poverty and societal inferiority, and a sense of having moved beyond the realm of experience and agency inhabited by most people we count as human. From that place, a person can neither define nor assert themselves in reliable ways. Perhaps they can articulate preference but maybe not, and certainly they can't make happen most things they want. In all-too-common worst-case scenarios, all they can do is scream or cry, try to sleep away the hours, kick or bite—and when those things happen, they are called "bad" or "difficult." They are punished, abandoned, or institutionalized, and ignored, tied up, or sedated. Even people who have made arrangements in advance for a phase of such profound debility cannot be sure their wishes will be respected. How they are seen and treated—really, every aspect of their lives—is controlled by others. The only escape is death.

I have used the word *they* for people in this state, for people in the Fourth Age. In some ways, this is accurate—I am not (yet) such a person but likely will be. Most of "we" will become "they" in the future for days or weeks, months or years, unless we find a new way to think about and address the Fourth Age, one that itself becomes routine and institutionalized, structural and universal. One that is both innovative and unprecedented. We think we can do this by manipulating the biology of old age, and maybe we can; but just in case those efforts don't succeed, why not apply similar attention, funding, and creativity to our experience of the Fourth Age as well? Even if the Fourth Age is really a black hole as Gilleard and Higgs claim, a place visible only by its impact on other places, we could work to see and make that impact more positive with the expectation that the reflection remains accurate.

My mother says she'd rather be dead than live in very old age with significant dementia or disability. If she even nears that state and anything else happens health-wise, she doesn't want that other thing treated. She doesn't say "even if it kills me"; she says she doesn't want treatment in hopes that it *will* kill her. And she worries that she will arrive at that state and not get sick, that she will linger in a body that resembles her but isn't quite her. It doesn't matter that she might not know the difference. She finds that prospect horrifying, for herself and for us, her family, and she thinks the costs of her care at that point would be better spent on someone with the ability to appreciate it. I think of people who are happily demented but can think of far more who are in a state that might be called "lingering" in a life without any evident benefits. Most express misery; almost all appear to be suffering. But some families don't see it that way, and some religions advocate the sanctity of life in all situations, which makes policymaking tough, even as it makes discussing this phase of life critically important.

My father said he'd never want to live if he had dementia, but then he had dementia and was happy to be alive. "I've had a good life," he'd say, proud and self-satisfied, holding forth from his position as center of attention in his hospital bed and, in his usual good-natured way, forgetting all the bad parts, "but I wouldn't mind more." Yes, he said to various procedures and surgeries. Definitely do that. But when he got to the point that may have been the point he had been referring to when he said he didn't want to live with dementia— the point where he was quite clearly no longer having fun—he also could no longer articulate things like how he felt or discuss huge abstract concepts, like the meaning of life or when a person might have passed a threshold where they lose what matters most. It's likely that my mother is thinking of both my father's last, bad year and also the few before that and their impact on the rest of the family. That caregiving was hard in so many ways, but it was also the important, meaningful work that defines a family. I would do it all again, with love and without hesitation. My mother knows that, and knows I'll do the same for her, and still she fervently hopes it won't come to that.

### PATHOLOGY

In the spring of 2013 I was invited to speak at a conference organized by a physician and a medical humanities scholar. A daylong program was looking at how everything from disruptive technologies to storytelling could transform medicine in the coming decades. At the pre-dinner reception, a tall, lean man with graying hair approached me, introduced himself, and stuck out his hand. His name sounded familiar, but after a day's travel and a few sips of wine, I couldn't place it.

The conversation became awkward. He reminded me who he was— a cultural historian who focused on aging, the head of a terrific local medical humanities program, and the editor of at least one anthology on my office bookshelf. Unfortunately, I hadn't so much read his work as heard about it. At best, I'd read an article or introduction he'd written. In my scant free time, I didn't crave the pedantry of a scholarly social science text but the beautiful sentences of literature.

Our conversation plummeted from awkward to mortifying. It became clear that although I knew his name, I didn't know his work, that he could see I didn't, and was surprised and disappointed. After several minutes of pleasantries, we moved on to mingle with others.

A few weeks later, two books arrived at my office. There were so many reasons why, if I was who I thought myself to be and portrayed myself as, I should have read his work. I sent what I hoped was a suitably gracious and grateful thank-you e-mail. Still feeling guilty, I shelved the books.

What we know about aging depends on whom we look to for information. There are medical, developmental (biopsychological), institutional (socioeconomic), and cultural (stereotypes, perceptions) approaches. The sociologist Carroll Estes has examined the medicalization of American aging that began in the late nineteenth century and continues today. Until then, aging was seen as a natural process and survival to advanced old age as an accomplishment. With medicalization, medicine gained the power to define normal and pathological. Behaviors, body functions, and physical states were reinterpreted, and what had once been considered natural or cultural became amenable to diagnosis, management, and treatment. Popular magazines stopped discussing longevity in favor of articles on senescence and its medical symptoms. Old age began to be formulated as a social problem by people across sectors. The focus moved to its "pathologies": physical and mental limitations, poverty and dependency.

The problem with medicalization is that while it opens up opportunities in some ways, legitimizing aging changes by drawing on the authority of medicine and creating work for people who tackle that "disease," it also limits the types of responses we have to it as individuals and as a society. Not infrequently, we forgo the more helpful for the more medical.

The medicalization of old age defined normal in the image of those who deemed it so, the powerful and usually not-old (or not seeing themselves as "old" regardless of their actual chronological age). Others, meaning well and hoping to steer clear of the inevitable pathologizing of medicalization, assert that old age has different norms. It's normal for older people to have thinner skin than younger people, for example, even if such skin is clearly more prone to tearing, bruising, and breaking down. But although it's common to have trouble seeing in the dark or hearing high-pitched sounds in old age, does that mean they aren't challenges and pathologies? And though most eighty-year-old men will have an enlarged prostate, is that normal? Most people would answer no: everyone wants to see and hear and urinate with ease, and not doing so is not normal; it's pathological.

In his breathtaking cultural history of American old age, *The Journey of Life*, the insightful Thomas Cole calls this our "paradigmatic polarity of normality and pathology."

I know that now, and can quote him, since I finally read the fantastic books he sent me. I'm also asking better questions.

For thousands of years, scientists and philosophers have noted this blurring between normal and pathological in old age. In Terence's play *Phormio* from around 161 B.C., the following exchange: *Demipho—What kept you there so long then? Chremes—A disease. Demipho—How came it? What disease? Chremes—Is that a question? Old age itself is a disease.* If old age is a disease, then a medical approach logically follows.

But if old age and disease cannot be reliably distinguished, is the problem old age, or is it something far more fundamental, such as our classification system and our compulsion to classify ourselves and each other in particular ways? If that's the case, is normal versus abnormal a useful paradigm?

Old age is partly defined by illness, but it is also a normal, natural part of life. If we want to understand and optimize it, we must look not only at medicine but into all other realms of human thought and experience.


## COMMUNICATION


By the time I arrived at the emergency department, George had been there for several hours, and the usual late-afternoon busyness was in full swing. I scanned the monitor, found his name, and saw the telltale five-letter word beside it: ADMIT.

They'd put him in one of the smaller rooms, and his wife, Bessie, had moved out of the way just outside the door to make room for the admitting team. They were stationed around his bed, interviewing him as Bessie and I greeted each other. In the silence that followed, we listened while George explained the circumstances of the fall that had landed him in the hospital.

"He's always loved an audience," whispered Bessie.

Inside the room, a young man wearing the short white coat given to medical students asked, "And that was when you felt faint?"

"Right," George said. "I'd gone over to inspect the workmanship. Woodwork wasn't my job but I've always liked it, and I wasn't half bad at it back in the day either." He looked around for Bessie, and she nodded. He smiled. "I've never done that kind of work myself, you know, pews and altars and like that, but I sure do enjoy seeing it."

"Sorry," said a small woman who was clearly the team leader. "Can you describe exactly what you felt just before you fainted?"

Bessie glanced over at me, her face silently posing a question, but I held off from moving into the room. George looked good—better than I'd expected based on the phone call I'd received from the administrator telling me what had happened. Luckily, I'd been in a meeting the next building over. From the doorway, it seemed that he'd suffered no serious injury and was pleasantly surprised to be the center of so much youthful attention.

"Yes, yes, of course," he said. "So I leaned forward to get a better look, and the next thing I knew, I was on the ground."

Darkness, said George conspiratorially, had come over him all of a sudden. He made eye contact with each team member, waving his arms for emphasis.

"You know he told a completely different story to the first doctors," Bessie said, referring to the emergency doctors. "They understand he's making all this up, don't they?"

I shook my head. The intern and medical students were taking notes, and the resident was listening attentively. This was one of the main reasons I'd rushed to the emergency department. George's dementia was of a type and severity that although he couldn't remember how he'd fallen, he could still invent a darn good story and relay it convincingly.

"Did you have any pain in your chest?" asked the resident.

"Oh, no. Nothing like that."

"What about a feeling like your heart was beating really fast or irregularly?"

George squinted with concentration. "Maybe." He folded his hands in front of him and looked down at them pensively. "Yes, definitely. I almost forgot! It was a funny sort of feeling . . ." He smiled, ready for the next question.

Unable to recall actual events, a person with dementia may construct a new, plausible version of reality. From the thoughtful pauses before he answered questions and his attention to detail, I was fairly sure that George believed his own inventive story.

In the little crowd of doctors, the intern stood closest to the door. I touched his shoulder to get his attention and asked to speak to him for a moment in the hallway.

"Oh," he said when I explained that George was confabulating. Bessie relayed that he had not fainted but tripped. They had gone out for a walk and stopped at the church, as was their habit. Needing the restroom, she had left him seated on a bench in the foyer and returned just a few minutes later to find him on the ground near the side altar, bleeding from his head. A parishioner who had seen the fall told Bessie that she'd watched George trip over one of the raised wooden baseboards connecting the pews. His cane was still propped by the bench in the foyer; this wasn't the first time he'd forgotten that he needed it.

To their credit, the medical team regrouped swiftly and a care plan was made based on the accurate information provided by Bessie rather than on George's misleading and potentially dangerous account of events. This spared George the considerable risks of a hospital stay and evaluation and treatment of problems he didn't have.

If George had received a workup for heart conditions that cause fainting, he would have unnecessarily incurred all the risks of those tests and of treatment for any positive test results, which were more likely given his age but might not require management given his lack of symptoms and limited life expectancy. During a hospital stay, he also would have developed delirium with all its grave risks—he always did. Equally dangerous, the true reasons for his fall would not have been addressed, leaving him at increased risk for more injuries. Knowing the real story helped us get him home that evening, which was what he and Bessie preferred.

People hearing George's story might reasonably assume that his dementia was missed because the doctors caring for him were still in training. Or that the medical team hadn't seen the Alzheimer's diagnosis on the long list of his medical problems. In fact, every few years studies come out demonstrating that fully trained doctors of all types frequently miss dementia or misjudge its stage and severity. Those same clinicians rarely fail to properly diagnose or stage other, similarly common problems in vital organs, such as heart disease or kidney failure. Like dementia, each has many causes and at least one validated severity scale that starts with disease the patient can't yet feel or see and progresses to fatal illness. All these conditions become more prevalent with age, but dementia is the only one handled this way.

A man will say he's got kidney problems, but on the medical record it will say "diabetic nephrosclerosis" and "stage III kidney disease." A woman may tell her friends she's got breast cancer, but her doctors will know its cell type, receptor status, grade, and stage. In dementia, the medical record often lacks that specificity. This is partly because of what information counts in medicine. Most dementia diagnoses are based on constellations of symptoms and behaviors. That approach is considered less useful and definitive than tissue pathology from a biopsy. Yet diagnostic criteria can be quite accurate— in the hands of a trained clinician. They take time, however, and there's no more precious commodity for clinic doctors. Biopsies take time, too, but someone else's time, and the billing is high, so health systems are pleased by the profitability and appearance of efficiency. Never mind that biopsies carry risks of bleeding, infection, and injury, while clinical assessments allow relationship building and insight into key health- and wellness-relevant aspects of a patient's life. Thus patients often are noted to have "dementia," even though in the absence of a more specific diagnosis it's impossible to give them and their families good advice about what to expect and when.

Doctors do many things when it comes to geriatric syndromes like dementia that would be considered sloppy or unacceptable for other chronic conditions. We are taught how to approach toddlers in order to look in their ears, how to use translators when patients don't speak English, and how to make a woman comfortable in advance of a pelvic exam, but most clinicians receive no training in how to communicate optimally with someone with dementia. As a result, history, physical exam, and rapport suffer. Some clinicians resort to infantilizing patients with dementia, ignoring them and speaking to their family member or caregiver instead. Unless the patient is in a more advanced stage of disease, they will know they are being ignored, insulted, and infantilized.

Because so many health professionals don't know the techniques that aid in communication with people with dementia, families assume such techniques don't exist. In a sick twist on Tolstoy's "each unhappy family is unhappy in its own way," millions are left to struggle independently, enduring years of frustration and misunderstandings with their loved ones. Fortunately, many community organizations offer online information and in-person trainings, filling some gaps left by the health care system. But many families, well trained by medical culture, believe if a treatment was useful, it would be used by doctors themselves or come from a doctor in the form of a pill or procedure.

At least George's care team began by talking to him. Their mistake was in not assessing his cognitive ability early on to determine his ability to provide the information they needed. They proceeded as they'd been trained to do, following a time-honored sequence for hospital admission questions, a process that places cognitive evaluation late in the interview and considers it extra, not essential. A one-size-fits-all approach that only works on patients whose lives fit within the approach's underlying assumptions.

## FREEDOM

In her early hundreds, Sadie Delany said of herself and her sister, also a centenarian: "You know, when you are this old, you don't know if you're going to wake up in the morning. But I don't worry about dying, and neither does Bessie. We are at peace." And there was also this: "We've buried so many people we've loved; that is the hard part of living this long. Most everyone we know has turned to dust." Roger Angell concurs: "Here in my tenth decade, I can testify that the downside of great age is the room it provides for rotten news."

But then again—in old age, there is always not only an "on the other hand" but a third hand, and a fourth, and so on—there was this, too, from Angell: "A majority of us people over seventy-five keep surprising ourselves with happiness. Put me on that list." His take echoes that of the physician-writer Oliver Sacks's thoughts on his eightieth birthday in a *New York Times* article titled "The Joy of Old Age. (No Kidding.)." The title captures the essence of the piece, which includes this reflection: "My father, who lived to 94, often said that the 80s had been one of the most enjoyable decades of his life. He felt, as I begin to feel, not a shrinking but an enlargement of mental life and perspective. One has had a long experience of life, not only one's own life, but others', too."

What these writers say about old age echoes what is told to me by my patients—educated and illiterate, rich and poor, immigrants and American born. More than old age itself, it's the insults and exclusion from conversations, buildings, and activities, and the threat or reality of life in an institution that deprives them of autonomy and humanity that transform ordinary hardships into the miseries and suffering we associate with being old.

Consider these casual degradations known as "microaggressions" routine in the lives of old people: *You're still up and around! You're not old! How are you, really?* Or: *She's so cute! What can we do for him today? Hello there, young lady! I know it's awful to ask, but how old are you?* Consider, too, the many nonverbal microaggressions against old people: Discounting. Ignoring. Assuming. Condescending. "Helping" without asking. Pushing by on the street. Stairs without rails. Chairs without arms. No clothing that fits. Technology made for different fingers, eyes, ears, preferences. Laughter. Eye-rolling. Speaking over. Looking through. Baby talk.

If we don't much like the idea of aging, certainly we don't want to be old, or associated with the portion of later life we think of as "old." In youth and adulthood we dread and in old age we lament the lost functions, faculties, and friends, occupational redundancy, social trivialization, societal marginalization, and isolation that eventually accompany old age. We don't want to have to constantly contend with what doesn't work and isn't attractive. And uniformly we don't want to end up dependent, hopeless, helpless, and institutionalized.

Most of us will experience at least a few of those fates in our lifetimes. But to look at old age and see *only* those situations is equivalent to looking at parenthood and seeing only the months of sleepless nights with a screeching, colicky baby or the midnights waiting and worrying about an increasingly distant and reckless teenager. Although the concerns are real, they represent just part of a much larger picture.

Glance at cartoons or quotes about the human life span, and you're likely to come away with two mistaken impressions: first, that half our years are spent in the transit from infancy to early adulthood, and second, that life is great fun until sometime in early midlife, when it becomes unpleasant, serious, and confusing, and then heads unremittingly downhill. Such portraits are fairly accurate appraisals of middle age, but completely wrong about old age in America. To most people's surprise, a large study of the United States found that midlife is the time of least happiness, greatest anxiety, and lowest life satisfaction for both men and women. Things begin looking up around age sixty—and not because the "younger old" are skewing the curve. The Gallup World Poll, which studies countries large and small, poor and rich, agrarian and industrialized, finds that life satisfaction assumes a U-shape across life in wealthier countries but different patterns elsewhere. Data from the United States and Western Europe confirm that most people are around sixty before they achieve levels of well-being comparable to those of twenty-year-olds, and rates climb thereafter.

The increased well-being of old people seems made up of both declines in negatives and increases in positives. In one recent study, anxiety marched steadily upward from the teenage years to its greatest heights between ages thirty-five and fifty-nine. In the early sixties, it dropped markedly, falling again at sixty-five, then staying at the life span's lowest levels thereafter. Conversely, sixty- to sixty-four-year-olds were happier and more satisfied with their lives than people aged twenty to fifty-nine, but not nearly as happy as those aged sixty-five and over. Even those over age ninety were happier than the middle-aged. As the poet Mary Ruefle has said, "You should never fear aging because you have absolutely no idea the absolute freedom in aging; it's astounding and mind-blowing. You no longer care what people think. As soon as you become invisible—which happens much more quickly to women than men—there is a freedom that's astounding. And all your authority figures drift away. Your parents die. And yes, of course, it's heartbreaking, but it's also wonderfully freeing." In sum, depending on the measure, by their later sixties or early seventies, older adults surpass younger adults on all measures, showing less stress, depression, worry, and anger, and more enjoyment, happiness, and satisfaction. In these and similar studies, people between sixty-five and seventy-nine years old report the highest average levels of personal well-being, followed by those over eighty, and then those who are eighteen to twenty-one years old.

Such findings are equally remarkable for their near universality and how they confound common lore. Ironically, it's the in-betweens, those generally thought to have the most power and influence in society, who are actually the unhappiest and least satisfied among us. It may not be coincidence, then, that this is the group most responsible for the nearly ubiquitous false messages about old age.

People's experience of old age varies widely, and always has. For most, it's not the facts of being old that bring suffering—often, quite the contrary—so much as the threat or reality of socially contrived accompaniments such as lack of purpose, poverty, exclusion, and isolation. That the answer to how to create a better old age lies in the gap between hard data and dearly held beliefs isn't new. Plato's *Republic* opens with the elderly Cephalus telling Socrates that some of his contemporaries

> harp on the miseries old age brings. But in my opinion . . . they are putting the blame in the wrong place. For if old age were to blame, my experience would be the same as theirs, and so would that of all other old men. But in fact I have met many whose feelings are quite different.

This is good news for old age. While human legs and skin, hearts and brains, change with age, they are pretty much the same now as they were in classical Greece. It's our beliefs, feelings, actions, and policies that can and do change, and that we can shape to support and celebrate old age in all its varieties.

### BACKSTORY

To cut into another human being's body and remove or rearrange parts takes a confidence that I do not possess. To take charge in a crisis and issue orders to other highly trained people secure in one's near-instantaneous assessment of a complex situation requires hubris, speed, and the psychological, emotional, and cognitive ability to trust that one understands the situation well enough and that well enough is good enough. I don't have those things either, or, more accurately, not enough of them to want to make crisis management my career.

In kindergarten, I was playing four square with friends when our ball rolled into the middle of our public grade school's huge asphalt playground, packed full of other kids. The smallest in my friend group, I usually held back until someone else went to fetch it, but this time they all looked at me. I walk-ran into the swirling fray of older children, and then, perhaps with the ball in hand and perhaps not (I don't recall), I crouched down and pulled my coat over my head to protect myself from the blows of passing legs and bodies. The bigger kids weren't trying to attack me—they just didn't think about me—and as their team game moved across the playground, I felt vulnerable and unable to escape their threat. Luckily an older girl rescued me.

As a girl, climbing trees also scared me, but I thrilled in it too. The problem was that I couldn't get down. "Jump!" my friends would call, or "Slide!"—strategies they used to move down quickly. I couldn't or wouldn't. Both seemed too fast, too dangerous, too risky, and too terrifying. ER docs, I have heard, are the ones most likely to parachute from planes. That holds no appeal for me, no thrill, only terror and a question: Why?

In high school, taking the PSATs, I was about halfway through when they called time. In those days (and still now), when people said a book was a quick read, I changed their hours into my days, then multiplied by two, three, or more, depending on the length and difficulty of the material. I read slowly. When I say this, sometimes people respond, "I do, too, but this one's a quick read." Not for me.

In college, I tried out for the new women's rugby team, but found I could not run full force into another woman for sport. I'd like to think I could do it if the other person was trying to kill herself or others, but I've never been in a situation that allowed me to find out. It's not that I never feel the urge for violence. As a child, such urges were almost always directed at my younger sister; as an adult, they take the form of diatribes and fantasies of retribution against people who have harmed my family, patients, friends, or vulnerable strangers, and on occasion people I feel have slighted me. But although I sometimes hit my sister when we were little, I've never actually been violent with another person as an adult, except if you acknowledge that certain actions and activities of doctors qualify as violence.

Some things scare me. Doing even a minor task badly disturbs me to a point that I'm told is extreme. Also, while I sometimes make mental connections quickly, I struggle with coordination and can be slow with decisions. If a person is trying to die and the doctor needs to be thinking through protocols plus the particulars of the situation and moving the various parts of the patient's body to positions and for procedures all at the same time, I'm not the best doctor for that job. I've done it—any trained doctor has. But it doesn't draw on my strengths or passions. I prefer having enough time to do a good job sorting through complexity. Also, where some feel a rush of affirming adrenaline that carries them for hours, I cannot separate my actions, however well executed, from the ethics of what was done, how it might have been done better, and its consequences in the lives of patients and families.

On the other hand, some things that scare other people don't bother me a bit. For years, I packed a backpack and set off for places most Americans didn't go, certainly not by themselves or with an equally young female friend. I went to the Thai-Cambodian border, to remote areas of Indonesia, Senegal, Mali, Guatemala, and Nicaragua. I took trains and buses across China to the Pakistani border, standing up to officials who told me there was no train and sleeping in spit-stained hallways when necessary. I hitchhiked through Scotland and hid my companion and myself from a group of drunk men who'd followed us from a bar to a local farmer's field where no one would have heard our screams. On an island off the coast of Belize, I asked a young man about his family and future plans and told him about mine so he saw me and my friend as human beings and did not rob us as he did all the others on our boat that day.

Similarly, for years, I did housecalls, working on my patients' turf without missing the power and control a doctor has in a hospital or clinic. I don't need that, which may be why I haven't owned a white coat since residency. In their homes, even during a doctor's visit, people are human beings first and patients second. I love that. I went into neighborhoods and residences I would not have come to know had I not been a doctor. "If we see a gun," I would tell residents rotating with me, "we keep driving." Often, I learned more of clinical relevance from seeing how people lived than from hospital discharge notes or my physical exam. I'd rather creatively negotiate those complex realities over weeks or months or years in relationship with another human being than use a new surgical tool or adjust the dials of a machine. Like most people in a position to do so, I have chosen work that makes the most of my interest, values, and strengths.

Chances are this is not every geriatrician's truth. But it's a big part of mine, for worse sometimes, I know, but also I'd like to think, more often than not, for better.

Five months after my snap and burnout, I returned to work—sort of. I didn't go back to my main leadership roles or to my housecalls clinic, though I got updates on my former patients from colleagues. I missed my patients, felt guilty about my hasty departure from their lives, and also was not yet ready to again take on responsibility for any part of other people's lives. I was still sorting out my own life and medications and trying to figure out whether I could still be a doctor and remain healthy, mentally and physically.

For the rest of that academic year, instead of returning to the places and patterns that had led to my ill health and burnout, I worked part-time on grants and projects. In what had once been my clinical and administrative time, I did various teaching jobs and started this book. As months passed, I felt better and better except when I thought about the roles and systems that had contributed to my burnout. Clinical practice in the second decade of the twenty-first century seemed to demand too many of the things I didn't enjoy or believe in and too few of the ones I did. I suspected that I would need to do what so many other doctors have done lately: stop practicing forever and find a completely different sort of work inside or outside medicine.

At all ages and stages, life changes. A year and a half after the snap, in the spring of 2017, I was feeling much better—really good, in fact—when a colleague told me about a job on a new hospital unit for old people. It seemed the perfect solution to my practical and moral quandaries about outpatient medicine—I could again care for patients, but those patients would be in hospitals, one of our health system's preferred settings. It wasn't an ideal solution, but it was an option that might make it possible for me to see patients without compromising their care or my values. They told me the job would open in the fall. The idea of stretching my clinical muscles again made me nervous but also, especially, excited.

## LONGEVITY

We live decades longer than we did throughout most of human existence—and, in recent decades, mostly better, with less poverty than previous generations of older adults, and fewer years of disability for people without obesity or significant chronic disease. In 1750, only one in five Americans lived to age seventy; now more than four out of five do. This longer life expectancy, combined with dramatic declines in birth rates, has made old people a steadily increasing percentage of the population. In 1800 they accounted for 2 percent of the U.S. population; in 1970 they were 10 percent; in 2017 the number had climbed to 15 percent. As often happens with minority and feared populations, as the numbers of older people grew, so, too, has society's animosity toward them. Although almost one in six of us is old, aging remains the subject of jokes, fears, discrimination, and denial.

Part of this is the natural response to change, as well as mixed messages and legitimate concerns. We hear often of "senior moments" when a person can't access the word or information they want. We only rarely hear of the equally if not more numerous moments when older people call on well-documented insight and emotional intelligence to make smart decisions. Conversely, we don't blame age when a younger person can't bring up the word that would complete their thought or sentence. Meanwhile, the Stanford economist John Shoven has made the case that "the current practice of measuring age as years-since-birth, both in common practice and in the law, rather than alternative measures reflecting a person's stage in the life cycle distorts important behavior such as retirement, saving, and the discussion of dependency ratios." He argues that if we define old age by the percentage of an age group that dies annually, old age may be getting older. Yet there is no evidence that the once anticipated "compression of morbidity," a decrease in the number of years a person spends with disease and disability, has come to pass despite our much-ballyhooed health and medicine progress.

Shoven suggests we become *old* when we have a 2 percent or higher chance of death in the next year, and we become *very old* or *elderly* when that figure reaches 4 percent or higher. Using that criteria, in 1920 men and women became old in their mid- to later fifties, respectively. Now it's age sixty-five for men and seventy-three for women—on average, with, as usual, whites doing best, blacks doing worst, and brown people in between. The implications of Shoven's work are considerable. Is it reasonable to work for forty years and retire for thirty or forty? Almost certainly not, especially if we're not "old" and all the more so because purpose, social engagement, and money are key contributors to well-being. Working longer, even (perhaps especially) if we work different jobs or fewer hours in our older years than in our younger ones, is likely to increase our life satisfaction while decreasing our rates of chronic disease and disability. This is just one of the societal and public health interventions that, unlike disease treatments offered by medicine, might move us toward true compression of morbidity—in other words, toward lives that are both longer and healthier.

We speak of the "silver tsunami" as if the unprecedented and permanent increase in both the numbers and proportion of older adults came about suddenly, without warning, and portends destruction and devastation on our society. But people in developed countries have panicked about their aging populations for a century. Americans worried in the 1930s and '40s and again in the 1960s and '70s, spawning ageist ads, books, movies, and lamentations (much like the ones of today) about how the aging population would ruin our country and the world. Fifty years ago, alongside movements to eliminate discrimination against women and African Americans, scholars and citizens' groups like the Gray Panthers worked to enlighten the public about aging myths and to offer more positive images of old age. They advocated for the rights and needs of old people, just as so many groups today do, meeting similar support and resistance. At times that pushback was warranted, as when the activists seemed to assert that old people differed from the young only in age—an obvious falsehood. Those were the years, too, in which the notion of the Third Age originated, in part to signal the potential of the longer human life span but primarily to distinguish the functional old from their debilitated peers and elders. All these groups differed in specifics and strategies but not in basic arguments and intentions from similar arguments throughout human history.

All societies have included old people, even ones in their eighties, nineties, and hundreds. At times, older adults have represented a significant portion of the population in some countries, not the 15–20 percent or more we see today, but around one in ten. Even past societies with far less technology, money, and other resources than we have now often supported large numbers of older people. What is new are the numbers and proportion of older people in the population. In the late twentieth century, living into old age became the norm in developed countries. In the United States in 1900, the average life expectancy was forty-six years; by 2016 the average had reached age seventy-nine. If you make it to eighty, you have a good chance of making it to ninety or beyond. Still, although more and more people are living into their second century, it's rare for humans to live past twelve decades. Anthropological evidence suggests our species' life span hasn't changed over at least the last ten thousand years.

Still, once upon a time, most people were young. If you created a graphic representation of the population, you saw a pyramid: lots of young people on the broad bottom of a triangular structure below progressively narrower bars for each subsequent period of life, indicating declining numbers of people alive at older ages. Lately, the pyramid has taken on a more rectangular shape, with increasingly similar numbers of citizens in most age groups.

The biggest increases in longevity in human history occurred over the twentieth century. Most people believe this was because of medical progress, but, more accurately, most of the credit goes to increased global wealth and public health: sanitation, better nutrition, and immunizations. You can still see the impact of those factors on world maps of longevity. In places that have those things, people live far longer than in the places without them, a reality that existed before most of the great advances of modern medicine. You can see it, too, among the subpopulations of the United States. While many of our poorest citizens have access via Medicaid to modern treatments not available in Afghanistan or sub-Saharan Africa, they still get sicker earlier and die younger for reasons of environment, social stress, and lack of access to healthy foods, hope, and opportunity.

The longest-lived humans today live in Okinawa in Japan, Sardinia in Italy, or Loma Linda in California, so-called blue zones. Okinawans eat healthy, low-calorie diets and maintain low normal body weights, with average BMIs around twenty. Isolated, inbred Sardinians seem to have a genetic advantage, since men are as likely as women to become centenarians, and people who move away in young adulthood still live exceptionally long lives. In Loma Linda not everyone achieves unusual longevity, just the large numbers of Seventh-day Adventists who outlive their neighbors by five to ten years. They abstain from alcohol, cigarettes, and other drugs, have strong spiritual lives, a close community, a vegetarian diet—and lower levels of stress hormones. Similar to worshippers of most faiths, they live longer than people who aren't religious.

In the United States there is much talk of a "baby boomer blip," as if that generation were moving through an enduring population pyramid like a mouse through a snake, creating an aberrant bulge as it passes. But older people will make up a larger percentage of all populations for the foreseeable future. A more accurate image of population trends shows the admittedly abundant boomers as the lead edge of an enduring shift in who and how old we are as a species.

The old people of today must inform our future planning, but they cannot be our sole guides. Right now, most old people are white. They also have less education than boomers. Both of those things are changing: since 1985, the share of older Americans with college degrees has tripled, to about a third of sixty- to seventy-four-year-olds. Medically, "the old" are changing too. The current oldest generation, members of the "greatest generation," tend to minimize pain. Sometimes, to get them to admit to it, clinicians have to use euphemisms like *discomfort* or *ache*, and even then many are reluctant to take strong medications. Contrast this with the baby boomers, most of whom don't hesitate to say what they're feeling and what they need. And drugs don't scare them: they were young in the 1960s. Because I have mostly cared for the oldest and frailest patients, I haven't had to ask about use of cocaine, heroin, acid, or mushrooms in years. I expect that to change in the near future.

In response to this unprecedented demographic transformation, the organization and priorities of every sector of life have shifted. But fundamental change, and particularly change that upends established beliefs and societal institutions, is slow, even when the need for it is obvious.

Unlike life expectancy, which changes from year to year, the human life span (maximum longevity) seems fixed throughout history. Despite the claims made for the exceptional longevity of Russian Georgians or Bolivian mountaineers, there is no reliable record of any human surviving past the age of 122. Age-related mortality increases from maturity then plateaus in advanced old age. And still people die—all of them.

There are scientists and think tanks working on that challenge, but the jury is still out on whether they will succeed and also whether extending human lives further would constitute progress. On this one, for the time being, I'm inclined to agree with a comment the comedian Sarah Silverman made to Jeff Bezos the day his company introduced technology that would eliminate all cashier jobs across the United States. The combined income for American cashiers that day was about $210 million, or less than 1 percent of the $2.8 billion Bezos made that day. In the announcement about the new technology, there was no mention of what would happen in the lives of the already poor and now potentially unemployed citizens affected by its introduction. Silverman tweeted: "Your scientists were so preoccupied with whether or not they could, they didn't stop to think if they should."

The same thing happens in science and medicine every day. Lifesaving advances sound like a good thing, something definitely worth funding. Often, they are—at first. What is not funded are the downstream consequences, the consequences geriatricians try to help people live with every day.

## CHILDPROOF

Partway through *Five Flights Up*, a movie about an aging couple who decide it's time to sell their Brooklyn walk-up, Morgan Freeman's character tries to open a pill bottle. He pushes, pulls, twists, and shakes, but the white cap remains resolutely in place.

Just as it seems he will find no pharmacological relief from the stress of strangers touring his treasured apartment, a child finds him struggling. She is nine or ten years old, with pigtails and the eyeglasses Hollywood puts on kid characters to indicate preternatural intelligence.

Quickly appraising the situation, she takes the bottle from him and opens it with ease.

"Childproof," she quips, handing it back. He shakes his head.

The humorous scene touches on one part of a larger, decidedly unfunny problem with how we do and don't regulate medication safety in the United States. As is often the case, well-intentioned efforts to protect one group end up hurting other groups when regulations take a widespread approach to a situation problematic for only a minority. Without question, that minority—in this case, children—deserves protection, but, as is often the case, the intervention's impact was studied almost exclusively in the minority target population (kids) and not the rest of us, the adult majority.

Anyone who has been around toddlers knows of their tendency to touch everything, insert their bodies everywhere they might fit, and put anything they come across into their mouths. That's why we childproof homes, putting plugs into electric outlets and gates across stairs, and making slats between railings too narrow for even the smallest human heads. In the 1960s pediatricians documented alarming numbers of child deaths from medications. Not just toddlers but older kids as well would come across colorful pills and capsules when exploring their homes. Either assuming they were candy or just curious, they ate them. In 1970 the Poison Prevention Packaging Act was signed into law to protect kids from unintentional drug overdoses, and pharmaceutical companies began using "child-resistant" bottles—no one ever actually claimed such containers were entirely childproof. As a result, poisoning deaths of children under five years old were nearly cut in half.

For almost fifty years now, child-resistant containers have been standard. Unfortunately, such containers offer little deterrent to older children, and even children as young as two and three can open many of them. Early benefits have been lost. A key reason for this is the protective medication packaging. Because child-resistance makes it hard or impossible for the people who need medications most—the sick, disabled, and elderly—to open their pill bottles, they leave them open, accessible to all.

The Consumer Product Safety Commission has addressed these problems in multiple ways. In 1995 revised requirements mandated testing not only on children between forty-two and fifty-one months but on "seniors" ages fifty to seventy. While this was an improvement, they added middle-aged and young-old testers and still left out most old people.

It's true that the people most likely to be stymied by childproofing are harder to study than their healthier, younger counterparts, but that's at least partly because the same challenges that render bottles inaccessible make the personal costs of research participation higher for them. Getting into child-resistant bottles often requires a combination of grasping, pushing, squeezing, and twisting. Such efforts may be fun for a small child but can be painful, difficult, or impossible for a person with impaired or feeble hands. If that person also has arthritic joints, weakness, or mobility challenges, as many old people do, getting to and from a testing site might require more of their energy or considerable discomfort.

More inclusive testing groups weren't the only consumer protection intervention. Manufacturers were again allowed to make easy-opening versions of products with labels specifying "for households without young children," and pharmacies could dispense medications without child-resistance packaging if requested by the prescriber or patient. Over twenty years later, many people, clinicians and patients alike, don't seem to know about these work-arounds, and the default remains adult-proof child-resistant packaging. Clearly, these efforts have been insufficient, or a recent movie featuring a septuagenarian actor wouldn't include a gag about a pill bottle he can't open.

To get a sense of the number of people affected, consider the prevalence of just one common health condition. According to the Centers for Disease Control, in 2012, 52.5 million adults—23 percent of the U.S. population—had been told by a doctor they had some kind of arthritis. Fully half of adults over age sixty-five were given that diagnosis. While not all arthritis affects the hands, a multitude of other conditions also affect general strength and manual dexterity. And for some Americans, wrestling with pill bottles isn't just an inconvenience; it can be life-threatening.

When I made a posthospitalization home visit to Nina, a widow who lived alone and had just had a heart attack, I found all her discharge medications unopened. Those medications are so important that hospitals are evaluated on the percentages of heart attack patients who receive them. But they were dispensed in child-resistant and thoroughly Nina-proof bottles.

When I met Edward and Carmen, they explained that they had their son empty their child-resistant bottles of medications into bowls each month when he visited from out of town so they didn't have to contend with the annoying containers. Their system worked fine until Edward developed dementia and took the wrong pills.

This is not just an issue for older people. An Internet search on the topic yields dozens of sites with instructions on how to change childproof bottles into "easy open" ones. Regrettably, my patients are not the target demographic for such websites.

Public health measures are necessary to save lives. But the facts of widespread circumvention of child-resistant bottles and the country's growing numbers of multigenerational homes indicate a dire need for better public safety strategies—ones that consider the safety and well-being of patients of all ages. The key question is whether we can decrease medication poisonings in children without preventing adults from accessing the drugs they need.

New approaches should look beyond containers to the entire pill-to-person trajectory and take advantage of how our lives and world have changed since the 1970s. Potential solutions include targeted rather than universal use of safety lids and dispensing systems using the same fingerprint, face, and voice recognition software already being used on smartphones. Equally important going forward, we must learn from the flawed assumptions that made the "child-resistant" packaging policy less effective—and more harmful—than it might otherwise have been. The original legislation stated that packaging should be "not difficult for *normal* adults" (italics added), discounting those adults most likely to take pills.

Forty-five years after the Poison Prevention Packaging Act, new packaging is still not tested on the oldest Americans, the age group with the highest per capita pill consumption. Maybe more shocking still: we have no idea how many adults of any age have been harmed by medication safety caps; we don't count those events the way we count poisoning events in children.

### RECLAMATION

Many Americans near or past fifty remember their first solicitation from the organization once known as the American Association for Retired Persons. It's not quite up there with one's first sexual encounter, first paycheck, or first child, but it has the feel of a momentous life initiation.

My AARP solicitation arrived in a stack of largely useless mail: unwanted catalogs, a journal renewal notice, a bill. The logo's wavy red, white, and blue lines caught my attention. Then I saw the name.

I wrote "OMG" on the white envelope and left it propped on the front hall chest for my spouse to see. We were forty-eight years old that year, so, really, we only met *old* by Silicon Valley or Hollywood standards. Also, AARP is actively trying to be the voice of the Third Agers and those, like us, in middle age headed toward Third.

Another truth cannot be denied: it was one of those moments when the world reminded me that I, too, would become old. Not only was I was shocked; my first reaction was one of distancing and denial.

Simone de Beauvoir captured this stance in *The Coming of Age*: "When we look at the image of our own future provided by the old we do not believe it: an absurd inner voice whispers that that will never happen to us—when that happens it will no longer be ourselves that it happens to." This divorce of the current self from the future self distances us from the biological and social diminishment of old age. Such actions are essentially human. Almost everyone can relate to them. We cleave toward those like us and toward those who make us feel like our best and most powerful selves.

The people who push back most ferociously against the label "old" are people in their sixties, seventies, and eighties who don't (yet) conform to stereotyped associations with that word. They make comments along the lines of: "I am still active and looking forward to the future so find having the word *old* attached to me disconcerting." Their argument is that they are not ill or disabled, despondent or dependent, and therefore not "old," their chronological age notwithstanding. Since the definition of "old" is having lived a certain number of years, usually sixty or seventy, it seems we have created a society in which carrying that label is so awful that octogenarians leaning on walkers adamantly assert they are not old. Clearly, the human life cycle isn't the problem. Societal prejudice is so strong, and the category old so stripped of respect and social worth, that old people feel compelled to argue against the obvious.

They also inflict violence on their future selves. A typical anecdote from continuing care communities goes like this: A couple moves in. Healthy and active, they easily make friends and join in social activities. Then something happens to one of them: a stroke, dementia, cancer, heart failure, and suddenly one of the two is "old." Now they have a problem at mealtimes, because they can't eat together at their usual table. Their limitation is not the result of the ill spouse's medical condition but of policies passed by the community that say only healthy people can eat in the independent-living dining hall. Thus the healthier half of the couple may eat in the dependent residents' dining room but not vice versa. Or each must eat without their partner. In this way the hale, who are more likely to hold governance positions in such communities, protect their current selves from reminders of their potential future. They also maximize the chance that they, too, will be ostracized and treated without compassion when they reach the later substages of old age.

Imagine a forty- or fifty-year-old saying, "I don't like to think of myself as an adult. I'm just a kid who's been around a few extra years." Or a children's hospital that eschews the term *child* because of its association with immaturity and instead markets itself as serving short, unemployed people. It's ludicrous.

Too often, the world gives considerable credit for what young people might do in the future and little or none for what old people can do or have already done. Too often, it assumes old people can do nothing and are good for nothing. This lose-lose equation is applied to anyone who lives past middle age, compromising both their individual life and our collective social potential. It also conflates vastly different substages of old age, devaluing the envied years while creating a hostile world for anyone who survives to advanced age.

With current generations transforming what it means to be in one's sixties, seventies, eighties, nineties, and hundreds, it's time for elderhood to take its rightful place alongside childhood and adulthood. Each of life's three acts is made up of many scenes. If we can accommodate infancy and adolescence under the umbrella of childhood, we also should be able to accommodate the young-old and old-old, and all those in between, under the umbrella of elderhood. Routinely using this long, varied stage of life's name is a small but essential step toward recognizing and optimizing the full trajectory of our lives.

A revised version of the life cycle, including its expected phases of dependence and independence, might look something like this:

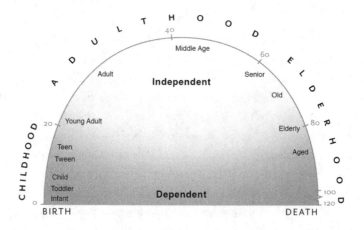

Given the variety and opportunities of twenty-first-century elderhood, anyone already in Act III and all of the rest of us who hope to avoid a premature death would do well to begin following the examples of the civil rights, women's, and LGBT movements. Each reclaimed, created, or repurposed simple words to redefine themselves and their place in society: *black* was reclaimed as beautiful; *chairman* became *chair* and *stewardess* became *flight attendant*; *queer* is so popular that young people keep expanding its reach and inclusivity. Despite the backlash against those changes in some social sectors, those reclaimed words give me hope. I'll be old in another ten years, more or less, and I'd like an elderhood as long and varied and hard and happy and legitimate and acknowledged as my first two acts.

# ELDERHOOD

*For age is opportunity no less / Than youth itself, though in another dress*
—Henry Wadsworth Longfellow

# 11. OLD

The year my mother turned eighty-one, not long after I dropped her off at the airport she got into a kerfuffle with a Homeland Security officer. Having put her bag and jacket in bins and on the moving platform, she was waiting her turn in the line for the body scanner when the official pulled her from the line.

"Ma'am," he reprimanded, "you need to take off your shoes."

"No, I don't," replied my mother with a smile.

He insisted. Shoe removal was required for security purposes. No exceptions.

"But I'm old," my mother argued.

"Ma'am," he said, "you have to be seventy-five or older to keep on your shoes."

She matter-of-factly informed him of her age.

He stared, muttered, "That's incredible," and waved her toward the body scanner, shoes still firmly on her feet.

This Homeland Security officer assumed old age signaled infirmity without exception, and perhaps his views were consistent with what he had seen until that day. He didn't check my mother's ID, presumably because, like many, he saw old age as so undesirable that a person would never claim to be older than she actually was. Unlike a young-looking twenty-five- or thirty-year-old who must produce an ID with a birth date to buy alcohol, older people are rarely carded. So sixty-year-olds get into movies by saying they are really sixty-two, betting that no one will ask for proof. After all, who in their right mind would pretend to be old?

\* \* \*

Health, appearance, and function are more varied in our later years than at any other period of life. Age alone isn't the issue; it's as much about appearance, behavior, experience, and expectations.

The "successful aging" movement celebrates true stories about incredible resilience and accomplishments in old age. Its message is accurate, helpful, and sometimes nefariously counterproductive.

In fairness, the notion of successful aging started out as one thing and became another.

In 1997, in their landmark MacArthur Foundation study of successful aging, the physician-researchers John W. Rowe and Robert L. Kahn found three key ingredients for a high quality of life in old age. People who felt and functioned the best maintained (via healthy behaviors) a low risk for disease, a high level of engagement with the community, and high physical and cognitive function for longer than the average person.

If the only way to describe older adults who are active, engaged, accomplished, or attractive is either to say they don't look or act their age or to add words like *successful* or *exceptional* to the word *aging*, then we are implying that being old, by definition, means a person is none of those things—an obvious falsehood.

The notion of successful aging is ancient. In Western cultures, it might be said to have its origins in the Fall in Eden, a perspective that sees a difficult old age as one consequence of humankind's moral failure, being cast from the Garden of God. Christianity held that God created man as perfect and possibly immortal, but illness and death were introduced after the Fall. This view implies that life span is preordained by God—not amenable to human tampering. It promises the possibility of longer health and life by spiritual redemption through Christ.

In *Rhetoric*, Aristotle used the word *eugeria* to mean a good old age—*eu* means in a good manner, and *geria* refers to the treatment of old age. A good old age might include what Rowe and Kahn defined as successful and also advanced years where none of their three factors are maintained, yet the person is comfortable and cared for.

\*   \*   \*

By any measure, Britain's Queen Elizabeth is an "exceptional senior." Around the time of her ninetieth birthday, the palace announced that she had had 341 engagements in the previous year, a record for a British monarch of any age. But while that accomplishment may make her exceptional among English royalty, it isn't what puts her in the exceptional senior category, the label commonly used to describe a healthy, active, and engaged old person.

My octogenarian mother is also an exceptional senior. She exercises six or seven days a week, volunteers as a docent at a science museum, takes several classes in every enrollment period at a university lifelong learning program, and has a social schedule of meals, movies, theater, and group walks that makes me feel like a recluse. She became "exceptional" in equal parts by inclination, effort, and good luck.

Decades before the constituents of an optimal diet became the subject of books, videos, scientific papers, and government public service campaigns, my mother ate huge quantities of vegetables, fruits, lean proteins, and nuts. She liked them and was sure they were good for her. But she wasn't equally prescient in other areas. She only took up exercise at age sixty when, in the span of just a few months, she found herself struggling to open jars and unable to make it back up the Grand Canyon without help on a family hike. Still, many people would have shrugged and said, *What do you expect? I'm not getting any younger.* My mother took up walking and joined a gym where she could do strength and balance training.

Even more impressive than these accomplishments, however, has been her attitude as she becomes less "successful." Planning a dinner party for a younger friend's eightieth birthday and acknowledging that she was slower than she used to be and tired more easily, she spread her preparation over a week, doing one key task each day. The next year, recognizing that at some point she would need to stop driving, she often took buses, walked, and got rides to her activities. She told me her friends said that the worst thing about giving up their cars was the sudden loss of the easiest way of getting places. She was practicing so she'd be ready when the time came, as it inevitably did.

The degree to which this approach is smart and sensible is remarkable. I'm less psychologically resilient than my mother, so I probably won't do as well as she's doing, though I'd like to try.

If only that were enough.

These anecdotes make my mother's successful aging sound exclusively like a matter of willpower and wise decisions. In reality, although those elements are fundamental and she excels in both, the lion's share of her success comes from several other attributes she shares with Queen Elizabeth. Both are lucky in three critical ways.

First, they were born into privilege: white, citizens of developed countries, wealthy (far more so in the queen's case than my mother's, but, from a global perspective, both qualify), and educated. Second, women live longer than men almost everywhere, and since each has at least one relative who lived into their nineties or hundreds, they may be genetically advantaged for longevity. Finally, both have had the good fortune of not having been assaulted, abused, felled by an advanced cancer, or in a debilitating car accident, to name just a few of the random insults that can derail a life.

These advantages are not a matter of character. Indeed, willpower and capacity for wise decisions are often by-products of fortunate lives.

Different people use the term *successful aging* to mean different things. For health professionals and researchers, it's the absence of disease, maintenance of physical and cognitive function, and a full engagement with life. For psychologists and social scientists, it has more to do with life satisfaction, social functioning, and psychological resilience. Finally, when older adults themselves invoke this concept, they generally mean independence, spirituality, comfort, coping, meaningful relationships, and contributions to society. The first definition focuses on the body, the second on the psyche, and the third on the experience of life. An optimal life at any age would include all these attributes.

Although some of how we age is determined by personal choices, much of the aging process is the result of genetics, social situation, and the public policies that shape our day-to-day world.

Technically, of course, anyone who is old has succeeded at aging. And anyone, from any background, can become an "exceptional senior." But if we step back far enough to look at ourselves as a population, it's clear that while healthy habits, effort, and attitude matter, many older adults who earn the "exceptional" and "successful" labels look very much like the people who earn those labels at other ages: born into privilege, bred in safe neighborhoods with access to healthy foods, able to lead lives absent many of the stressors known to accelerate aging.

I understand the appeal of successful aging and the vibrant, exceptional senior concept. We all want that scenario for ourselves and those we love. But we need to beware the deceptive implications for those who acquire the label and the harmful blaming of those who don't. Our society equates disability with lives not worth living and aging with bad news. Yet their presence doesn't necessarily deprive people of happiness.

A few years ago, a video of a 103-year-old playing the piano went viral. Some of this was the usual exceptional elder fascination: She's ancient! She's still playing! She's really good! But of equal note was Alice Herz-Sommer's life story: a fortunate childhood, studying piano with Franz Liszt, marriage, a son. Then came Adolf Hitler. Her husband and most of both their families were killed. Her son survived but died suddenly at age sixty-five. She remained alive, living in a one-room flat in a country to which he had moved her when she was already quite old. Look closely at her expressions. Watch her play. She looks happy, relaxed.

We can't all accommodate loss and hardship as well as Alice, nor do we fully understand why some among us remain optimistic despite tragedy, while others, even people with lives that might be described as fortunate, suffer and feel defeated in the face of far lesser life stresses. The Puritans believed the right attitude would lead to happiness, health, and prosperity. Failure to achieve those in life indicated sin and distance from God. Many people today similarly believe success and happiness are solely the product of effort and character, the "born on third base, but thinks he hit a triple" mentality. We provide universal early childhood education and school lunches because it's clear the foundations are laid *before* we control any aspect of our lives; hunger impairs learning. Attitude helps— centenarians are more likely than the rest of us to handle stress well and have a good sense of humor; conversely, people with fatalistic views of old age are more likely to develop disease—but attitude is just one piece of a complex reality.

FUTURE

In 2016 Facebook's CEO Mark Zuckerberg and his physician wife, Priscilla Chan, announced a three-billion-dollar investment "to cure, prevent or manage all disease in our children's lifetime," and some months later the first of their Biohub grants was announced. This was great news for science and medicine, but not necessarily for American health and health care.

In his remarks at the Biohub's launch, Zuckerberg stated that we, too, often tackle diseases once people are sick and don't do nearly enough to prevent them from getting sick in the first place. That's right, but their project goal—disease eradication over the next century—isn't the fastest way to make prevention a bigger part of health care. It may not even be the best way.

Well-studied, proven-effective, and cost-effective strategies already exist and could be preventing illnesses and injuries right now if only we sincerely supported and actively disseminated them. In the face of this considerable evidence, the Biohub venture claims that scientific progress is the single best key to helping more people live healthy lives. Advancing science advances health—sometimes. It can also lead to the replacement of one set of problems with another, as happened when recent advances generated our current epidemic of chronic diseases. Anyone who has ever received or provided health care can tell you science is just one part of human health's more complex equation.

The list of strategies known to prevent disease or improve its management is long. It contains such disparate measures as exercise, education, access to primary care, antismoking campaigns, availability of food, not building factories and toxic chemical waste sites near poor communities, intolerance for racism, taxation of sugared drinks, home health care, reduction of added salt, and particular communication styles, among many, many more. Although I applaud the Chan-Zuckerbergs' generosity and ambition, I question their decision to categorically accept that science is the best means to their laudable end. Curing disease is an important and inspiring goal, but we could make huge strides toward better health and health care for people on this planet right now by focusing less on the pursuit of what isn't known and significantly more on making better use of what is. That's the approach the Gates Foundation has taken, with remarkable results.

Some will argue that I have missed the point; advancing science and technology is the mission of the Biohub, and others can work on the issues I raise. True, except the larger Chan Zuckerberg Initiative mission is "advancing human potential and promoting equality." Ignoring all the many proven approaches to prevention and valuing future generations over current ones does little to promote equality.

A second overlooked failing of this venture is its assumption that disease eradication is an unequivocal positive. If we focus on diseases affecting particular individuals—if you have cancer or your parent has heart disease—it may be. But we must not confuse the elimination of disease with the eradication of suffering. Whenever we have fixed one problem in the past, others have become prominent. Critically, too, for our species and planet, if eliminating disease means that all humans live longer, then surely a project with that aim should invest a considerable proportion of its resources into considering how communities, countries, and the environment will handle so many more people, however healthy they are.

What will happen if humans begin living our full life span of 125 years, give or take? If the years of childhood and parenting are just the first third of the whole? If there are even more people and we're alive for three times longer than humans have been through most of history? It's not as if our doubling of the life span is going so smoothly. What happens to jobs, food, housing, war, competition, greed—to all those things we already have either too little or too much of today? Shouldn't medicine be thinking rather more about the consequences of its strivings instead of continuing its myopic investment in a single strategy?

The prospect of a species with little or no disease raises significant philosophical questions. Is no disease really possible or desirable? How would a life cycle progress, or end? What might this goal mean for our species, other species, or our planet?

Such theoretical and philosophical questions are light-years from the laboratories where the genome gets sequenced and a cell atlas elucidated. But continuing to ignore or underfund known tools for preventing disease and improving health is a moral and political decision. We have seen far too often in human history the dangers of pursuing scientific and technological advances without consideration of their social and practical consequences. Certainly, Mr. Zuckerberg is familiar with that scenario.

I am not anti-science-and-tech or antichange or antiprogress. Like many people, I routinely use science and technology to work for change and toward progress. My hope is that we might try to advance in each of these areas in ways that don't just pursue what can be done but also consider the potential consequences of each innovation for our cities, country, planet, and, most important, for people. Not just a select few people either, but all of us.

That's unrealistic, I know. But we won't begin to have an ethical, humane future if we don't at least try to create one.

There are many ways to make the world better, now and for the future. In medicine, I can't help wondering whether the most radical move of all would be a leader, investor, or institution with the courage to tackle the policies, biases, and structural incentives that are sickening the health care system itself.


DISTRESS

I started my new clinical role, as the geriatrician on our new hospital geriatrics unit, in October 2017. I had mostly been an outpatient doctor in my career, but after more than two decades on the literal and metaphorical other side of the medical street, I walked straight toward the sliding glass doors I had first crossed twenty-five years and four months earlier as a nervous, excited new doctor.

Inside, everything was at once familiar and strange. The building was pretty much as it always had been: linoleum floors, pale walls, harsh light, people in scrubs, white coats, or uniforms. Those in ordinary clothes looked serious, scared, dazed, or lost.

At the end of a hallway, I waited for an elevator. My floor was the last one, the top. I had been up there just twice before. My inaugural visit to the fifteenth floor had taken place over a half century earlier, when the floor was still obstetrics and my mother gave birth to me. In 2015 obstetrics had moved to our medical center's new, state-of-the-art, LEED Gold–certified "next-generation" hospital complex in a part of town that once upon a time was a marsh and lagoon.

My second visit had been the previous month, when I'd gone to see what the hospital and my colleagues were calling "the new ACE unit," that word connoting expertise and success serving in hospitals as an acronym for Acute Care for Elders.

The ACE unit concept dates from the early 1990s, when a group of doctor-researchers at the University Hospitals of Cleveland decided to test whether a hospital ward geared to the unique needs of older adults might improve outcomes (and therefore lives) in much the same way as children's hospitals had already been proved to save and better the lives of children. The idea made good sense, and it worked. The ACE unit improved function and independence on hospital discharge, decreased institutionalization, reduced readmissions to the hospital, lowered costs, and improved patient and family satisfaction with care. The first few items in that list tend to be what older adults care about most, and the last few capture what matters most to health system leaders. In the more than twenty years since the initial research came out, studies had continued to show benefits, and hundreds of ACE units had opened across the country. Now, at last, our hospital was starting one too.

Just a few years earlier our medical service chief had said he didn't see any point in starting one unless we could do something original with it, something we could study and publish. The patient benefits alone weren't enough. Now the tune from on high was changing; for the first time in my twenty-five-year association with this institution, words like *old* and *aging* appeared in the hospital and medical school's strategic plans. This wasn't because our center lagged. There are over five thousand hospitals in the United States, and most don't have ACE or other geriatric-specific units.

On the wards of the old hospital, things looked pretty much as they had when I was a trainee. The fifteenth floor was a long rectangle, with patient rooms arranged along the outside walls on three sides, and the nursing station, medication room, kitchenette, resident workrooms, and offices at the center. The wing had been given a new coat of paint, and I could see the recently installed handrails running down the corridors. There was also a multipurpose room with soft chairs in one far corner, although no signage to let patients and families know it was there for their use. Nor was there anything green there, either literally or environmentally, and certainly nothing interactive, high-tech, playful, or inviting—those much-lauded attributes of our new hospital. Also, unlike the wards across town, this unit offered no natural light, no clues about whether it was day or night, and no chairs in the hallway for people who might need to rest while making their way down its long expanse.

The art was standard-issue institutional with the ironic exception of a bulletin board featuring photographs of "exceptional seniors." There was a centenarian runner and an ancient woman doing the splits, one leg on the sidewalk and the other extended upward along a lamppost at 180 degrees, something I couldn't do at age eight or eighteen and certainly wouldn't attempt now.

Medical professionals clustered around computers, and the nursing station was populated by administrators and nurses who didn't look up when I stood on the other side arranging my face into the sort of pleasant, expectant expression I hoped would inspire their attention. (I like to do this in facilities; it gives me a sense of how patients and families are treated.) Walking down the hall, I heard one patient cursing, another moaning, and many beeping machines. I also had my usual response: it amazed me that anyone got better in such a noxious environment.

ACE units were designed for frail older adults, people in the Fourth Age, not the Third. They can be run as primary or consult services (ours was the latter) and have four defining features: elder-friendly surroundings, independence-promoting design, early discharge planning, and interprofessional team oversight to reduce complications of hospitalization.

The specially designed hospital environment usually includes carpeted floors, and a common room for both meals and family visits. Feet don't slip or stick on carpets and they are quieter, allowing for better sleep, as well as more homelike, which might reduce patients' fear and confusion. People eat more and better in social environments; it's more fun, reduces isolation, and makes eating the expected activity. Our unit didn't have any of those features, but it had a few of the other design elements that promote independent functioning: those new hallway handrails to enable safe walking; large signs in patient rooms showing the day and date and whiteboards with large print listing the day's treatment plan; and some rooms also had raised toilet seats to facilitate self-transfers.

In the studies, discharge planning began immediately, with the team's social worker or case manager working to identify what needed to be done to get the patient back home. On my first day on our unit, I discovered that case managers didn't come to the ACE team meetings, and their primary goal was getting patients out of the hospital as quickly as possible. Whether the person went home or to an institution seemed to matter very little.

The last proven trait of effective ACE units stipulates that interdisciplinary teams of nurses, doctors, aides, dietitians, social workers, and rehabilitation therapists meet regularly to review patients' medical care and reduce avoidable hospital complications. We did this. Sort of. The rehab staff wasn't allowed to attend, the nurses often refused, and no one seemed to expect the other disciplines to show up at all. For all our academic emphasis on evidence-based medicine, our institution apparently didn't feel the need to apply that standard to its oldest patients.

"It's new," my colleagues told me. And: "It's a huge step forward. Give it five years." I knew they were right, and also that none of the new units for cancer patients or kids or pregnant women were opened so far below established standards. We weren't the only hospital approaching the care of old people this way—and our outcomes are far better than most—but I suspected mine was one of the few specialties that expressed such profuse gratitude for inadequate facilities, staffing, adherence to evidence, and control over the care of their patients.

I loved my first day. I loved our patients and loved working with the dedicated, elder-friendly occupational and physical therapists, even if they couldn't attend our team meetings. Everything was new and exciting, the start of something needed and wonderful.

The second day brought an awareness that no one I was dealing with seemed very happy about the new ACE consult service except the physical and occupational therapists. Only two of the many floor nurses I interacted with seemed interested and engaged. The case managers had to be tracked down and didn't see why they had to speak to someone not on the primary team. Several of the doctors on whose patients we consulted responded by protecting their turf; the majority didn't respond at all. The clear message from almost everyone I interacted with was that although people had heard of the new service, it had been started over their objections and they resented its presence and intrusion. They didn't recognize the problems ACE needed to address; instead, it was yet another bureaucratic sinkhole sucking their precious time.

On the afternoon of that second day, a nurse asked if I could do anything for a woman in evident discomfort whose care plan made no sense. She walked me down the hall and pointed at a tiny semiconscious woman moaning and writhing in her bed, her brown skin pale yellow and draped like loose tissue paper over what remained of her.

From the doorway, it seemed obvious to me, as it had been to the nurse, that Georgia was dying. I went to the computer and looked her up. She'd been in the hospital for months, mostly in intensive care. At one time or another every organ had failed, but because Georgia had said she wanted "everything done," that was the approach being taken. Her family, who hadn't been to visit for some time, wanted to respect her wishes. So now, instead of palliative care, she was slated to get a big intravenous line and a course of dialysis. I called the hospitalist, who said it was worth a try and they didn't want to "give up" just yet. I offered another perspective but to no avail. Each time I passed her room, Georgia was moaning and writhing. Late that day, they inserted a catheter and cleaned her blood. Two days later, her family arrived and said she'd never want to live "like that," meaning the way our hospital "care" had made her. That afternoon, Georgia moved to the hospice suite, where she quickly and comfortably died.

On the third day, I arrived at the windowless residents' room and sat down at one of its computer terminals. As had been the case the previous morning, across the hall a young patient was screaming and cursing with pain. Cancer was eating away at his organs. As I had done the day before, I went out to see what I could do and was told it was under control. Back in the residents' room, I changed to my computer glasses and still had trouble reading the electronic record. Feeling more settled in my new role, I decided to address the issue. I called IT and was told there was nothing they could do. I called Facilities and learned that my unit could request a different terminal that might arrive in six months. I called my disability contact, who told me his work-around; but when I tried it, it didn't work on those terminals. The young man across the hall was still screaming and cursing. Through the residents' room's little window, I could see staff in his room and also that his gown was partway off, revealing some of his death-blackened parts. They seemed able to make him comfortable later in the day and I hoped they were working on a strategy for mornings too. I went back to my terminal, squinted, and got to work.

Later that morning I had a new consultation. Rafael was in his late eighties and a huge baseball fan. After a nice conversation that included mention of his daily walks in the park across the street from his house, I moved on to the physical exam only to find Rafael couldn't lift his right leg at all. I phoned the primary team, told the hospitalist what I'd found, and offered to help with the many tasks that needed doing. "No!" she snapped. "I'll take care of it." And then she hung up. Ten minutes later, in the hallway outside Rafael's room, I introduced myself. She shook my hand and walked away.

By my fourth day on the ACE unit, I was heartsick, a term that has gone out of favor but seems apt here. I read the overnight reports on the patients I'd been following and chatted with the rehab therapists as they did the same. Residents came and went, mostly ignoring us. The young man across the hall moaned. I looked up a few ACE research papers trying to find criteria for patient selection, since our unit didn't yet have any. Then I picked several new patients to see that morning, reviewed their charts, and walked down the hallway to a small, dark room with a locked door and telephone. Since the unit's director was out of the country, I called the next person up the chain and told her I was sorry, really and truly so very sorry, but I couldn't work on the ACE unit; I just couldn't.

She was kind and helpful, and the nicer she was, the more I unraveled. Suddenly, I didn't know why I'd become a doctor. I felt the full trauma of every horrible thing I'd ever seen or done as a doctor and all the ways people suffer—even, or perhaps especially, in a place where everyone was working hard to help. As a person who had most recently been in such places as a patient and patient's daughter, the sounds, sights, odors, and emotions seemed like those you'd expect in a place designed for low-level torture, not healing. Either my burnout wasn't quite over, or in middle age I no longer could suppress my normal human responses to such concentrated misery.

In addition to that personal reaction to the hospital, I was also struggling ethically and philosophically. It was great that our medical center was finally taking an interest in old patients. And I was pleased that the higher-ups had started using jargon like "age-friendly health system," which the World Health Organization defines as one that meets the needs of older people:

> As people age, their health needs tend to become more complex with a general trend towards declining capacity and the increased likelihood of having one or more chronic diseases. Health services are often designed to cure acute conditions or symptoms and tend to manage health issues in disconnected and fragmented ways that lack coordination across care providers, settings and time.
>
> Health systems need to be transformed so that they can ensure affordable access to evidence-based medical interventions that respond to the needs of older people and can help prevent care dependency later in life.

Although I appreciated that our institution was finally at least paying some attention to old patients, I feared the ACE unit's unwelcome status and narrow focus would reinforce people's prejudices about old people and geriatrics. Our consults were largely limited to geriatric syndromes and the collation of data obtained by others into a plan of no apparent interest to primary teams.

Those last sentiments didn't go over very well with my colleagues. They kept telling me how envious people were at other institutions where geriatrics still got no attention at all. I agreed wholeheartedly with their very good points about the need for patience with culture change. But I couldn't help but think of a different metaphor. To me they sounded like a battered woman saying, *Things are so much better now: he still hits me but hasn't knocked me unconscious even once this year.*

I finished out the week, and the next week a colleague took over. At an academic medical center, there are always other roles to play and jobs to do. My first brief stint on our ACE unit wasn't my finest moment as a doctor or human being, but it would turn out to be the sort of "midlife crisis" that moved me closer to the joy of elderhood—that period of life when a person is clear about who she is and what she values. I'm an outpatient doctor with a low tolerance for patient distress who works best in a supportive, creative, collaborative environment. I wasn't sure at first where I'd find that. But I did find it, and I didn't have to go far. I just had to look at the world, at my medical center, and at medicine, from a slightly different angle.

## WORTH

My octogenarian mother is cutting cheese. Always short and even shorter since a fall and vertebral compression fracture, she is having trouble getting enough height and leverage to cut through the huge, hard triangle of Gouda. I worry the knife will slip and she will cut herself. I consider that I could dispense with the rind more quickly, easily, and cleanly. Then I remind myself that I am more often absent from than present in her kitchen, and she is neither starving nor covered in cuts and bandages. I take a deep breath. We are not in a rush, and since the cheese will simply be part of a midafternoon family snack, it doesn't matter whether the slices are elegant or even of similar sizes. In this scenario, I'm the one with a problem. Sometimes speed matters, sometimes things need to be done just so. This is not one of those times.

Modern life is so focused on time and speed and doing multiple things simultaneously that old people often are called "out of touch" or "behind the times." But emerging data on social-media-related anxiety combined with the amount of money spent on spas and relaxation apps suggest we could just as easily say the rest of us are rushing and stressing ourselves to misery and premature aging. Relative to young people, old people may do $x$ and $y$ more slowly, but it might behoove us as individuals and society to consider which situations truly require speed and which require only that a task is done well. What problems need solutions and which do not?

Although older adults as a group hold a disproportionate amount of wealth, the average older adult of today, often no longer generating work income, is not wealthy. While those in upper income brackets tend to over-save, people with less to begin with get poorer by the year. Both are working in increasing numbers, albeit for very different reasons, to the point where the so-called encore career may become the new normal. Recent studies show an increased risk of death in the two years after retirement for men in their sixties and that over 40 percent of older people, fitter than those of previous generations in their age group, are "unretiring." In our society, increasingly dominated by the tech industry, where thirty is old and forty is ancient, people in their seventies are the fastest-growing segment of the working population. Some return to the same work; others do something new. Many work fewer hours than they did in middle age. This is often by choice—one of the benefits of being old—but sometimes it's enforced by a culture that simultaneously laments the "burden" of old people's unemployment and prevents them from working. Most unretirees looked forward to retirement or accepted the social mandate for it only to find that their lives lacked purpose, social engagement, or needed income.

"Nothing hastens old age more than idleness," wrote the sixteenth-century French physician André du Laurens. A useful vision of aging, he believed, had to go beyond biological destiny to include the need for purpose and activities. A century later, even advocates for the care of old people often made their case not by arguing for a different view of old age dispositions and function but despite them. In 1627 the physician François Ranchin argued that medicine needed to pay more attention to the health and care of old people. He admitted it was a hard sell, since "not only physicians, but everybody else attending old people" were "accustomed to their constant complaints and [knew of] their ill-tempered and difficult manners." Caring for them, he insisted, was therefore "noble and important . . . serious and *difficult* . . . *useful* and even *indispensable* . . ."

As director of the New York City Farm Colony in the 1930s, Ignatz Nascher "tried to promote incentive to work, stimulated pride in appearance, tried to improve attitudes on life, created reading and games rooms, made workers' clubs, stimulated competition with private clubs, etc.," among aged public dependents. Around the same time in San Francisco, Lillien J. Martin, the child psychologist, realized that disturbed behavior in children was often the result of the presence of an older person at home who was upset and unhappy, not because of physical discomforts or ailments, but by a loss of purpose and self-worth. The work of psychotherapy in old age, Martin advised, required "the double task of breaking down a prevalent social misconception [that old age means only decrepitude and misery] and rebuilding a person-ality that has accepted that misconception and all the misery that goes with it." Her work implied that the "ill-temper" of old people so upsetting to fami-lies and physicians over centuries was manufactured by social expectations that stripped them of opportunities to meet essential psychic needs that don't change across human lives.

Here are words often used for old people today: *Irrelevant. Useless. Burdensome. Ugly. Inferior.* The same has been said of babies, disabled people, various races and nationalities—for most people at some point or other and for some nearly constantly. Let's examine these words and concepts one at a time.

Whether something is relevant or irrelevant is a matter of who and where you are and what you value. It's different for different people: the same person can be irrelevant in one arena but relevant to another. This concept of rele-vance is most often invoked by people who believe their own work, world, and worldview to be more important than others' and inherently implies conceit on the speaker's part. In San Francisco, young techies often lob the word around, setting up an us-versus-them, hip-versus-"old" dichotomy into which all humans are segregated. Perhaps the average ninety-year-old isn't designing the latest technology, but neither is the average twenty- or forty- or sixty-year-old. Most people aren't in tech, even if they regularly use it, which means by the prevailing techie logic of relevance, most of us are irrelevant.

(So, for whom are these relevant techies designing?) And then there's this: Silicon Valley is scrambling to "capitalize on the silver economy," as the *Economist* magazine has phrased this booming business opportunity. From job search sites and ride-hailing apps to assistive robots and smart hearing aids, tech for older adults will not work unless designed with and refined through testing with older adults, which makes old people active participants in the tech economy.

The label *useless* similarly depends on what counts, and one's values. If usefulness is defined as contributing to society by working, huge swaths of the population are useless: children, homemakers, many disabled people, most homeless people, and the unemployed. Families often provide for the needs of people in at least the first three categories. We accept that; many people even applaud it. So that version of "useless" can't be right. Ideally, families take care of whichever members need care at a given time, and who that is varies throughout most lives. Some people argue that children are different because we are investing in their future. But all children grow into adults, and many adults don't meet the expectations implied by this rhetoric. On the flip side, many older adults have already made contributions. One could argue they are a better bet than children, offering opportunities both to repay society's debt for their contributions and to create an incentive system for others to "earn" a good old age in earlier years. But there again, we'd have to judge what counted as a contribution; those who didn't make the cut would be in dire straits.

Burdensome. Anyone who has ever been a good friend, a spouse or partner, a parent, an engaged adult child, or an employee knows burden is one component of every relationship of any significance. Sometimes we take on the burden because we have to, because we need a job or want to be a good person. Other times the burden is just one part of an overall satisfying relationship. Eliminate everything that qualifies as burden, and there's little of life left.

As for "ugly," one person's ugly is another's cute, if not handsome or pretty. Other times, ugly is an accurate descriptor. Some categories of people are more famous for their looks than others—Ethiopians, Scandinavians, Southeast Asians—but in all peoples and all age groups, some people are better looking than others. Many babies are ugly. Ditto many teenagers. In old age, people are far less likely to have the attributes associated with beauty and so are sometimes seen as ugly.

Inferior suggests a hierarchy, and in any hierarchy, there is only one superior position. If we are looking at the entirety of the human race, or even just the citizens of one country, it will be hard to identify, much less agree on, who holds that one superior position. By definition, the rest of us (most people) are all inferior, regardless of what attribute or scale we choose. Could we say that older adults are, as a group, inferior at generating income and maintaining the economy than middle-aged adults? Perhaps, if you count earned income, not wealth, and if you ignore the years they already put in generating income and maintaining the economy. Can it really be that entire generations earn no credit whatsoever for services rendered?

Judging lives based on utility and contributions creates a slippery slope: What then of kids, the lazy and less productive, the less talented, the less fortunate, the sick, the less wily and ambitious? What of the "weaker sex" and the "inferior races"? Put together the full panoply of human prejudices and what's left is a small percentage of people, with the rest of us in the worthless category, and that small group headed inexorably toward worthlessness. If a certain brand of productivity is our only standard of worth—or of worthiness for care and compassion—we're all in trouble.

## BELOVED

"I am more interested in the positive pathologies," declares Oliver Sacks in Bill Hayes's *Insomniac City*, a book that is a triple love story—to Hayes's first partner, Steve Byrne, who died suddenly in his sleep at age forty-three in their sixteenth year as a couple, to New York City, where Hayes moved after that unimaginable loss, and to his next partner, Sacks, who died at eighty-two when Hayes was in his early fifties. The centrality of these deaths to the story might give the impression that the book is sad. In fact, it's luminous, enchanting, and often funny. Similarly, the ages at which Steve and "O," as Hayes refers to Sacks in the book, die might make it seem as if the former were the greater tragedy. It was for Steve, given all the decades he didn't get to live, and perhaps for Hayes himself in the more immediate aftermath of

Steve's sudden death at what he likely imagined to be just the midpoint of his life. Yet, with the tincture of time and a generous curiosity reminiscent of O himself, Hayes portrays his two lost loves as merely different, neither greater nor less than each other.

When O makes the comment about positive pathologies, Hayes asks what they are, and I was relieved, since I wondered too. Sacks explains they are bodily excesses and "hypertrophies" or enlargements, not the losses or absences that are the more customary focus of medicine. That struck me as an apt description of how Hayes handles old age in this book. He makes mention of O needing or asking for certain sorts of help—a guiding arm for stability, the removal of socks, the fetching of nighttime pills. These are noted not as problems, lost abilities, or inconveniences but in passing as simple facts or as attributes that made Sacks even more himself, highlighting his fascinating idiosyncrasies and defining quirks.

Hayes's take is the opposite of the normal frame in which old age is viewed as accumulated losses. For him, every life is sculpture, a work of art defined by what is present and the surrounding negative space. The usual take is that what remains among old people is just a wisp not worthy of attention. Hayes doesn't articulate his alternative view; he shows it in his stories and photographs: all that once was but is no longer makes it easier for us to focus on and cherish what is present. Admittedly, Sacks lived what Hayes calls "a hypertrophied life," and while his presence in old age was duly impressive, at least as impressive to this geriatrician was Hayes's ability to present reality to the reader without apology or fanfare.

While both Hayes and Sacks might reasonably have expected Sacks to die first, since he was thirty years Hayes's senior, Sacks considers himself healthy and hale just weeks before his terminal diagnosis. It surprises and saddens them profoundly, and no less so for his age. Not that his age doesn't matter. He is clear with his doctors: he's had a good, long life and it's not quantity of time he's after but quality, days and weeks and months in which he can continue to do those things he loves best. He wants as much of that as he can get. Being eighty-two might mean he no longer rides motorcycles or sees patients, but it doesn't mean he doesn't have a meaningful, enjoyable life.

The best part of how Hayes relays this important message is that he doesn't narrate or explain or expound. He lets simple facts—basic, universal, ageless facts—speak for themselves. O's age is present, not paramount. The death of a beloved is the death of a beloved is the death of a beloved.

## PLACES

"Linens!" exclaimed Emile and Lilly's daughter. "And fresh flowers. The place is gorgeous. I could practically live there myself."

I took a deep breath and carefully chose my words. Karen was a hands-on daughter, and I hated to disappoint her. She also was just right about the assisted living facility's beauty and its attention to a certain sort of detail. I knew because I had cared for several people who lived there. But I wouldn't want my own parents to move in, so I couldn't in good conscience recommend it for hers.

"Why not?" she asked.

I explained that I had been to dozens of eldercare facilities and this one was of an increasingly common type that I think of as long on aesthetics but short on the sort of care that matters most.

"Walk around at different times of day," I advised. "Not when you have a scheduled visit with the marketing director, but randomly. Look at the residents and the staff: Are people talking to each other and smiling at meals and during activities? When residents meet in the hallways, do they stop to chat and discuss their plans for the day?"

I paused, giving Karen time to take in these descriptions of normal life. Normal, that is, in our family homes and in communal settings like workplaces, cafeterias, and colleges. I could see that she didn't like what I was implying. It's time-consuming and difficult to find a decent place for an old person to live if they can no longer stay in their own home or with family and friends. Karen thought she had found the right place, and I was suggesting she reconsider.

"Okay," she said, finally. "What else?"

I continued. "Does the staff talk to the people who live there, or only to each other and on their phones? And how do the residents treat the staff?

Do their interactions seem to be part of an ongoing personal relationship?" Basically, I wanted her to look at whether the staff seemed to know and like the people they assisted, or whether they treated them like widgets and tasks on a to-do list. Equally important, in the best places, residents greeted staff people by name, asked about their kids or what they did on their day off. They never demanded help as if addressing a servant or spoke to their helpers as if they were interchangeable or subhuman.

I knew Karen didn't want her parents living in a place where half the people felt they were in prison for the "crime" of growing old and frail and the other half acted as though they were doing time on an assembly line of decrepitude.

Like most people, Emile and Lilly also would be happier in a place with people who shared their interests and some of their life experiences. It wasn't that they all needed to come from the same background, just that there had to be enough people there with whom they'd feel an easy kinship and ideally some others who would extend their life experience in interesting ways. The place she'd chosen fit that requirement, except the people in it were so demor- alized, they lost much of the potential benefits of their shared values and interests. The bottom line, I said, was that her parents needed a place not only where they'd be treated well but where they could make friends. ("My friends are all gone," Emile said to me during a recent visit. "I don't know what I'm supposed to do to get new ones.")

"So," Karen said. "Are there any places we can afford that do all those things?"

If it was sad that she had to ask, the answer I had to give was even more disturbing. Too many places meant to care for old people do too few of the things that make for a meaningful, happy life, and the monthly fees at many of the better places mean they are only available to the wealthiest Americans. Emile and Lilly had money saved, but they weren't rich.


In a TED talk that has garnered over eleven million views, the Harvard psychiatrist Robert Waldinger used data from the longest study of human happiness to answer the question, "What makes us happy and healthy as we go through life?"

The Harvard Study of Adult Development began in 1938. They have eighty years of data. What Waldinger found was simple. Relationships are the key to happier, healthier lives, though not just any relationships. Quality matters more than quantity, and the happiest among us have one or a handful of close relationships and stable, satisfying marriages.

In old age, as at any age, once basic survival needs like water, shelter, and food are met, people's well-being comes down to two things that are commonly overlooked by almost everyone, including those who operate senior living facilities, policymakers, families, and our health care system: engagement (i.e., relationships) and meaning (i.e., purpose). Often, though not always, the two are related, and a well-appointed facility doesn't guarantee either.

Only the most economically fortunate can afford assisted living, continuing care communities, and the sorts of nursing homes with linen and flowers. Money improves lives across the life span, but it doesn't guarantee meaningful relationships or a reason to get up in the morning. People can be socially isolated and lonely even when they are not alone, and in older adults, loneliness leads not just to unhappiness but also to functional decline and death. Even living in communal settings, older adults who feel lonely or isolated think, feel, and function less well, are less physically active, and are more depressed. The health impact of social isolation is equivalent to smoking fifteen cigarettes a day. All else being medically equal, loneliness increases mortality by 26 percent.

Human beings seem to have a deep-seated tendency to prefer those like us to others. But older adults don't usually choose the segregation of a facility; they lack other options, since most homes and communities aren't built with consideration for old people. Or they "choose" to go for the sake of their children or spouse. There are other groups we force into segregated living situations: criminals, the mentally ill, the disabled, the young. Often, such places replicate life elsewhere. But they differ from workplaces, social organizations, and religious groups because of the participants' involuntary or mandated presence.

Old age homes also have other traits rarely present elsewhere. As Emile noted after he and Lilly moved to assisted living, "What they don't tell you when you move into a place like this is that you'll see so much death." At most residential care facilities for the elderly, or RCFEs, scarcely a week passes without someone going to the hospital or not coming out of their room. People die fairly regularly; sometimes once a month, sometimes several in a week. With time, more and more of the people who were healthy when they arrived become forgetful or need canes and walkers. These transitions impair relationships when the changed person isolates him- or herself for reasons ranging from anxiety to inadequacy and shame or is shunned by former friends who don't want to be seen with people with disabilities. And if long-standing, meaningful relationships are the key to human happiness and you live in a place where people are constantly changing, disappearing, and dying, what are you supposed to do?

The lucky still have friends on "the outside." But those elderly contemporaries tend to vanish as well—between the walls of their homes, into hospitals, into nursing homes and assisted living communities and other facilities, and away to other cities and states, closer to their adult children, anticipating what will come next. Those people gain some security and proximity to people they can count on, but at the cost of their social networks, familiar haunts, and personal history. In some cases, those losses are compensated for by new adventures, places, people, and opportunities. In others, the accumulated losses and effort of forging new relationships takes a toll. At all ages, some people adapt better to change than others. In old age, dementia, loss of hearing or vision, or the ability to walk with confidence or significant distances makes these transitions more arduous.

Moving into an institution, however nice, is among people's greatest fears as they grow old. As we age, we don't stop wanting control over our lives and schedules or enjoying the familiar objects and rhythms of our own homes. "Eldercare" institutions represent the opposite of adulthood and freedom, and their social and personal implications are mostly negative. People can be deemed no longer safe at home, safety being the primary and too often the only factor considered, and sent to one against their will. In nursing homes, almost everyone has the sense of being removed from society and warehoused as punishment for doing the very thing we all do: living.

People vary in their ability to express their distaste for this transition. A wheelchair-bound woman in her eighties whose cousin was moving out of their shared apartment and into a son's home in Southern California said she would take the risk of ending up on the floor in pain for hours or days just so long as she could remain in her home. A childless nonagenarian refused to see doctors because they tended to put her in the hospital or tell her she couldn't continue living alone in her apartment. When her grand-niece somehow convinced her to let me do a housecall, she denied all symp-toms, though some were evident despite her efforts to conceal them. Only when I was seated on the kitchen floor cutting toenails she hadn't been able to reach for over a year did the truth come out: she'd rather die than go into one of those places; in fact, by comparison, having visited some friends after they'd been moved into facilities by their families, death looked pretty good.

But then there was also this: the thin, unkempt woman who blossomed at a board and care home with regular meals, help with bathing, and people to talk to. And this: for years, my father said the only way he'd leave my child-hood house was feet first. He said something to that effect the day we went to some friends' housewarming party in a particular assisted living apartment complex—the same one he thrived in a few years later.

Homes are always better than institutions. Not all families are supportive, interactive, respectful, and loving, and not all nursing homes, hospitals, group homes, and other institutional settings for older adults are Dickensian horror factories. But homes are structurally more likely to be inviting than institutions. Although some people do terrible things to their relatives, most people reserve the majority of their love, generosity, and kind-ness for their kin. Institutions are bureaucracies, impersonal by definition and structurally focused on cost and efficiency. Those priorities affect resi-dents both directly and indirectly through the procedures and people tasked with getting them through their days. It's both a matter of what is present and what is missing.

There's one last, critical problem with institutions. They deprive not only their residents but also everyone else of the cross-generational interactions essential to a full human experience. Confronted with another person's reality, we can less easily make assumptions about them and fill in the blanks with our own beliefs and prejudices. Living in communities of people of all ages, we form relationships that inspire learning, anger, ingenuity, discomfort, frustration, love, and creativity—normal, human relationships. In those bonds and battles, we imagine our own futures, relive our pasts, and recognize our shared humanity.

## COMFORT

We got the call from our friend Ping on a Sunday afternoon, and by Tuesday evening Cathy was dead.

Ping was distressed, concerned about her friends: a family who had lived next door to hers for over thirty years. The wife was dying, her husband was devoted but unprepared, their youngest daughter was very pregnant, and their two sons lived on the East Coast.

"They need help," said Ping, "and hospice isn't cutting it." Although not in health care, Ping had cared for each of her dying grandparents and knew what a family needed to make that happen.

Cathy's cancer diagnosis had come five years earlier. She'd had rounds of treatment that helped enough that she'd been able to keep working for a couple of years. After her first relapse, she began working part-time, and when the cancer spread and she began feeling ill, she stopped altogether. That was a year or two earlier, and a few weeks before Ping called us, Cathy had been put on hospice.

When she could no longer climb the steps up to their bedroom, Cathy's husband moved their bed into their large, sunny kitchen. The previous week—just a day or two before we got the call—Cathy had still been able to talk with her family and walk a bit in the house with help, although already she wasn't eating much.

Friday the pain worsened. Her hospice nurse started her on morphine around the clock. Cathy got weaker and sleepier but seemed more comfortable. Now they were having trouble caring for her.

"There's nothing there," Ping said. "I went to the pharmacy and bought diapers, mouth swabs, all that. And I'll show them how to turn her and clean her, but they might need more help."

Once upon a time, a hospice would have provided all that. They also would have come out when things got worse so quickly—to reevaluate, provide essential supplies, adjust medications, educate, and prepare and console the family.

In many cases, they still would, but since hospice transitioned from vocation to industry, you could no longer reliably count on any of the many hospice agencies in San Francisco to do the right thing. Some were trying to make money in a burgeoning industry; others were just trying to stay viable as regulations forced them to choose between doing what they knew their patients needed and not having their bottom lines turn red. The care a patient received increasingly seemed to depend on luck: which nurse was assigned, how busy the hospice was, who was on call during a crisis. I couldn't tell what was going on with Cathy's hospice, only that they weren't meeting her needs or her family's.

Cathy's worsening pain and need for morphine meant her situation had changed. The family's many phone calls to the hospice that weekend meant the lead-up to her death had arrived.

Each time they called, they were told not to worry and that their regular nurse would visit on Monday. Because Cathy's family had never helped anyone die before, they accepted that advice. Until her diaper was wet and they couldn't figure out how to clean her up and change it. Until her lips cracked and her tongue looked shellacked and they didn't know whether that was to be expected or a problem they needed to address. Until Cathy was writhing and they didn't know how to help.

Having called the hospice, and called again, and been told the nurse would come Monday, they thought they couldn't call back, that they'd already been helped. Both the hospice's regular nurse and the ones on the phone seemed harried, with too many patients and not as much patience in answering their questions and calls for help as the family would have liked. Nor did they consult her longtime cancer doctor; he'd made clear that once Cathy moved to hospice care, he was done. Unable to bear seeing her mother so uncomfortable, her daughter had gone next door to ask Ping for help.

It's a rare family in which at least one person doesn't know how to care for a child. Yet, though birth and death occur in human lives in a 1:1 ratio, and human mortality is holding steady at 100 percent, it's common for no one in a family to know how to help someone die. This wasn't always the case: for millennia people died at home. With the medicalization of aging and dying after World War II, that changed. By the 1980s, five out of six deaths took place in hospitals. Generations grew to and through adulthood without seeing or helping with a death. In the 1990s the trend began to reverse. In 1974 there was a single hospice agency in the United States; by 2013 there were 5,800. Now one in three deaths occur at home, and over 80 percent of hospice patients in the United States are over age sixty-five.

When it comes to death, patients and families often don't know what to expect; not having been to medical or nursing school, they rely on their nurses and doctors for guidance. Ironically, despite the medicalization of dying, most doctors have little training in death.

Medicine still largely sees death as its adversary, instead of positioning itself as a tool to help ease that inevitable transition. Education about how to talk with patients and families about difficult decisions, bad news, and death only became standard in medical schools in the 2010s. It still isn't a required part of residency training in most specialties or subspecialties.

When we arrived at Cathy's home, it was clear she had entered the phase known as "active dying." Fortunately, it didn't take much to make Cathy comfortable. It took recognizing that she could no longer swallow and moving to liquid medications that could be absorbed through her gums. It took knowing that giving her pills or food would only cause choking and suffocation, and that she no longer needed them. It took knowing to fold a flat bedsheet in half under her torso so she could easily be repositioned without any of her family members hurting her or themselves. It took knowing how to change a diaper on an adult by rolling her to one side or another. It took knowing that she probably was not thirsty but that her dry mouth and lips were uncomfortable, and glycerin sponge mouth swabs and lip balm could make her feel better quickly.

It took experience and comfort with death. Not an advanced medical degree. Not liking death. Not looking forward to it. Just understanding that it's a defining part of life and approaching it accordingly.

TECH

On each housecall, I stay longer than I should, longer than I want to, and longer than planned for by our home visit scheduler. I can't leave because Dot is holding my hand, or because she won't stop talking—telling me, not for the first time, about the time Aunt Martha cut off all her hair and they called her a boy at school, or how her daddy lost his job and the lights went out and the babies cried and her mother lit pinecones and danced and made everyone laugh. Sometimes I can't leave because Dot just has to show me one thing, but getting to that thing requires that she rise unsteadily from her chair, negotiate her walker through the cluttered kitchen and narrow hallway, and find whatever it is in the dim light of her bedroom when I know she can hardly see in the bright fluorescence of the kitchen where I usually examine her.

I can, and do, write prescriptions for Dot's many medical problems, but I have little to offer for the two conditions that dominate her days: loneliness and disability. She has a well-meaning, troubled daughter in a faraway state, a caregiver who comes twice a week, a friend who checks in on her periodically, and she gets regular calls from the Friendship Line.

It's not enough.

And she, like most older adults—like most of us—doesn't want to be "locked up in one of those homes." What she needs is someone who is always there, who can help with the everyday tasks she now finds so challenging, and someone who will listen and smile and hold her hand. What she needs is a robot caregiver.

In an ideal world, each of us would have one or more kind and fully capable human caregivers to meet our physical, social, and emotional needs as we age. In an ideal world, the many people who need jobs would be matched with the jobs in need of many people. But most of us do not live in an ideal world, and a reliable robot may be better than an unreliable or abusive person and better than what most people get, which is no one at all.

Caregiving is hard work. More often than not, it is tedious, awkwardly intimate, physically exhausting, and emotionally challenging. Sometimes it is also dangerous or disgusting. Almost always it is 24/7 and unpaid or low-wage and has profound adverse health consequences for those who do it. It is women's work and immigrants' work, and it is work that we have made so undesirable and difficult that many people either can't or won't do it.

Many countries have acknowledged this reality by investing in robot development. In Japan, where robots are considered *iyashi*, or healing, the health ministry launched a program designed to both meet workforce shortages and help prevent injuries to humans by promoting nursing care robots that assist with transfers. The robots help with mobility and lifting, and they are programmed to be emotionally expressive, polite, even charming. There are also "socially assistive robots" that do things such as lead exercise classes, even recognizing their regular attendees, greeting them by their names, and engaging them in conversation. A consortium of eight European companies and universities collaborated on a programmable, touchscreen-toting, humanoid-appearing "social companion" robot that offers reminders and encourages social activity, nutrition, and exercise. In Sweden researchers have developed a robot that looks like a standing mirror–cum–vacuum cleaner, monitors health metrics such as blood pressure and activity, and allows virtual doctor visits.

Although investigators in the United States are developing robot caregiver prototypes as well, we have been slower to move in this direction. The reaction to robot caregivers in our press, in professional journals and conferences, and among some of my medical colleagues has included skepticism, concern, and occasionally outrage.

As Jerald Winakur, a San Antonio internist and geriatrician, puts it, "Just because we digitally savvy parents toss an iPad at our kids to keep them busy and out of our hair, is this the example we want to set when we, ourselves, need care and kindness? When we need to know we are loved, that our lives have been worthwhile, that we will not be forgotten?"

Robot caregivers raise fundamental questions about what and who matters in society, how societal priorities are created and reinforced, and how we define progress. Although Winakur mentions screens as babysitters, we already have abundant evidence on the harms of that approach to kids' social, emotional, intellectual, and linguistic development. Tech has adverse health consequences in adults, too, including increases in insomnia, vision and hand disorders, anxiety, narcissism, distractibility, and the need for instant gratification.

Hesitation about robot caregivers among some health professionals is not because American medicine eschews robotics. We have robots to assist in surgery, and basic "walking" robots—usually faceless or, in children's hospitals, with decorative humanoid features—that deliver medications and other supplies. Some long-term care facilities are testing robots that help with lifting or cleaning, and robots increasingly are used in rehabilitation after strokes and other debilitating events.

Of course, a robot that carries linen along hospital corridors, or cleans out your arteries as you enjoy an anesthesia-induced doze, or even one that helps transfer you from bed to wheelchair, isn't the same as a robot meant to be your friend and caregiver. For most of us, it makes sense that a robot might address certain physical and functional needs. But could a robot—a machine— possibly play a role in the most human and existential parts of our lives?

My initial response was *no way*. Yet, while the jury is still out, it seems increasingly likely that the answer will be yes. Search YouTube, and you can watch elderly Japanese people with dementia smiling and chatting happily with a robot that looks like a baby seal and responds to petting and talking. You also can see developmentally delayed children doing therapy with a cute, colorful robot that also collects information about their performance.

Walk down any street, or sit in a restaurant, or enter a workplace, and you cannot miss the ubiquitous people fully engaged with the machines in their hands or on their desks. Admittedly, some are interacting with other humans via their machines, but nevertheless the primary interaction is human-and-machine. Despite compelling protests that such interactions do not constitute meaningful, empathic relationships, they seem to provide stimulation and satisfaction to billions of people. Maybe you are one of them, reading this on a device.

Those who say a robot cannot provide the same comfort and caring as another human being are not considering three important facts. First, not all humans provide comfort, care, and stress relief to their relatives or the people for whom they provide caregiving. Indeed, many have the opposite effect, sometimes despite good intentions, and other times in willful acts of negligence or abuse. Second, robot caregivers and human caregivers are not mutually exclusive. We are not choosing from a menu of two options but developing ways to use both the humans and the robots to optimize care. Robots must supplement, not replace, human care. Third, we do not have enough caregivers for the current numbers of older Americans. Of course, we could change that by providing a reasonable wage, education, training, rewards, and recognition for this critical work to make it more attractive and interesting to the many millions of people who need jobs or currently choose other types of work. With a rapidly aging population and declining birth rate, we need creative solutions to this urgent workforce crisis.

In the next decade, scientists will refine current applications of robots and combine their physical assistance and social support functions to meet at least some of the complex needs of frail, older adults. According to James Osborne, director of the Quality of Life Technology Center at Carnegie Mellon, the current limitation is not the technology but finding a viable business model. Still, he adds, "I really expect there will be a robot helping me out when I retire. I just hope I don't have to use all my retirement savings to pay for it."

In that new world, my patient Dot's lonely life would be improved by a robot caregiver.

Since the robot caregiver wouldn't require sleep, it would be alert and available 24/7, perfect for Dot, who reads late into the night and wakes after noon. It would be there in case of crisis. Because Dot does sleep, the robot could do cleaning, laundry, cooking, and other household tasks during those hours. And when Dot awoke, she would be greeted by a kind, humanlike voice, a smile, and a "being" able to help her get out of bed and to the bathroom without injuries to either of them. After she washed her face, the robot might hand her a towel, wipe any water up off the floor so she wouldn't slip, and make sure she was clean after she used the toilet. It would ensure she took the right medications in the right doses. At breakfast, the robot might cook a warm meal or bring in the freshly delivered meal and heat it for Dot as they chatted about the weather or news, both of which the robot would know or could provide by turning on its internal radio.

And then, because Dot's eyesight is failing, the caregiver robot would offer to read to her. Or maybe it would provide her with a large-print electronic display of a book, the lighting just right for Dot's weakened eyes. "What does *durian* mean?" she might ask, and the robot would say it's a South Asian fruit that smells like old socks and tastes like perfume.

"No wonder she's making a face," Dot might remark of the story's heroine, and they would both laugh.

After a while the robot would say, "I wonder whether we should take a break from reading now and get you dressed. Your daughter's coming to visit today and we want to be ready."

This reality is both disturbing for the human abdication of social responsibility it represents and a portrait of a safer, more pleasant life than Dot's current one. It's perhaps not surprising that most of the engineers of robots of all kinds come from the demographic groups least likely to provide actual human-to-human care. The more we use their devices, the more rich and powerful they become. In society, their ascendance has paralleled increasing income inequality and social strife. In medicine, it has ushered in the era of burnout and a time when patients describe their pain and suffering to the side of their doctor's face as he or she types, and types, and types, into the electronic medical record. We forget that technology is not necessarily mutually exclusive with compassion, equity, and justice—unless we allow it to be.

When someone becomes ill or frail, they usually also become less public. Perhaps they are mostly homebound by sickness or fatigue or debilities. Perhaps it is a choice. But sometimes, too, getting out requires help, and that help isn't forthcoming. Or going out provokes stares or their twin, the deflected gaze, so they stay home, sparing others discomfort and themselves shame and humiliation. We throw a party and don't invite them—it would be too much trouble; they probably couldn't manage anyway; it would show up their current embarrassing state. So often by the time we might, through our own hardship, learn to fully appreciate the unnecessary hurt we've caused others, it's too late.

Allowing us to further abandon caregiving roles isn't the only risk of technological caregiving. Other technologies, many already in use as part of the "quantified self" movement, and more in the pipeline, often reinforce the paternalism and lost autonomy of old age. Tech companies, sometimes trying in good faith to address the concerns of adult children of frail or cognitively impaired old people—and sometimes preying on them in terrifying ways—have created an array of devices to alert family and caregivers to old people's health status and activities. Some monitor pulse and blood pressure, blood glucose, and sleep patterns. Others check whether the person got out of bed or opened the refrigerator.

Some of these actions violate the privacy and rights of old people in ways that would spark outrage if done to middle-aged adults. Different generations have different notions of privacy, so this may change with time, but those who are old now and who will become old in the next few decades tend to see distant monitoring of their body and behavior as a violation of their privacy. If an older person can access and understand the message—that is, if they are literate, digitally literate, and do not have dementia, as most older adults do not—then why is someone else being informed about what is usually considered personal health information and no one else's business?

We must distinguish between this sort of infantilization and benevolent help in a life stage when people cannot always adequately care for themselves. Too often younger people assume incapacity in old people until proved otherwise, instead of the other way around. Too often, too, we assume the young way of doing something is the best or only way. Adding to the confusion is the interpretation of *adequate*, which often enough is in the eye of the beholder. It may look one way to a person who has never taken medications except when she feels ill and to her son who always follows directions. Here again, we hold old people to a different, higher, and sometimes unjust standard compared with younger adults.

"You mean to tell me," began a horrified, furious alcoholic former nurse, "that when I was sixty-four I could drink as much as I wanted and it was nobody's business, and then overnight people can call Adult Protective Services if they don't like how I choose to live?"

Yes, I had to say. That's just how it works. There are some good reasons for this, including that old age comes with physical and cognitive vulnerabilities not present in earlier decades and that acquired impairments in those functions rise significantly in the eighth decade of life onward.

At the same time, the dividing line of sixty-five is historical and in many lives outdated. And there is the problem that reasonable people often disagree about the right approach to various situations. One person's good decision is another's bad decision. It's hard to tease out judgments we may disagree with from ones that are simply wrong, and there's also a huge gray area. A hard line can and should be drawn at harming others. But what about harming oneself? Often enough, drinking too much, eating too much, not washing, living in a filthy home, and taking risks are behaviors we allow once people reach adulthood. If a person has always lived a certain way, the sixty-fifth birthday seems an arbitrary moment in which to punish them for socially disapproved activities.

Particularly as digital technology enables programming of household functions from afar and relaying of medical and personal information to family, caregivers, and health professionals, older adults will be at risk of losing autonomy and privacy. Too often tech innovations seem designed to assuage the anxieties of adult children at the expense of their parents. Innovators consider what old people actually need or want too infrequently. Whereas tech for younger adults focuses on self-monitoring and tracking, tech focused on older adults often pulls in one or more others, without controls that can enable or refuse sharing, or guidance about the sorts of conversations families need to have to best balance the needs and worries of different members. It also focuses on the far end of old age, doing little to increase tech access for old people in the first decades of that life stage or even acknowledging the large numbers of tech-using old people.

Some technology shows tremendous potential. In no age group are people consistently able to remember to take medications, especially when they are needed several times a day. Reminder systems make sense for old patients not only because they are more likely to take medications, and to take many medications, but also because they have a higher likelihood of cognitive impairment. Exercise and activity apps appear to motivate people fairly effectively, and it's worth considering how regimens can be made useful across ages and generations and levels of fitness, as well as what rewards provide the most motivation.

Of course, for some people, monitoring may simultaneously lessen privacy and increase safety and independence. If a person can't quite manage on their own, but a device and the help of distant others allow them to stay at home and manage better and more safely than without the device, that may be an attractive option.

Different people value privacy and safety differently. It's well known that adult children generally put safety first, while their parents often are willing to take risks in exchange for remaining at home or retaining control over their bodies and lives. A patient of mine complained that his son wanted him to wear monitors and install grab bars because he'd fallen at home, but when the father told the son he thought his motorcycle riding was dangerous, the son said, "That's my business."

In old age, as at all ages, tech has previously unimagined benefits and terrifying harms. Acknowledging the moral range of potential applications is the first step toward using it to improve our elderhood, not replace nursing homes with virtual control and manipulation.

## MEANING

Zeke Emanuel—brother of both Chicago mayor Rahm Emanuel and the Hollywood talent agent Ari Emanuel, the latter made famous by the program *Entourage*—is an oncologist, bioethicist, and one of this country's leading public physicians. In an *Atlantic* essay called "Why I Hope to Die at Seventy-Five," Emanuel said he would stop most medical care at age seventy-five. He would do things like get a hearing aid and take pain medications but would not try to prolong his life with preventative or heroic medical treatments.

Emanuel isn't going to kill himself. He has opposed euthanasia and physician-assisted suicide for decades. Instead, he argues that past a certain point, medical care that once might have been helpful becomes counterproductive, with treatments more likely to prolong time people don't want and less likely to provide them with more of what they do. I, too, have seen this, again and again, as have so many doctors. He wrote:

> Here is a simple truth that many of us seem to resist: living too long is also a loss. It renders many of us, if not disabled, then faltering and declining, a state that may not be worse than death but is nonetheless deprived. It robs us of our creativity and ability to contribute to work, society, the world. It transforms how people experience us, relate to us,

and, most important, remember us. We are no longer remembered as vibrant and engaged but as feeble, ineffectual, even pathetic.

The article combines important truths about old age with a very particular worldview, and it has several blind spots. Emanuel appears to assume decline and disability cannot co-occur with contributions to "work, society, the world." He cares so deeply about his legacy of public achievements that he denies the possibility of meaningful relationships with people who are or have become enfeebled and further devalues the majority of human lives, ones in which his notion of "legacy" is irrelevant.

In a later interview on the same topic, Emanuel claimed that if you talk to experts in Japan, you will learn that everyone has dementia by age one hundred. (Unless the Japanese are very different from Americans, this is false, although with age the brain, like everything else, changes.) If dementia terrifies him—as it does so many, and if, given his values, it's his worst possible future outcome—then he's entitled to hedge his bets, changing course medically as he ages in hopes of dying before he might get it. His approach both makes good sense and assumes a life worth living is always mutually exclusive with cognitive decline or frailty. After decades spent caring almost exclusively for very old, frail people, I know three things: lives can have meaning despite significant decline and disability; different people draw the line in very different places as far as where they would like to die; and because of medicine's shortsighted approach to "progress," too many aged people are forced to go on once they've passed their natural and preferred thresholds as a result of medical "care."

For Zeke Emanuel, meaningfulness has to do with the ability to do a certain sort of work, the sort of work he has always done and values most. That's fine—for him. In the interview, he notes that few people are productive in their work after age seventy-five, a comment that isn't completely accurate and doesn't adequately take into account how longer human lives have begun to change our relationship to work as we age. It also discounts the value to society and in individual lives of the same sorts of work that often go unpaid or underpaid—so-called women's work, most particularly caregiving and volunteering of all sorts. (A quarter of America's forty million unpaid caregivers are themselves over age seventy-five, and most are women.) To Emanuel, "meaningful work" implies a paycheck and perhaps even an influence on the world. The sort of work he does, in other words, though not the sort done by most women and men. He also adopts the modern industrial notion that what counts most is productivity, raising the question of whether learning or art or relationship building qualify as productive activities.

His value judgments continue: "a life where the dominant thing is only fun or play, doing a crossword puzzle, reading a few books, seeing the grandkids once every month or something. That's not a meaningful life. I don't want that life. I don't think anyone should find that life fulfilling." Emanuel is entitled to his vision of his own life, but he gets himself into trouble with that last sentence. It judges others in ways that deprive them of what he is asserting for himself: the right to assign value to their own lives. It also discounts the daily reality for the majority of humans of all ages who are less economically and socially fortunate than he and the millions who take pleasure in such lives. Disturbing, too, from a life course perspective is this statement: "I would challenge them whether that really is meaningful or what they have done is narrowed down what constitutes meaningfulness for them to accommodate their limitations physical, cognitive and whatever." If such adaptation were a problem, we'd all have to kill ourselves by age forty.

When someone with Emanuel's authority and influence makes statements without also acknowledging his cultural vantage point or the social disparities and policy failures that have created the circumstances in which such sentiments seem reasoned and reasonable, he then constructs, allows, and enables the old age he wants to avoid—and not just for himself but for all the rest of us, especially those who aren't in a position to judge or shape the lives of tens and ultimately hundreds of millions of their fellow citizens.

What Emanuel does to old age in his essay is what medicine does to old age in American society. Contrast that biology-as-destiny approach with the view of Linda Fried, the geriatrician head of Columbia's School of Public Health. Writing in the same magazine just a few months before Emanuel, she said:

> Too many of my patients suffered from pain, far deeper than the
> physical, caused by not having a reason to get up in the morning. Many

of my patients wanted to make a difference in the world but, finding no role for themselves, were treated as socially useless and even invisible.

Fried echoes Marjory Warren, who transformed medicine with her mid-twentieth-century Middlesex hospital old age ward. Fried has worked to accomplish something similar, starting the Volunteer Corps and leading other societal and policy changes that take advantage of older people's experience and skills while creating opportunities for them to do meaningful work. At all ages, biology is but one part of a human being's experience of the world.

Adaptability is generally considered evidence of an open mind, creativity, and resilience. The anthropologist Margaret Clark reframed aging as an ongoing process of simultaneous adaptation—not only to one's changing body but equally to one's specific social and cultural situations.

Interviewing both healthy community-dwelling older adults and ones admitted to a psychiatric hospital for late-life mental health problems, Clark found the two groups agreed on personal goals in old age: having independence, social adaptability, adequate personal resources, and the ability to cope with external threats of changes; maintaining significant and meaningful goals; and having ability to cope with changes in self. Where the two groups differed was in how they thought they would achieve those goals. Healthy participants used values that would allow attainment even as they became frail (congeniality, using resources wisely, calm self-acceptance), while the hospitalized ones set themselves up for failure by judging attainment based on external factors including power, status, and recognition. Successful adaptation to old age, Clark concluded, required renouncing middle-aged and culturally dominant norms in favor of ones better suited to late-life abilities, resources, and roles.

The work of the medical anthropologist Sharon Kaufman further clarified the transition: "The old Americans I studied do not perceive meaning in aging itself; rather, they perceive meaning in being themselves in old age."

She explains that people continue to revise and create their identity, that people's self-perceptions are independent of age, and that distress ensues when self-image and others' perceptions are in conflict. She also discusses that people are best able to maintain a sense of meaningful self when they continuously restructure their identity to unify who they were with who they now are. People often say they didn't feel old until they had a fall or were hospitalized or several of their closest friends died in a short span of time. In response to those realizations, some people feel resigned or hopeless. Others reconstitute who and what they are.

Two patients of mine had to start using a walker in the same short space of time. Neither was particularly happy about it. Helena refused to go out. She didn't want to be seen as old (something that seemed obvious to me, walker or not). Esther asked if we could reschedule our appointment. She was going to the movies with a friend; it took her a bit longer to get around, and she wanted to be sure to leave enough time. Later, she told me she now needed an aisle seat with a wall nearby to prop her walker and that I should definitely go see the movie. The aging body matters in what people can and cannot do, but identity, additions and modifications to how a person sees themselves, and social context are no less important in determining a person's well-being.

We revise our behaviors, expectations, and self-image throughout life. In that regard, old age isn't different from earlier stages.

### IMAGINATION

It was to be my first commencement speech, so I did what most twenty-first-century people do when facing a situation that calls for insight, humor, and, especially, originality: I went to Google and YouTube to see what others had done.

That, as I later admitted to my audience, was a mistake. Some of the best graduation speeches have been given by people like Steve Jobs, J. K. Rowling, Ellen DeGeneres, and the Dalai Lama. Naturally, my reaction to those cultural icons' funny, moving, insightful speeches was to check my e-mail and Twitter accounts and to realize that, although our dog appeared to be sleeping, any fool could tell he needed another walk. I couldn't possibly work on my speech.

On the walk, I got lucky. Perhaps because exercise stimulates creativity, I realized that I should talk about the very thing those famous people, with their disparate accomplishments, had in common—not only with each other but also with most people who make a difference. They hadn't succeeded simply because they were smart and hardworking. Success came because they saw the world in new, interesting ways. It came from imagination.

But I still had a problem. Although imagination had the right mix of import, surprise, and universality to make an ideal topic for a speech intended to launch young people into their adult lives, I worried that it would be a hard sell to my intended audience of graduating health professionals and medical school faculty members.

To some people, including many doctors and scientists, the need for imagination in medicine and science is obvious. It may be that such people themselves have powerful imaginations. Others, often also doctors and scientists, require more convincing. This isn't because they lack the capacity for imagination so much as because they don't always apply that word to their work when it's warranted or because their own imaginations have grown weak from disuse in the years since they decided on their "serious" health science careers. Because imagination is hard to see or measure or test for, it has increasingly been associated solely with the humanities and arts, those second-class citizens of twenty-first-century life, and rarely discussed or cultivated during medical and scientific training. That parsimonious view of imagination couldn't be further from the truth.

By *imagination*, I don't mean fantasy or make-believe but something close to and necessary for creativity, insight, innovation, and empathy. For hard-core scientists and others who see themselves as not in need of imagination in their work or lives, it's worth considering the wisdom of Albert Einstein, who said, "Imagination is more important than knowledge. For knowledge is limited to all we now know and understand, while imagination embraces the entire world, and all there ever will be to know and understand."

If a person bases their work on knowledge alone, it will be limited; but if the same person engages their imagination, anything is possible. Imagination is the progenitor of hypotheses, new ideas, and original ways of seeing. It helps organize information, shaping what we think and feel about other people. Imagination isn't just a tool used by writers, artists, chefs, designers, and advertisers. It's the faculty or skill that led Steve Jobs to look at the ugly collections of metal and plastic then called computers and ask: *Why can't it also be beautiful, and fun, and small enough to fit in my jeans pocket?* And imagination led Sidney Farber, a groundbreaking physician, in the 1940s to suppose that lessons learned in treating nutritional anemias might be applied to treating leukemias as well. Now most kids with leukemia are cured.

An intellectual use of imagination is essential for scientific and medical progress. But it's not the only use of imagination that matters for health and in health care or for happy, successful lives.

Sometimes, it's not even the one that matters most.

My cousin's son, whom I'll call Marc, is a college student who plans to go into medicine. He spent a recent summer working in a lab at a medical center where he also sometimes shadowed doctors. One August evening, at a family birthday dinner, Marc said he'd seen the most incredible thing in the emergency department that day. He was really excited, so we all put down our forks and leaned in to hear his story.

Apparently, a young man had been brought in from a local prison because he'd fallen from his bunk bed and could no longer move or feel his legs.

"It was the lower bunk," Marc said, shaking his head.

The emergency department doctors stuck the patient with pins, poked and prodded his legs. Nothing. No response. "I can't feel it," the man kept saying. He was visibly upset. Then one doctor distracted him while another went behind him and jammed something really sharp into his back. He jumped, screeched, and moved his legs. He'd been faking. The doctors and nurses filed out of the room laughing.

"The whole thing took less than five minutes," Marc said with a grin.

Now, this story has many lessons, and one of them is that you might not want to invite me to your birthday party. Here's why: I was outraged. I told Marc the doctors had behaved unprofessionally and dangerously. I asked him to consider the harm they might have done if the patient had truly been injured. Next I suggested he imagine a different young man, perhaps a university student like himself rather than a prisoner, reporting a similar fall and complaint. How did he think that scenario would have played out? Might they have followed standard procedures rather than jumping to the conclusion that he was faking? I thought so.

Finally, I asked Marc to think of reasons why the patient might have faked an injury. Maybe he'd accidentally angered a gang member and feared for his life. Maybe he had a mental illness and a voice had told him to jump from the bunk and next time would tell him to do something far worse. And maybe, in a tough situation, he exhibited traits that someone paying attention might help him harness so when he left prison he would have the agency and know-how to put them to use building a life for himself on the right side of the law.

And maybe he was just a scammer. We'll never know, since his doctors failed to engage their clinical, empathetic, and ethical imaginations.

But they weren't the only ones. Hearing Marc's story, I responded in just the same way, leading with my own dearly held biases and goals, and without thinking about the needs of the other people in the room, particularly the youngest one, who was telling his story to people he was supposed to be able to trust. I failed to use my imagination, and I should have known better.


I am an unlikely doctor. For the first twenty-some years of my life, I went to great lengths to avoid math and science. Early on in high school, I got permission to take one course over the normal load so I'd have as many As as other good students, even when I got a bad grade in algebra, which I was sure to get.

Years later, after the first day's lectures at med school, I phoned home and explained to my parents that I understood about one of every four or five words uttered by my professors, and too often those words were articles or conjunctions. I suspected I might perform nearly as well if the instruction was being given in Cantonese, a language I do not speak.

I also soon discovered that I had all the wrong instincts. In my case-based learning small groups, the other students would all, swiftly and uniformly, offer up identical questions and next steps: How does that work? What's the mechanism? What tests do we need? My responses were different: How are we going to tell his family? Or: What do we need to do to get her on the transplant list? The problem wasn't that their reactions or mine were wrong, but clearly theirs were the ones desired by our course directors and teachers, and mine were not.

And then, I began—insidiously at first, but soon with increasing frequency—having similar responses to my peers. I asked the right questions and proposed the right next steps for scientifically rigorous clinical care. Thinking like a scientist was fun, and not just because I'd mastered a skill essential to my survival. I realized there had been entire sectors of life and thought that I'd been missing. What's more, this new way of thinking gave me meaningful skills with which to make a difference in people's lives.

I became a doctor, and that role has been one of the great pleasures of my life. But it has also been the source of some of my greatest frustrations. Because alongside medicine I learned that there were things a doctor did and things she did not do, things that should interest her and things that shouldn't. Too many of the things in the *didn't* and *shouldn't* categories were the things I loved.

That made me sad. Once I finished my decade of medical training, I started doing some of those things, like reading literary fiction in my free time. Eventually, I got a master's degree in creative writing. Now, you might think, as I did, that fiction writing can have nothing whatsoever to do with doctoring, but it transformed my career.

It wasn't just that writing skills helped me get grants, though they did, or that learning to put myself into other people's minds made me a better clinician, though that happened too. It was also that, by combining my particular interests and skills, I was suddenly getting published in leading newspapers and journals, giving me access to tens of millions of people. Suddenly, I wasn't just taking care of my patients; I was also influencing health care. And once I saw how owning up to my nonscientific interests and engaging my imagination actually helped my medical career, I gained the courage to write about things that I saw differently from the medical establishment.

Finally, I became what only I could be, and that made me very happy.

I said all these things in my commencement speech, defining my terms like a good scientist and using stories to make my case like a good humanist.

I concluded the talk by mentioning that the word *imagination* comes from the Latin for "picture to oneself." I told the new graduates that their education had given them a certain set of pictures; yet, as Einstein said, those pictures were limited to all we now know and understand. To make a difference in health and health care, they needed to use all they'd learned and their imaginations too.

That afternoon, I flew back to San Francisco, where it occurred to me that medicine and old age might just be related in more than the obvious way of medicalization of aging. Maybe the problems with American health care and the challenges of elderhood were both consequences of failures of imagination, of how we picture ourselves, our lives, and our work, and how we don't but could.

BODIES

You don't have to be a doctor to recognize that the body changes with age, and you don't have to be officially old to know from personal experience that many of those changes are unwelcome. The physical and physiological changes that accrue to "old" begin subtly and early, in a person's thirties or forties, and at some variable point in our sixth, seventh, or eighth decade, we pass the physical, social, and legal thresholds of old age. The negative parts of this transformation—the losses—initially require adaptation, then limitation, and sometimes, finally, renunciation or the need for work-arounds. None of us want a cane, much less a walker, or help with finances or driving or grocery shopping. And uniformly, we don't want to end up hopeless, help-less, and institutionalized—most people's image of advanced old age and, often enough, at some late point, its reality. If you also consider that—unlike the terrible twos, a traumatic adolescence, a squandered young adulthood, or a midlife crisis—what follows being old is death, it becomes clear how old age achieved its current reputation.

Healthy, able-bodied people often say they wouldn't want to live with grave disability. Meanwhile, a majority of people who become disabled— after an adjustment period—report good and, not infrequently, very good quality of life. Yet, when I suggest to friends in their seventies and eighties that a good part of the suffering in old age is manufactured by our policies and attitudes, they work hard to fill their expressions with nothing but curiosity and interest. In their eyes, I see suspicion, disbelief, and several unspoken retorts: *She's too young to understand. Facts are facts, biology is biology, and we are all destined for more or less the same downward slide to oblivion.*

Their reaction depends a bit on what kind of day or week or month they're having. Being sick or in pain or the recent death of a friend colors everything, and each of those things is increasingly common with age. People who are relatively healthy but have the pain or limitations of chronic diseases wonder what will happen next, and when. They worry about suffering and dying, about the loss of the people they love best, about being alone and about being gone. Those who are frail and sick or heading that way worry they won't die as soon as they'd like to. Others, with lists of ailments and medications long enough to unfurl like scrolls, fight to stay alive, even as ever greater proportions of their days are devoted to the basics of body tending: hygiene, and food, and medications.

People with highly restricted lives—the sorts of people in our house-calls practice, for example—lament less their lives' small stages than the accompanying isolation. The official term for the space we move through in the world, whether large or small, is *life-space*. Mine extends to continents; theirs is often limited to their home, a single room, or a bed. They would like to get out, to again be the sort of person who could or would go more places. But that's not the source of their greatest hardship. What they miss most, what they are starved for, is engagement, touch, conversation, and connection, those basics of being human that come in just above our needs for food, shelter, and safety on Maslow's hierarchy. Much has been made of what missing touch and connection did to Romanian orphans. The impact of isolation in old age, of never or rarely being touched or talked to or loved, is less formative but no less profound. Social isolation and loneliness worsen physical and mental health, leading to nursing home placement and premature death. In the UK, a young man spent a week alone in an apartment as part of the Loneliness Project, and although he started out okay, over the week he became increasingly frustrated, bored, despondent. He focused on small daily tasks, little things gnawed at him, he tried to turn off his brain, and he watched TV or went to bed for lack of other options.

On FaceTime, my mother, in the lobby at her gym, holds her phone midway between her mouth and ear. In public, she doesn't want it too loud, but in each of the last two years, she has consulted an audiologist, wondering whether the time for a hearing aid has arrived; on her most recent visit, they agreed she was getting close. I'm on my computer. Her cheek, one eye, and parts of her nose and lips fill its large screen. This close, the softness of her skin seems visible. It has a laxity, a slight droop, creases and texture. It is subtly colorful, a canvas of tans, pinks, and off-whites. She has blemishes, too, darker patches hinted at beneath the makeup she has put on to hide them. At the corner of her lips, I see an irregularity, and the doctor in me considers diagnoses to explain it. I smile at the sight of the small pale pouch under her eye; she hates it, just as her father in his old age hated his. For fifteen minutes, I talk to my mother while watching this video of the side of her face. It's no less captivating than the several art films I have recently seen, and no less beautiful.

Do I imagine I see the softness of her cheek because I have kissed that cheek and know the feel of it on my skin? Is it because her cheek is so familiar—likely the first skin I kissed over a half century ago—and because I love my mother? Or is it because I know in some essential way that if something looks as her cheek does, it's soft to the touch, warm, yields on impact with a gentleness that is inviting and comforting. A younger cheek, taut and smooth, is more like a trampoline; a touch doesn't sink in so much as bounce off. Later than night, climbing into bed, I realize that, for me, faces are like bedsheets in winter. My favorites are our oldest, soft and welcoming from years of use. When we use the newer ones, my heart sinks. They are nicer to look at but crisp and cold on my skin.

There is a photo of me at age twenty-two, stretching before a run. I remember the orange tank top, my favorite at the time, and the now exquisitely dated white shorts with blue piping. I recall the feel of that lean, fit, youthful body, how I could simply take off running with no thought to anything beyond loosening up my hamstrings. I didn't have to consider ominous tweaks of tenderness in my lower back, searing foot pain, a catching hip, cramping muscles, or the *snap-crackle-pop* of joints. I never gulped air on inclines or worried that my pace, never fast enough to make a school team, might appear pathetic. Instead I looked at myself in that fitted tank top and those hideous shorts and felt simultaneously exultant in and dissatisfied with my body. I wanted it to be leaner still, faster, and more graceful. At all ages, we interrogate and shame our bodies. We always want something more than or different from what we have. I often look at straight hair and think: How great would that be? And most weeks someone approaches me to say, *I love your hair; I wish mine would curl like that.* But wanting to be other than you are isn't the same as feeling that either the body you inhabit lies about who you are or that, because of features beyond your control, people looking at you see not you but a stereotype of the category that includes you.

At a party where the people present ranged from their late twenties to early eighties, a woman with pink-streaked white hair and considerable wrinkles took the makeshift stage, five huge badges with photographs on them pinned to her shirt and sweater. She explained that in order to get people to really see her, she'd made the badges to show pictures of herself at different ages. Each told part of her story, and together they offered a more complete portrait of who she was than people got from just looking at her. At any age, it's interesting to look back and learn how a person has, and hasn't, changed. It's also often helpful to have a physical object and story as a conversation starter among strangers at parties. And still, her badges made me sad. Here was this clearly interesting woman with a body that moved easily around the room and whose clothing and grooming playfully expressed her big personality, yet she was convinced that her current face did not represent the real her. With it as her only introduction to strangers, she felt unseen or inaccurately perceived. She wore her giant badges to prove she hadn't always been old, as if to say: *See me, I, too, was once a person who counted.*

## CLASSIFICATION

Many stakeholders determine who and what counts in medicine. How we approach vaccines provides insight into how we handle many other aspects of health (and life) as well. Doctors determine which shots patients should get, and when, based on the Centers for Disease Control's recommendations. The CDC guidelines are presented in two "schedules": one for children, the other for adults, both divided into age subgroups based on developmental biology and social behaviors common at different stages of the life span.

The 2018 schedules included seventeen age-based subgroupings for kids from birth through age eighteen. This makes sense: a six-month-old has had little time to develop immunity, weighs far less than an eight-year-old, and is exposed to different people and places than a teenager. There were five subgroups for adults. All Americans age sixty-five and over are lumped in a single subgroup, as if our bodies and behaviors don't change in any meaningful ways over the half century of life from the mid-sixties forward. Like so much in medicine (and society), the CDC guidelines acknowledge the diversity in two life stages while ignoring equivalent diversity in the third.

It's not difficult to distinguish sixty- and seventy-year-olds from the nonagenarians and centenarians a generation ahead of them. These two groups—the young-old and old-old—don't just differ in how they look and spend their days; they differ biologically.

Aging progressively affects the function of our cells, tissues, and organs. With advancing years, both innate and acquired immune functions gradually decline, people develop more diseases, and the body's ability to fight infection and respond to immunizations decreases. As a result, older adults are more susceptible to infections—more likely to get sick from them, more likely to require hospitalization, and more likely to die.

Our one-size-fits-all approach undervaccinates some older adults whose immune response can't keep pace with their longevity or whose behavior doesn't conform to stereotypes, and it gives others vaccines that do little or nothing to help them. The infections most likely to sicken and kill us in old age differ from those that do the most harm in earlier decades. While the current approach acknowledges some of those differences with its recommendations for flu, pneumococcal, and zoster vaccines, the approach is far less targeted and comprehensive than it is at younger ages.

Given our waning immunity with age (a phenomenon known as "immunosenescence"), coupled with increasing longevity, some researchers are exploring novel strategies of infection prevention. These include "priming" immune systems of younger adults to stimulate responses that will endure into advanced old age, developing vaccines for infections that preferentially affect old people, use of adjuvants to boost the response of older adults to current vaccines, and not just vaccinating against individual diseases but enhancing the aging immune system itself.

Optimal vaccination requires recognition that immunization and other medical decisions cannot be based on age alone. They must also factor in health and physical function. Most healthy eighty-year-olds will outlive frail seventy-year-olds with multiple diseases, and many of us will reach a point toward the very end of our lives when even annual flu vaccines either don't work because our immune systems can no longer respond to them or when getting vaccinated is inconsistent with our end-of-life preferences.

Human diversity reaches its apex in old age. There is no set age when we transition from adult to elder, and both the speed and extent of aging vary widely. As geriatricians are fond of saying: "When you've seen one eighty-year-old, you've seen one eighty-year-old."

A large and growing literature illustrates why age differences matter, both for immunizations and in health care more generally. Older bodies respond differently to vaccines and treatments, and disease biology can differ among different age groups too. In a series of recent studies of treatments for common urologic conditions, so-called minor procedures such as cystoscopy, bladder biopsy, and transurethral resection of the prostate that help healthier and younger men not only had no efficacy in frail older men but caused functional decline and death. In lymphoma and breast and lung cancers, cellular alterations and tumor behavior often change with increased age. In acute myeloid leukemia, studies report significantly lower treatment responses in older patients. (In part, this is because treatments target the biology of younger adults' cancers.) Additionally, changes in the kidneys, heart, skin, and other organs as people move through elderhood steadily increase their risk of toxicity and decrease their ability to tolerate chemotherapy and radiation.

Biology matters in other ways too. The older-old have more functional impairments than the young-old. From prevention to intensive care, old people with greater debility and shorter life expectancies often incur all the immediate harms of treatments developed for younger adults without living to see the benefits. Although older adults are getting more attention now in many sectors of health care than previously, they are still primarily presented as variants of a middle-aged norm, an exception or outlier, even in management of diseases like cancer where the majority of patients are old.

Even in studies when treatment of the oldest-old is specifically addressed, outcome measures frequently reflect the priorities of the (younger) researchers, not their old patients. Studies of hip, knee, or aortic valve replacement in the very old, for example, assess length of hospital stay and mortality, when most old people are at least as interested in staying out of nursing homes and retaining the ability to think and walk. In the twenty-first century, when numbers of older adults will surpass numbers of children globally, we need to target elder health with the same life-stage lens we have already used for adults and children. Failing to fully acknowledge the ongoing human development and diversity of older Americans is bad medicine and flawed public health.

There has been much discussion lately of how poorly equipped and organized our health care system is to address the needs of the chronically ill and old. That's changing—slowly, reluctantly. Look at the advertisements for most medical centers, and you'll find their messages still emphasize the acute care save—lives brought back from the brink. Those stories make great marketing, but these days a health system not focused on treating chronic disease and old people is like an education system that can't handle children.

There is one easy step that would not only help the CDC correct the deficiency in its vaccine recommendations but would increase structural equality throughout medical science and our health care system: whenever we apply something to people by age and are tempted to divide the life span into just childhood and adulthood, we should add elderhood to the list as well.

# 12. ELDERLY

## INVISIBILITY

Often, people's worst nightmare about old age looks like this: a bent old woman with wild hair, missing teeth, a hooked nose, and bulging, unfocused eyes—a crone, a hag, a witch. This is the stuff of the original fairy tales collected in the cold north by the Brothers Grimm, considered on their first printing to be unsuitable for children.

That was why I tried to schedule my housecalls to Betty Gallagher on days when I didn't have medical students working with me in our geriatrics housecall practice.

As if following the fairy-tale script, Betty lived at house number 666 on a flat street in a neighborhood that looked postapocalyptic. In place of front gardens, most houses had cement driveways, scruffy shrubs, and lawns of pocked, dead grass. Even the well-tended homes registered as drab and worn. On days dark with San Francisco's famous fog, I sometimes wondered whether the area's absence from tourist maps and most local news reports meant the lives lived inside those homes mirrored their exteriors. In our rapidly transforming city of techies, foodies, start-ups, and Silicon Valley multimillionaires, Betty lived in one of the few areas that had failed to capture anyone's imagination or interest.

Betty wasn't rude or dangerous. She never hit, swore, yelled, bit, kicked, spat, leered, or grabbed, as disturbing patients of all ages sometimes do. Although blind, she always smiled when she heard my hello, never failed to ask how I was, patiently answered my many questions, and put up with my ministrations without complaint. When I stuck her with needles to monitor the progression of her diabetes and kidney disease, undressed her and turned her over in bed to inspect her skin, or poked and pushed in other ways that even if they don't hurt aren't much fun, her most evident complaint would be a silent grimace.

For the first half of the almost decade I knew her, our appointments took place in her living room, Betty seated in a faded armchair using an exercise device that consisted of bicycle pedals without the rest of the bike—just foot pedals on a stand. As I unpacked my equipment or typed my visit note into my laptop, she would move her feet around and around while discussing her family or listening to talk radio.

Her radio stayed on from morning until she went to sleep at night, usually playing the sorts of programs that reveled in the denigration of entire categories of human beings. Since those categories described not only the vast majority of California residents but also all her caregivers and many of our medical students, I sometimes wondered what our appointments might have been like if Betty could have seen. But that wasn't the reason I hesitated to visit Betty on my teaching days.

The problem wasn't who she was so much as how she looked. Her appearance didn't qualify as outright grotesque, but with lost eyesight, worsening debility, out-of-town children, and poorly paid caregivers, she looked as any of us might, given enough decades in old age and care that prioritized the bare necessities. Betty could neither do for herself nor ask her caretakers for the extras that often come to define us: things like a good haircut, a flattering shirt, and, for many pale-skinned women by midlife if not sooner, some foundation face cream and a little rouge or lipstick. In appearance, she embodied people's deepest fears and prejudices about old age, even if once you knew her she was just Betty: widowed wife, former mother's club leader and guild president, proud grandmother, and enduring local team sports fan.

Ironically, Betty was a terrific student "case." From the perspective of medical science, it was remarkable that she had lived into old age. For as long as anyone could remember, her body had needed insulin injections to keep her blood sugar from surging into the territories of coma and death. Diabetes claimed her vision, a good bit of her kidney and heart function, and much of the feeling in her feet and fingertips. Around the time I met her, the first studies had come out showing an association between diabetes and dementia, so even though we didn't yet know whether it would help, as Betty's cognition worsened, I worked hard to keep her sugars fairly normal in the hope of slowing her intellectual losses. That strategy worked really well—until it didn't. One winter, for no apparent reason, she kept landing in the hospital with astronomic blood sugar levels.

I should back up. For several years before and after I took over her care, Betty was one of the most stable patients in our housecalls practice. Although I occasionally spoke to her out-of-town family by telephone, mostly I dealt with her live-in caregivers. Then one day, the surly Filipina who often disappeared downstairs to her room behind the garage after letting me in was replaced by a Tongan woman. Her name was Tokoni, and her personality was as expansive as her tall, soft body. By my second or third visit after her appearance in Betty's life and house, Tokoni was hugging me hello, smiling, joking, and squeezing my arm when I commended her work. Betty seemed to like Tokoni too. She smiled more and began gaining weight.

The only time I remember discussing Tokoni's work situation was the second time I met her, when I asked a few questions in order to update the caregiver section of Betty's social history in our medical record system. For frail patients, it's essential to know the names and contact numbers of the people playing important roles in their lives.

"Who else works here now?" I asked.

"No one," Tokoni replied, grinning and slapping her big thigh. "I am the only one."

We looked at each other. It's illegal to have someone work twenty-four hours a day, seven days a week. Given the state of the house, I doubted Tokoni was paid overtime, though she obviously got room and board, and the twenty-four-hour rule can sometimes be finessed if the caregiver lives in the same house or apartment and isn't technically working at all times. At the very least, caregivers need to be allowed to sleep, and it seemed to me likely that Tokoni slept most nights, since Betty slept a lot even during the day. Still, I could only think of one reason why someone would take such a job. Clearly, Tokoni was not only a woman in later middle age with great intelligence but little education; she was also undocumented.

For a second or two, neither of us blinked while we silently took stock of each other's priorities and position. The facts were these: Betty needed care, her family didn't have much money, and they either couldn't or were unwilling to provide that care themselves. Tokoni needed a job and a place to live and knew how to take care of people, but her legal status left her with few options, and she was satisfied, if not pleased, by her current situation.

While there may be sectors of the economy in which undocumented workers take jobs from Americans, in twenty years of geriatrics, I had only met a handful of working- or lower-middle-class families who had been able to find an American willing to care for their aging relative for a salary they could afford. Even the upper and upper-middle classes, with enough money to pay the going rate or more, struggle to find caregivers. Often, when they do, they pay higher rates, most of which go to agencies, while the caregivers themselves—those people in whose hands a loved one's life and well-being are placed—still receive minimum wage.

My role, it seemed to me, was to make sure my patients got what they needed and that neither they nor their caregivers were endangered. In an ideal world, caregivers would get paid a living wage with benefits and protections, and more people would want to do that work. In the real world, if Betty's family could not hire people like Tokoni, they would put her in a nursing home—a fate she, like most older adults, dreaded. From what I'd seen of the places Betty could afford, and given her complex medical diagnoses and total care needs, it seemed likely she would suffer, then die within a matter of months. If she didn't, the family would need to sell her house to pay for her care, and when the money ran out, Medicaid would take over. Those simple realities made my decision easy. As long as Betty was adequately cared for, I had no intention of making trouble.

Tokoni read my mind. She put her broad, warm hand on my wrist and nodded, sealing our unspoken agreement.

But there was one other question I had to ask. Betty could not be left alone. Lately, when she tried to get up unassisted, she fell. At the same time, it wouldn't be good for either of them if Tokoni was a prisoner in Betty's house.

"Do you ever get out?" I asked.

Tokoni laughed and clapped her hands. "Of course, of course! My sister works just there." She pointed south with her lips and nose. "Just two houses away."

We were both grinning. Tokoni's singsong English and mirth were charming, and I was hugely relieved by her answer.

"Her patient cannot think but can walk. They walk every day, all day long. When I go out, they come here and watch Betty. That way, I go shopping. I go get the medicines. I go wherever."

"Good," I said, trying to make a point indirectly. "You need fresh air and exercise and time off too. If you aren't healthy, Betty won't be either."

Tokoni squeezed my shoulder, a look of delight on her face. "Yes, yes! You are right! I do that. You don't worry."

I couldn't tell whether that was true, but clearly I had pushed far enough. And the rest wasn't necessarily any of my business as long as Tokoni seemed healthy enough herself and continued to take good care of Betty.

Over the next few years, I would sometimes encounter Tokoni's sister, Elenoa, and her charge at Betty's and marvel at how different the sisters were—practically opposites physically and in terms of personality. Elenoa was shy, reserved, and surprisingly slight for a Tongan. I wondered whether they were actually related or merely "sisters" in the sense of compatriots who had bonded to get through the disappointing and difficult realities of life for the undocumented poor in the United States. Then one late winter afternoon a few months after Tokoni told me Betty was less and less able to walk, I arrived for a visit to see if the physical therapy I'd ordered had helped, and Elenoa answered the door. The sisters, she informed me, had traded jobs.

Without elaborating on the when or why of the job exchange, Elenoa stood aside for me to enter the house. On past visits, if she and her former charge had been present, she had always vanished quickly into another room or left the house. Now I noted that—unlike Tokoni, who always wore loud, loose, mismatched shirts and pants—Elenoa had combined similarly bright-colored clothing into an artful, understated outfit.

Her eyes studied the carpet. She seemed uncomfortable and a bit sad. When it became clear she wouldn't speak spontaneously, I asked how Betty was.

"I show you," she said, turning to walk toward Betty's bedroom in the back of the house.

Although considerably smaller and fitter than Tokoni, Elenoa moved in slow motion. She also struggled to answer even fairly straightforward questions. Later in my visit, she took five minutes to get a pill bottle I needed from the next room. I couldn't tell whether she was bored, not fluent in English, not very smart, nervous, depressed, or some combination of all those factors.

After I finished with Betty, I asked to see her blood sugar log. Elenoa looked at me and picked up the phone. A few minutes later, Tokoni showed up.

"Sorry, sorry!" she said, laughing. "Now Betty is too much for me! She need more help. My sister is younger. So we make a trade. Good for everyone, no?!"

I could see her point. The neighbor woman's dementia was more advanced and she no longer spoke, but she was thin, agile, and fit appearing, perhaps because she was constantly in motion. Betty had become voluptuous, and although she could still sit up, she could no longer walk, dress herself, or get to the commode. She went into the living room every day and periodically used her pedal exerciser, but she needed a sling lift to get her out of bed and a wheelchair to get around the house.

"I teach my sister the insulin," Tokoni said. "You no worry. Look, look—how good is Betty?" And she straightened Betty's hair, patted her arm, and grinned.

A few months later, on an early summer's day, Elenoa called to say that Betty was sick. She couldn't sit up or get out of bed. She wouldn't eat. Elenoa couldn't wake her up completely. Maybe Betty was coughing. Maybe she had a fever, or maybe her urine had an unusual odor—potential signs of infection. Though vague on specifics, Elenoa made clear that Betty was sick.

One of my colleagues took the urgent call, then spoke to Betty's grandson, and they sent her to the hospital. Blood tests found her sugar level—less than 110 in healthy people and generally kept at least under 200 in people with diabetes—was over 500. Other blood test results and kidney function were also significantly abnormal. Illness raises the sugar level, even if the person takes their usual medications, pushing them into a cascade of dehydration, higher sugars, dangerous levels of blood salts and acids, coma, and death. Betty had bacteria in her urine and blood. She'd developed a bladder infection, but perhaps because older people usually don't have the same symptoms as younger people with such infections—they are more likely to feel sleepy, fall, become confused, or lose their appetites than to have painful, frequent urination—Elenoa didn't notice. The infection spread to Betty's blood, becoming life-threatening both directly and because of its effect on her diabetes.

Betty was admitted to the intensive care unit. Although she had two serious conditions, she responded well to careful adjustments of fluids, antibiotics, and insulin. Three days after arriving at the hospital, she went home.

The next day, I added her to my morning housecalls schedule.

After I arrived, Elenoa and I exchanged pleasantries, and then she walked not left into the living room but through the dining room toward Betty's bedroom.

"How is she?" I asked.

When people have enough dementia that they give unreliable answers to questions about anything other than that moment in time but not so much mental impairment that they can't tell they are being discussed, I talk to their caregiver or family in another room before seeing them. That's what I would have done with Betty, except I'd already learned that Elenoa didn't feel comfortable with that approach. If I asked her about Betty's eating, sleeping, and other activities in the hallway, she gave answers that suggested she thought her role was to guess what I wanted rather than provide me with facts.

"She is okay," Elenoa said.

"Has she gotten out of bed?"

"Not yet."

By this time, we were almost at Betty's open bedroom door. I had time for just one more question.

"Has she eaten?"

"Last night."

What I really wanted to know was whether Betty was back to herself. Often when older people end up the hospital, even for a few days, the focus is on fixing the medical issue—in Betty's case, out-of-control diabetes, and bladder and blood infections. Little attention is paid to what illness and a few days in bed can do to the person, and too often people who didn't know a frail older person before their hospitalization will assume they couldn't walk or think clearly in the first place. And sometimes they couldn't, but everyone has a functional baseline. It's hard for hospital doctors and nurses to assess whether someone is back to a baseline they've never seen. In the days when the same doctor took care of a patient in clinic and in the hospital, that doctor would know. Now hospital staff must rely on family or caregiver reports, but what two different people mean by "He walks normally" or "She's totally with it" can differ dramatically.

Betty was asleep. At least, I hoped she was asleep.

I put down my bags and said hello. No response. I touched her shoulder and shook her gently, knowing full well that I wasn't trying very hard.

Her eyes opened.

"Hi," I said using *Ms.* and her last name, and then *Dr.* and mine.

Her lids fluttered and her lips parted into the best smile she could muster with a dry mouth.

"Hello," she said. "You're here early."

It was morning but no longer early. On the other hand, how could she know that when she didn't have enough vision to tell day from night?

Betty's tongue moved inside her mouth and along her lips.

"Would you like a drink?" I asked.

She nodded. Elenoa and I exchanged a glance, and she left the room.

As I asked Betty questions—Was she in pain? Where had she been the last few days? Who was the president? What was her favorite football team?—I turned on my computer. By the time the hospital had sent her home, Betty's blood sugar and salts had returned to normal and a specialized diabetes test had come back. Unlike a blood sugar level, which measures a single moment in time, the Hemoglobin A1c test gives a sense of the sugar levels over a six-week period. If you think of blood sugar level as how a student does on one quiz, then A1c is more like their grade for the semester.

For the first that we knew of, not only had Betty badly failed the quiz, but her grade for the entire term was also in jeopardy. Her A1c wasn't awful, but it was higher than it had been in all the years I'd cared for her.

The hospital doctors said she needed more medicine. They recommended increasing her long-acting insulin and maybe adding a second type of insulin, suggestions they made with a familiar, irritating confidence. If you're a primary care doctor and work mostly in clinics, not hospitals, the tone says they are smarter than you and that you have screwed up and that's why your patient is in the hospital.

But in caring for Betty, they were more like the blood sugar level and I was more like the A1c, so I knew they were treating a symptom and not the underlying problem. Yes, Betty's sugars were higher, but why?

Though she had bruises up and down her arms from hospital IVs and blood draws, Betty seemed back to normal mentally and, for the most part, physically. Looking at her, a person from a distant land might think the hospital staff had beat her up, not saved her life.

After Elenoa set Betty up with water and the start of her breakfast, I asked her to join me in the kitchen. A person's blood sugar can go up for many reasons, the most common being a change in diet, activity, or medications. Elenoa assured me that before the hospitalization Betty had been eating the same amount of the same foods she always ate and nothing else about her routine or activity level had changed. Although it was possible she was deceiving me, it seemed unlikely. While Elenoa had still been in with Betty, I'd had a look around. There was fruit in a bowl and the refrigerator had a good range of foods, including two prepared meals wrapped in cellophane. That meant I needed to review Betty's medications.

Elenoa produced a stack of papers from the hospital. The one that mattered listed Betty's medications. I compared it with the list I had and Elenoa's, which was years old with a few lines crossed out and added over time. I was relieved to find complete concordance among the three, something that should happen every time a patient goes home from the hospital but which is too often the exception not the rule.

Next, I asked Elenoa to show me the bottles for Betty's medication and tell me what she gave her and when.

She opened one bottle and turned it until a pill dropped onto her palm. "This one in the morning only," she said.

She closed that bottle and opened another. "Morning and after dinner," she said.

Watching her hands, and the little lines that appeared around her eyes as she stared at the pills, I realized Elenoa was older than I'd always thought, probably in her late fifties or early sixties. I'd been fooled by her graceful movements and lovely skin.

She continued dropping pills into her palm until she'd been through each bottle, both the prescription medications and the over-the-counter vitamin D. At no time did Elenoa consult any of the medication lists, nor did she read the pill bottles. And she didn't look at me once as she did this or when she finished.

Oh, I thought, maybe Elenoa can't read. At the very least she couldn't read well enough to do it in front of me. Trying to pretend I hadn't just realized what I'd realized or noticed her shame, I said, "Terrific. It looks like you're doing everything just right, and we don't need to change any medications, so you're all set. Can you show me her insulin too?"

Elenoa went to the refrigerator and showed me the vials lined up on a shelf in the door. Betty took two types, and Elenoa knew which was which and how much to give of each.

Then something occurred to me. If Elenoa couldn't read, maybe she didn't know numbers either. I hesitated for a minute, not wanting to make her feel worse. But then I did what I had to do for Betty's sake. I made my tone warm and supportive, knowing full well Elenoa would not be fooled.

"Can you show me how you draw up the insulin?"

Moving even more slowly than usual, she picked up a syringe from the stack of them in a bowl on the counter and took a vial of insulin from the refrigerator. She placed them side-by-side on the countertop. Then she walked across the room and returned with a small square I recognized right away as an alcohol wipe. She tore it open, wiped the top of the vial, then paused. She seemed to be considering crossing the room again to discard the wipe and its wrapper. To my relief, she instead plunged the needle through the rubber lid. Turning toward the ceiling light, she pulled back on the plunger. For a moment, she didn't move at all. She adjusted the plunger a last time and, without looking at me, handed me the syringe.

I looked at it and again worked to soften and neutralize my tone. "So this is what you'll give her now, with breakfast?"

Elenoa nodded.

As gently as I could, I said, "Can you show me where the twenty is on the syringe?" I held it out. She took it and again turned toward the light. She squinted.

"Here."

Elenoa was pointing at the right place on the syringe, but the clear insulin was way below that line, and there was a huge air bubble in the middle of the fluid. By my estimate, the syringe would give Betty ten to twelve units of insulin, not twenty.

I don't remember how I responded in that instant. I do remember thinking, Aha, and Oh, my God.

Whether or not Elenoa was literate remained unclear, but one thing was certain: she couldn't see well. And she couldn't do much about the problem with no health insurance and a poverty-level wage—most of which, I would later learn from Tokoni, Elenoa sent back to her children and mother in Tonga.

"The insulin isn't right," I said. Then I took off my glasses. "Without these, I couldn't get it right either."

She looked at me and we both half smiled.

If Elenoa couldn't read the amount of insulin, she could give Betty too little, raising her sugar and increasing her risk of infection, heart attack, confusion, incontinence, and a variety of other problems. If she gave too much, she could kill Betty. I wanted to be kind and a bit funny to lighten the situation, but it was serious, and Elenoa knew it as well as I did. I tried to think through work-arounds. After all, Betty's family could not afford standard, agency-based in-home care, and Elenoa needed a home and a job. While she couldn't see well, she could provide most of what Betty needed. Maybe, I thought, I could find a pharmacy that would pre-fill the syringes, and Elenoa could give the injections. But that would be expensive.

We had a big problem, and then, in the same instant, Elenoa and I had the same idea.

"Tokoni," she said, and with relief I nodded my agreement.

## DUALITY

"I seem to have entered a new phase," my mother informs me two months before her eighty-fourth birthday. "There just aren't men anymore." The evening before, she had been with a large group of friends, all women. One was divorced; another still had a husband, but he was quite ill. Every one of the others, herself included, was a widow. She's not looking for romance, she clarifies, just normalcy. "It's unnatural," she adds. "This huge part of life is missing." She found it strange and sad to think that the rest of her life would have this significant absence.

Across locations and racial, economic, and ethnic groups, my mother's experience is typical. Old age is profoundly gendered. Its skew hurts both men and women, though in different ways. Women are 51 percent of the population overall but 57 percent of people over sixty-five, 68 percent over eighty-five, and 83 percent of centenarians. The gender imbalance of advanced old age dates back to at least the twelfth century in western Europe. Women haven't outlived men in all countries and decades since then, but they almost always have. Some people think this makes advanced old age a women's health issue.

Surely, it also makes it a men's health issue—or, more accurately, a men's health crisis. Why do men so consistently die sooner than females? If men can live into very old age but most don't, and if the system is designed with them in mind, then is the problem that more care does more harm or that living into old age depends on more than biology? When I mention this glaring imbalance in public, people always call out certain facts: men are less likely to go to doctors; we raise them to be stoic, to endure, to not show weakness, so they wait longer before seeking help; men don't like to follow someone else's direction and are less likely than women to adhere to medical recommendations; men still carry the societal expectation of excellence and providing, and those stresses erode their health; men take more risks. The list goes on, but these are the possibilities that always come up. The answer is likely a mix of these and other social and biological factors. Given how consistently men die before women, you'd think addressing this disparity would be a major goal of medicine. It isn't.

The relative longevity of females has long confounded doctors, particularly in the years when menopause meant old age. They noted that common diseases afflicted women earlier than men, a phenomenon that seemed linked to menopause. For centuries, now debunked humoralism offered an explanation: the acquisition of diseases and debilities with age was unsurprising after bad humors ceased being expelled from the body through menstruation. Still, doctors didn't pay much attention to uniquely female aspects of aging. The prototypical patient in textbooks was male (good old "Norm," still in many medical schools today), and aging female organs received far less study or commentary than the aging penis and prostate.

Because men are more valued for their achievements, power, and money and less for their appearance, age can offer them benefits in a way it rarely does for women. This is less the case now than in past years, but the primary target demographic of the trillion-dollar cosmetics industry confirms the ongoing import of a certain sort of appearance for women, even those who have achieved the most prized sorts of professional success.

When we care about something, when we really need it, we usually pay for it. In medicine urologists make more than gynecologists, although both do medicine and surgery. In fact, urology patients are much older than gynecology ones on average, so it may be that gender trumps age in terms of value, or it did in the middle of the last century when specialty prices and prestige were established. When it comes to old age, we worry there aren't enough caregivers, yet as other jobs disappear with technological advances, we continue to pay caregivers—mostly women doing traditionally "female" tasks—nothing or low wages. These are among the ways we compound existing social inequities. Just as women make less money if they have kids but men do not, the mostly female people who are caregivers for older adults make less money immediately and over a lifetime, accruing less retirement and benefits because they must reduce the number of hours they work, take a leave, retire, or change jobs. Not surprisingly, women are more likely to be poor in old age.

Twenty-first-century elderhood consists of dying men and impoverished women. We must be doing something wrong.


CARE


"She's just screaming and saying her leg hurts," said the hospitalist when I responded to his page. "I can't get anything out of her, and the husband is nowhere to be found. Does she have a leg problem?"

Every month or two, I visited Inez's one-bedroom apartment in a run-down subsidized housing building just blocks from the heart of the Castro. Getting to her required surmounting a gauntlet of minor hurdles. First, I had to be buzzed in, at least in theory. It was never clear who, if anyone, was responsible for the main door buzzer, and as often as not, no one answered. Fortunately, people often milled in the entryway and common area just inside the glass front door. Many ignored me, but eventually someone would let me in. Sometimes that person appeared to be a rent-a-cop, an ever-changing cast of characters of diverse ages and races wearing an uncomfortable-looking uniform. The official would size me up and ask for identification. They didn't want my medical center badge but would painstakingly copy my name from my driver's license onto a sheet of paper used to log the visit date and time of entry and exit. Finally, they would nod, and I'd turn toward the nearby elevators.

But by then I would have attracted the attention of the residents in the common room. I never visited without being approached by one of those not necessarily old people sitting in wheelchairs in the lobby, watching the passersby on their colorful block midway between a huge Catholic church and a commercial intersection where businesses had names like Rock Hard and Does Your Mother Know. They seemed starved for conversation. Sometimes one would accompany me up to Inez's floor, chatting as the elevator lurched slowly upward. I then walked to the far end of a long, dimly lit hallway, passing the open door to at least one apartment where loud music, pulled shades, and glassy eyes suggested active drug use. It was for these reasons that Inez's husband, Esteban, needed to hear my voice before he'd open the door with a huge smile and a warm "¡Doctora!"

But two days before the hospitalist's call, there had been no smile. Instead, he had said, "Passa," and led me quickly back to their bedroom. There, Inez, obese and bedbound with moderately severe vascular dementia, lay propped up in her hospital bed, her mouth open and chest visibly rising and falling. A quick assessment revealed low oxygen levels, high pulse and blood pressure, and what might have been hard-to-hear breath sounds in one lung. Because of her size and inability to move in bed or take deep breaths on command, Inez's lung exam was always difficult.

I had Esteban give her one of her nebulized breathing treatments while I called an ambulance and the emergency department.

At her most healthy, Inez had a significant array of active and debilitating medical diagnoses and, despite my best efforts, an obscenely long list of medications. Now it seemed she had pneumonia, an asthma exacerbation, and—because of underlying conditions and acute illness—some heart failure and dehydration as well. However, neither that day nor previously in the two years I'd been her doctor had she had a "leg problem."

"If her leg hurts, that's new," I told the hospitalist over the phone.

"Did she fall at home?"

"She's been bedbound for years," I said. "Doesn't even try to get up at this point. Can she describe the pain?"

"She's just screaming. Won't answer questions. The resident gave her something, so I'll go by and try again in a bit."

"That's not her baseline," I said, meaning Inez's usual behavior and ability to communicate.

When she was well, Inez answered my questions to the best of her ability, speaking to that moment in time with accuracy even if she couldn't say much about the hours or days preceding it. She could list perhaps two of her medical conditions and one of her medications, and only in Spanish. She never screamed or hallucinated or behaved in the way the hospitalist was describing. Even on days when Inez didn't feel well, she greeted me with a smile and asked after my family. Sometimes, too, I got a glimpse of who she had been before her strokes and the dementia, the person she sometimes still was. If I happened to be wearing a colorful shirt or sweater, she commented on how nice I looked and had me turn or come close so she could inspect the fabric and tailoring. Best of all, a few weeks before her hospitalization, she had offered the Spanish equivalent of "va-va-voom" to me behind the backs of her husband and our clinic's new, tall, and broad-shouldered social worker as soon as the men's attention was elsewhere. Then she raised her bushy eyebrows and winked her good eye at me as if to say did I really think I could fool her into believing it was mere coincidence that I was wearing a skirt on the exact same day I arrived to see her accompanied by such a handsome man?

I quickly relayed some of this to the hospitalist, listening to the background noises of a busy hospital on his end of the line. He was probably standing at the nurses' station.

"Could be a DVT," he said, meaning a blood clot in the leg.

I had another concern. "She's big and deadweight. Something could have happened when the paramedics were moving her or since she got to the hospital."

I felt certain no injury had occurred at home. Esteban was a meticulous caretaker. He checked and double-checked Inez's pills, carefully arranging them in a large pillbox. When they were short on money, he gave her meat and ate only beans himself. Although also eighty years old, with his wiry body and easy grin, he sometimes seemed more like Inez's son than her husband. Still, if he had dropped her in a transfer from bed to wheelchair, he would have needed help to get her up, and I would have heard about it. By my estimation, he weighed about 140 pounds and she was well over 200.

"Right," said the hospitalist, his tone making clear Inez's home situation and cognitive and functional baselines were of no interest to him. "I'm thinking clot, fracture, dislocation, maybe even a large bruise or wound we missed when she came in."

I had entered the same list into my note as we spoke, with one addition: the need for repositioning.

"I can't explain this," I said, "but she always lies on her right side. If I move her during my exam, she's uncomfortable. Her husband says it's been like that for years."

The hospitalist made a sound that might have been an unsuccessfully suppressed sigh.

"I know it sounds crazy," I said, "but someone should check her position in the bed and put her on her right side if she isn't already." Imagining his eye roll, I added, "If it works, it'll save your intern time and the health care system the cost of X-rays she doesn't need."

"Let's walk through the plan," he said, and began outlining his thoughtful treatments for Inez's atrial fibrillation, pneumonia, and volume overload. Before hanging up, I repeated my suggestion about repositioning her as a first step for the leg pain, since, if successful, in addition to the benefits I'd already listed for him, it would relieve her pain and eliminate the need for the pain medications that were worsening her confusion and chronic constipation. Again, he didn't respond.

Here were the cultural divides between inpatient and outpatient care and between internal medicine and geriatrics. My colleague focused exclusively on diseases and X-rays and medications, not seeing that, for a frail older adult like Inez, information about her baseline function and home situation was equally important—particularly since, with sickness layered over her dementia, she was unable to communicate her norms and needs for herself.

After hanging up, I called Esteban. Having first cared for his increasingly ill wife over two days and nights at home and then waiting the better part of a third night with her in the emergency department, he had gone home to sleep but was heading back to the hospital shortly. No one had phoned to tell him how Inez was doing, so I explained that her breathing was better, but she was in pain. I asked him to move her into a more comfortable position if he could when he arrived, and he said he would.

That evening, Esteban left me a voice mail. He reported with obvious pleasure and relief that Inez was much better. Then he added that she'd had awful leg pain when he'd first arrived, but once he'd moved her onto her right side, the pain went away. He said the nurses told him that she could probably return home the next day.

I logged into our electronic record and read through the normal X-rays of Inez's pelvis, hip, leg, and knee. There was no mention of her bed position in any of the doctors' notes. I was reminded of a comment by a medical student after a visit to an impressive and all-inclusive site for the care for the elderly. The student, just months shy of his MD, had commented, "That's not medicine, that's just taking care of patients."

## EDUCATION

Less than two decades into the twenty-first century, medical education has changed in unprecedented ways. Pedagogically, we have shifted from *what we want to teach* to *what learners need to know*. In the digital age, "textbooks" are interactive, nonlinear, and multimedia. Students gather for active learning in small groups while lectures are podcasted or streamed; use of stories, gaming, videos, and other forms of so-called edutainment are often required. With the rise of the quality and safety movement, we have incorporated into every level of education attention to systems, interprofessional teamwork, and quality improvement. In response to society's need for more primary care physicians and in recognition that most doctors spend a majority of their work time in clinics, not hospitals, we have developed outpatient rotations for core clinical training. We increasingly ask learners to look beyond organ systems at common genetic, metabolic, and immune system pathways. For the first time in 2016, the licensing body for medical education in the United States required programs to ensure clinical competence across the entire human life span.

Still, much of what was taught and emphasized in my medical school days remains prominent. Most doctors in training still get intensive exposure to the populations that dominated health care a century ago, when most Americans died before becoming old. Students do the same core rotations I did twenty-five years ago—largely the same core ones my father did in the 1950s when the average age at death was sixty-eight. Today, a sixty-five-year-old can expect to live another twenty-five years (half will live longer than that), octogenarians are forty-eight times more prevalent, and "old" includes people two and three generations apart. That's why almost all doctors see old patients. People over sixty-five account for over 30 percent of patients seen in surgery, psychiatry, and neurology; over 40 percent in internal medicine, orthopedics, and emergency medicine; and more than half of patients in cardiology and ophthalmology. All those doctors learned about each other's specialties, and they spent months learning about the care of children and pregnant women, though most don't treat either of those groups. Only a small minority received specific training in the care of old people, and some of that training, even today, isn't really geriatrics at all. Instead, it's traditional education about diseases that occur more commonly with age. Geriatrics isn't just about *who* is being treated or *what* diseases they have; it's also about *how* and *where* they are cared for and *what* and *who else* besides usual medicine and doctors might help their health and well-being.

If you look at the curricular overview maps for schools from the perpetually top-ranked Harvard Medical School to the much-lauded newcomer, Dell School of Medicine in Austin, Texas, you will see the same things: required rotations in surgery and medicine, pediatrics and women's health, and psychiatry and neurology, but no mention of aging or geriatrics. Almost without exception, learning about the specialized care of old people is an elective endeavor left to each student's interests and discretion.

It's worth considering how and why a group with a growing social footprint and significant health care utilization and costs—one that an overwhelming majority of clinicians interact with regularly—might be relegated to a status other than required in medical curricula. And it's worth considering how bright young people can enter medical school intent on learning as much as they can in order to take good care of all patients but, after an average of about twelve teaching sessions about older patients, think they've learned enough.

There are some great innovations in med schools all across the country. Many of these new models may improve training and care, but most haven't questioned the fundamental structures and assumptions of medicine.

A randomized clinical trial found that medical students who completed a clerkship year containing a specialized rotation in geriatrics (as they already do in pediatrics and adult medicine) acquired more knowledge and skills in geriatric care than did students who did not—a conclusion that may seem self-evident. But something else about this study is disturbing: the specialized geriatric clerkship did little to improve students' attitudes toward old patients.

Another study illustrated how our definitions of medicine and medical care, as well as the structure and priorities of our health care system, put health professionals off old patients. Among the seventeen identified themes were despair at the futility of care, being unsure how to handle ethical dilemmas, and feeling depressed by the decline and death of their patients. Medical students also reported frustration at low reimbursement rates and low prestige despite fellowship training. Although they found communicating with older adults enjoyable, it was also time-consuming and challenging.

Their comments illustrate failings of medical culture, medical education, society, and our health care system. Taking each item in turn: *Care* is never futile, though *treatment* can be. Too often those two words are used interchangeably, though they have very different meanings. Given how commonly ethical dilemmas occur across medical specialties and how important they are, students must be given sufficient training to feel as comfortable with them as they are made to feel sticking metal and plastic into living human beings. If not, we aren't preparing them for medical practice.

Considerable evidence shows that a great many Americans do indeed receive futile or harmful treatment, particularly late in life or at the end of life. We should be relieved that young doctors want to avoid the moral and medical distress of futile care for their patients, and change the system that causes that kind of harm to patients and clinicians. Society and medicine both need to build better systems for dealing with aging and death. Those facts of life are not improved by attitudes and reimbursement policies that make them harder than they already are existentially. Almost everyone is happier doing work, no matter how difficult it is, if they feel able to do it well and appropriately recognized for their efforts.

We teach doctors in training that certain things are important and others are not. If medical education wants to produce clinicians able to provide safe, evidence-based, high-quality, high-satisfaction care to patients of all ages, we must do more than include the entire human life span somewhere in doctor training, as the 2016 mandate requires. We should instead retire the centuries-old adult-as-norm model. Children and old people are 40 percent of the population and over half of health care utilization—numbers likely to keep climbing. Treating them as exceptions is demographically and biologically inaccurate. A better approach would replace our current "normal

+ variants" approach to organs, diseases, and specialties with an equally weighted child-adult-elder lens.

Here's what an age-inclusive curriculum might look like: When medical students are taught normal anatomy, physiology, and pharmacology, they would learn the norms at all three major life phases. When they learn about diseases and pathophysiology, their curriculum would include classic presentations in patients of all ages, as well as conditions unique to each life stage. And when they do core rotations, their training would expose them to the full diversity of specialties, clinical settings, and approaches to care with the simultaneous goals of ensuring broad general competence in graduates, providing students with the necessary experiences to make informed career decisions, and producing a workforce that meets society's needs.

## RESILIENCE

Approaching her eighty-sixth year, my mother says to me: "There are just so many things I have to do in the morning. I have to put the drops in my dry eyes. I have to take my thyroid medicine right away so it's on an empty stomach but I can still have breakfast at a reasonable hour. I have to do the neti pot with my nose or it runs all day and I cough. I have to put the cream on my face for the rosacea. I have to do my stretches and exercises to loosen up my parts and get them going. I have to get my hearing aids in and then pin back my hair because I can't put it behind my ears anymore with my glasses and hearing aids already there. It's incredible to think I used to just get up, wash my face and start my day."

This is true of all parts of her life, yet in her old age, my mother never ceases to amaze me with her resilience. Widowed and with friends dying at regular intervals, some expected, others suddenly, she sometimes seems sad but never depressed, and she sometimes complains, but minutes later she's back to living her life and commenting on the world's larger issues. "I'm trying to be low-maintenance," she tells me. "Until I can't be."

I hope I'm like her in thirty years, and I feel certain that hers is a standard I will not attain. Some people are more resilient than others.

I'm making progress, but that particular form of toughness isn't one of my strengths.

In medicine these days, resilience is a popular concept. Some considered it the profession's number one weapon against burnout. Like many medical centers, mine now sends out e-mails touting opportunities for resilience training. I delete those e-mails. I'd rather learn my resilience outside the institutions that claim they want to help me cultivate it while continuing the structural injustices that jeopardize it. Nationwide, health care's medicine-as-business mentality, "death by a thousand clicks" electronic record systems, and antisocial priorities harm patients, waste money, and erode clinician morale.

Some of the techniques I've used to make myself healthier are addressed in resilience training: regular exercise and meals, enough sleep, days off, and replenishing activities. Of course, another way to describe these things is "a healthy lifestyle." But modern medicine doesn't support healthy lifestyles among its practitioners any more than it emphasizes health and wellness in patient care.

After I quit the ACE unit, I had trouble finding clinical work as a geriatrician in our health system. I could no longer drive reliably enough to do housecalls. I didn't seem to have the mettle for what passed as eldercare in the hospital, and my institution's sole outpatient geriatrics clinic was small, without room for another clinician. I could have changed systems, but there were wonderful colleagues, inspiring students, and many other parts of my job that made me eager to stay. In the end, I did what geriatricians do best: I took all my knowledge and experience, looked around at both what existed and what was needed, and came up with a creative, pragmatic, evidence-based, and socially useful solution. I decided to try and start a new clinic that would approach elderhood the way pediatricians approach childhood. It would combine the best of modern medicine's disease-fighting ability and the best of traditional geriatrics' function and personal priority-based care with the wellness and health promotion emphasis of the new specialty called integrative medicine. The new clinic's goal would be to help old people in all stages of old age optimize their health, lives, and well-being.

New clinics, even when they are just clinical sessions added into an existing practice in a thriving health system, don't take shape overnight. Before I could get started, I had to get support from institution leaders, develop a self-sustaining business model, learn more about prevention, health maintenance, and wellness, and decide how the new clinic could be most useful to older San Franciscans. That turned out to be a lot of fun. Clearly, I was coming out of my burnout.

It's impossible to avoid medicine's resilience evangelists. They are everywhere. At a continuing education training in another state, I was seated in the middle of a large auditorium of doctors when our next speakers announced they would be talking about burnout. One was a medical school dean, the other a program leader. Their presentation offered resilience-building exercises and tools.

After maybe half an hour, I went to the microphone and asked if they would be discussing any of the structural contributors to burnout. One of them assured me that they would be. As I walked back to my seat, doctors I didn't know nodded or gave me a thumbs-up. And then one of the speakers commented that there is lots of blame casting in the world and they wanted to take a different focus.

In my chair, I kept my face blank. It is typical in medicine to reduce complex problems to singular perspectives and solutions. As an educator, I know the most worrisome students are those who always blame others for their challenges, and as a professional I know that systems that similarly don't carefully examine their own assumptions and actions in contributing to problems will never solve those problems. What I was suggesting was not the abdication of personal responsibility but that burnout could not be addressed without looking both at individuals *and* at the structures and culture of medicine: the powerful doing what the powerful do; the culture following money, not values; the politics that shape so much of our lives.

Not everyone is burned out, so clearly individual factors matter. But if over half of doctors are, and if that was not always the case, and if in study after study people list the same systemic and cultural contributors, it seems fair to me to discuss those issues, as well as ones of personal resilience.

Next the two doctor-leaders showed a slide about leadership in the age of burnout. I look up their bios online. They were people who make institutional policies: well-meaning shepherds who think they can address cultural and structural problems by sheer force of will and good intentions. Despite being doctors, their slides suggested that they didn't realize their approach mostly palliated symptoms rather than addressing underlying causes. As the writer-photographer-critic Teju Cole has written about a human rights and social injustice journalist, "All he sees is need, and he sees no need to reason out the need for the need." In medicine, the need is burnout, and the need for the need is American health care's morally distressing norms, structures, and policies.

I have become more resilient since my burnout. I take better care of myself using many of the tools in their presentation, and others. But because it so often feels like doctor-leaders are themselves casting blame on those of us in moral distress, one of the most effective tools I use is the one that tells me when to be honest with other people about what happened to me and when to lie. That one is easy to apply: if a doctor asks, I usually lie; if anyone else inquires, I tell the truth. Among doctors, normal human emotions are still seen as evidence of weakness.

Cultivating resilience doesn't mean never feeling sad or angry. It's about contentment and the happiness born of connection, meaning, and purpose. With aging and in old age, resilience requires accepting you are still yourself despite changes, losses, and limitations and recognizing your ongoing personal and spiritual development. It means finding a purpose that may differ from prior goals and inspires learning or helping someone else or going somewhere new. It requires knowing what matters most to you, being clear with others about your priorities, and living in an environment that meets your needs, optimizing your independence and comfort. Resilience emerges when a solid dose of optimism is tempered with just enough pessimism to match goals with realities.

Anne Fadiman's father lost his sight at age eighty-eight. In the hospital after being told his one seeing eye could not be saved, he told her his life was no longer worth living. People feel this way for many different reasons. For Clifton Fadiman, a huge reader and critic, two reasons stood out: he didn't want to burden his wife, and he would no longer be able to read. Anne asked him to wait six months before doing anything about wanting to die. He agreed. A short while later he attended a program for visually impaired persons and described his first day there as perhaps the most interesting day of his life. The program gave him strategies for independence that helped him be less of a burden and do much of what he enjoyed most. He lived many more years, and after his death his daughter wrote:

> I believe the period between my father's first class at [the low-vision program] and his final illness was in many ways one of the happiest of his life. This was in spite of his age; in spite of his losses; in spite of the moment every morning when he awoke from a dream in which he was invariably sighted, and then remembered he wasn't. It is said that old people can keep their minds agile by learning how to speak Italian or play the oboe. My father learned how to be blind . . . He had considered himself a coward. Now he knew he wasn't.

A blind old man sitting in a chair listening to a book or the radio may not meet many people's criterion of courage. In these early years of the age of elderhood, a time when most people still fear and dread the label and reality of *old*, the failing seems less one in the concept of courage and more in the imaginations of those who can't see it in all its forms.

## ATTITUDE

In "Letter from Greenwich Village," Vivian Gornick describes encountering a short stretch of newly poured concrete on an icy winter's morning in Manhattan. Workmen had left a wood plank and flimsy rail for pedestrians. She was about to cross when she saw a "tall, painfully thin, and fearfully old" man at the other end. Wordlessly, she held out a hand for him. Wordlessly, he took it and came across. Face-to-face on the icy New York street, the man was the first to speak. This is how Gornick describes the entirety of their conversation:

> "Thank you," he says. "Thank you very much." A thrill runs through me. "You're welcome," I say, in a tone that I hope is as plain as his. We each then go our separate ways, but I feel that "thank you" running through my veins all the rest of the day.

At first, given the mundanity of this exchange, we can only guess at the source of Gornick's thrill. Maybe there was something about him—his looks, gaze, or manner—that she found unusual or surprising, sexy or familiar. She doesn't keep us in suspense:

> It was his voice that had done it. That voice! Strong, vibrant, self-possessed: it did not know it belonged to an old man. There was in it not a hint of that beseeching tone one hears so often in the voice of an old person when small courtesies are shown . . . as though the person is apologizing for the room he or she is taking up in the world.

This anecdote is equally remarkable for Gornick's insights into our cultural norms of old age as for the man's defiance of them. The traits she ascribes to his voice are ordinary in the larger realm of adult voices. What made them noteworthy was her expectation (and likely ours) that strength and self-possession are invariably lost by the time a person becomes frail and "fearfully old." The man's tone implies that the meekness so common in older voices is not intrinsic to their owner's chronological station. That means our usual social stance in advanced old age is unnecessary and, worse, that we who are not yet old are colluding with those who are to perpetuate this demeaning cultural behavior.

One centenarian, Diana Athill, whose most recent books were written in a care home, says that in old age "one's chief concern must be how to get oneself through time with the minimum of discomfort to self and inconvenience to others."

The man's voice, Gornick tells us, "did not know" it was supposed to beseech. It didn't believe the sort of person who occasionally needs assistance of others is faulty and culpable. It didn't subscribe to the human worth metrics of ability and self-sufficiency that have been revered since the Industrial Revolution. Immune to current social norms—rules based on assumptions that older individuals are burdens, that older adults as a group are a problem to be solved and a catastrophe of tsunami proportions, and that helping them is inconvenient—the man's tone divorced his frailty from its customary accompaniments of apology and neediness.

The exceptionality the old man displayed after crossing the icy plank differs fundamentally from the "exceptional senior" championed in the media—the octogenarian gymnast or custodian; the nonagenarian grocery bagger, assembly line worker, product designer, or CEO; or the centenarian marathon runner. Those supposed exemplars are indeed exceptions, often as much because of their abilities or courage to redefine work and who does it as because of their age. By contrast, the man in Gornick's anecdote did something ordinary, something any one of us could do: he retained his agency, self-respect, and perspective, assessing the scale of the help Gornick offered and replying with commensurate, rather than elaborate, thanks.

I suspect there is a second reason why the man's voice stuck with Gornick all day. Toward the end of the scene, she says that as they "stood together—he not pleading, I not patronizing—the mask of old age slipped from his face, the mask of vigor dropped from mine." Given the essay's date of publication, Gornick would have been in her mid- to later seventies when she played the role of the younger person in this scenario, the one lending a hand and making an effort not to flaunt her vigor or patronize the older person. That's unlikely the age most readers who don't know her would assume when reading these excerpts, making them all the more powerful. Directly and indirectly, Gornick reminds us that old age is only partially determined by biology. It's long, varied, relative, and relational. By contrast, our assumptions about old age often persist in the face of refuting evidence, which may be why so many people deny their old age until they are frail. Anecdotes like Gornick's demonstrate the physical changes of old age and the experiences we have as a result of them are not linked by some biological necessity beyond our control. It also makes me wonder how often I, intending to offer help and care, am actually contributing to what might be called "an attitude of frailty."

What, then, is the "right" attitude about old age? There are well-known positives of our third act beyond not being dead. Strengths. Joys. A satisfaction with the self as is. A lesser striving for external validation. Newfound freedoms. A clearer sense of what matters. Of course these aren't the case in every life, any more than the positives in younger years are. Since studies of life satisfaction in wealthy English-speaking countries show marked increases in old age, and also marked ageism, we can only imagine the potential satisfactions of aging in a culture that doesn't ignore or deride old people.

Importantly, a person's attitude about oldness doesn't just affect how they feel about growing or being old; it affects their health, how they spend their time, and how long they live. Preventive health measures improve health at all ages, yet older adults are the age group least likely to engage in them. In one study controlled for age, race, gender, education, self-rated health, and function, people with more positive attitudes about aging practiced more preventive health behaviors such as exercise, nutritious eating, and taking prescription medications as directed. In another notable study, people ranging in age from sixty-one to ninety-nine showed more improved physical function from an intervention that strengthened positive age stereotypes than from an exercise intervention.

Beliefs about aging are self-fulfilling prophesies; our health and wellbeing in old age often become what we imagine they will be, whether what we imagine is good or bad. Biology matters, but it's only one part of a far more complex equation that includes attitude, behaviors, relationships, and culture. That's a terrifying thought in a culture where ageism is more common than sexism or racism, and most people of all ages see old age through a window rendered dark and dirty by negative stereotypes. But there's hope—beliefs have frequently changed through history, and for individuals, they can change at any age. And when beliefs about elderhood change, the culture and experience of old age, in life and in medicine, will change too.

## DESIGN

I heard about the new building for months before I saw it. Part of a leading medical center, its "green" architecture and design were getting a lot of attention, as was its integration of top-notch modern medicine with health and wellness spaces inspired by cultures from around the world. My father's doctor had moved there, and driving to his appointment we looked forward to experiencing the cutting-edge new building firsthand.

Outside, I unloaded his walker and led my father through the sliding glass doors. Inside, there was a single bench clearly made of recycled materials but without the arm supports a frail elder requires to safely sit down and get back up. It was a long trek to the correct clinic, and I was double-parked outside. "Wait here," I said, hoping he would remember to do so long enough for me to park and return.

He nodded. We were used to this. It happened almost everywhere we went: at restaurants, the bank, movie theaters, the airport, the hospital, City Hall, and department stores. Like the new clinic, many of these places were gorgeous—historic City Hall with its wide steps and renovated dome; trendy restaurants where design features served as metaphors for food that could pass as fine art; a futuristic movie theater.

Not one of them was set up to facilitate access by someone like my father. That may have been intentional. A few years earlier, I'd heard about our supposedly ultra-welcoming city's new LGBTQ community center, where the older adult program was positioned so attendees entered via a nondescript side entrance in order not to "scare off" the younger people the center hoped to attract.

Such approaches may make sense from a business perspective—or might have, until recently. Philosophical arguments for less ageism aside, demographic realities are increasingly creating financial and practical reasons to build more senior-friendly homes, businesses, health care facilities, and public buildings.

Healthy, literate adults can successfully navigate any structure. There may be frustration with confusing signage and other inconveniences, but they manage. The same cannot be said for old people with one or more physical, sensory, and cognitive challenges, or for the frail elderly who have many. The

Americans with Disabilities Act's accessibility design standards help, but do not ensure access or safety for this unique and rapidly growing population.

To some, this may sound like a small issue, a special interest group adding its lament to the cacophony of gripes about modern life. It's not. Eleven million Americans—the fastest-growing segment of the population—are over age eighty. Over forty million Americans are sixty-five years old or older, a group that is accustomed to active, engaged lives and has considerable financial power.

Too often, current buildings turn impairments—a bum leg, less-than-perfect hearing, the inability to walk long distances—into handicaps. Ironically, this includes not just restaurants, multilevel houses, and large businesses but most health care structures. I heard about this regularly in my years as a housecalls doctor. While patients often end up in our Care at Home practice because they can no longer leave their homes, not infrequently the problem is at the other end: the hospital or clinic is too difficult to navigate.

It wasn't until I left my father at the much-lauded green clinic that it occurred to me the challenges he and my patients faced navigating medical facilities were symptomatic of a larger problem. Just as eco-friendly architecture and design came into being as a response to the energy crisis of the late 1980s, in the twenty-first century we must proactively and creatively build to meet the challenges of our aging population. Some architects and designers are doing this. Most are not.

*Green* is a natural label for environmental causes and eco-architecture. It was less clear to me at first what word might capture elder-friendly building design. A recent NPR survey indicated that no words used to describe old age have much appeal to either the old or the young. But *silver* has positive connotations of beauty and value, as well as associations with old age. *Silver architecture and design* therefore follows in the semantic footsteps of the green movement while invoking its unique mission.

A silver medical building would offer easy, safe access that doesn't require walking long distances, opening heavy doors, going to multiple locations, or standing in long wait lines. Its building materials would reduce noise, and design features would optimize lighting and minimize overstimulation, distraction, and risk of falls. Doors, rooms, and public areas would accommodate walkers, wheelchairs, and a person walking side by side or arm in arm with a friend, family member, or caregiver. Space use would prioritize navigation and accessibility, offering regular places to rest and regroup. Such changes would increase accessibility, nonpunitively acknowledge patient challenges, recognize old people as valued customers, and create a safer, more pleasant, and welcoming environment for all patients and families.

Architecture and design strategies that improve the safety, health, and well-being of old people are already in use in many long-term care facilities and in specialized areas of hospitals, such as geriatric emergency departments or ACE units. But they aren't nearly as prevalent and valued as they should be. Surely such design elements should be universal, at least in health facilities, present at entrances, exits, cafeterias, hallways, and other public-access spaces, as well as anywhere else an old, ill, or disabled person might be, which in a medical center is almost everywhere.

This isn't just an issue for public or health care buildings either. In an era when almost all of us grow old, shouldn't homes be silver too? Yet much home architecture seems based on the assumption that people should move into "special housing" or institutions when stairs become challenging. Doing housecalls, I frequently entered supposedly accessible apartment buildings where residents had to climb at least a few steps from street level to reach the elevators. And almost all bathrooms are designed without grab rails or shower seats. Perhaps the most important reason people don't install them until they need them is because they are so ugly. They don't need to be. Imagine what they might look like, how they could add to a home, if designers thought as much about their aesthetics and variety as they do for other functional household items, from cabinets to handles to sinks and stairways. Imagine if they were good-looking and as expected as a towel rack, so they'd be there when you needed them—if you break your leg, are very pregnant, or grow old.

Imagine, too, public spaces where you could have a conversation with the person you're with—an issue not only for old people. In San Francisco and many other cities around the turn of the millennium, restaurants intentionally became louder to seem more successful. This is a problem for middle-aged people, since hearing loss begins for most of us in our fifties, and for younger people who want to talk, not yell, and hear their companions without straining. Imagine movie theaters without steep steps, or where you can easily see the steps and seats, not just vague shapes in the dim light, or that can be accessed at multiple levels. A sixty-five-year-old eye admits only one-third the amount of light as a twenty-year-old eye, yet in places where we expect many sixty-year-olds, the lighting is set for twenty-year-olds. Imagine restaurants and bars with a degree of illumination that allowed for both menu reading and mood setting.

In health care design, prototypes already exist that could easily be applied or adapted to create silver hospitals and clinics. A 2018 magazine advertisement showed a labeled photograph of a kid- and family-friendly patient room at a newly renovated children's hospital. Accompanying text explained the features identified by numbered red dots on the photo. They included smart monitors that identified staff on a TV monitor as they came into the room, a service helpful to any patient but even more useful in a person with dementia, delirium, or impaired vision or hearing. Every patient room had a window with a planter box and outdoor view. No less important for the children of old patients as for the parents of young ones, each room also had a pullout couch bed, second TV, and privacy. Evidence-based design studies have shown that such patient-centered design features don't just increase patient satisfaction; they can improve hospital safety and health outcomes.

Architects, city planners, business leaders, and ordinary citizens should take note of what works best in hospitals and clinics. And health care leaders and designers should follow innovations in the new arena of aging-in-place homes. The most successful and competitive new buildings, homes, neighborhoods, and cities will help people remain where they want to be and continue living full (if changed) lives, usually in their homes and communities, through the stages of old age. When communities review plans for new or improved buildings, they should ask questions not only about job creation and traffic flow but about how well the design meets the needs of residents and consumers of all ages, prioritizing equal access, health, and safety across the entire life span.

Some might say that buildings can't cater to every group with special needs. But silver architecture and design aren't about indulging a special interest group. They're about maximizing quality of life and independence for a life stage most of us will reach.

Green architecture is good for the environment; silver architecture is good for humans. The best new buildings will be both—inside and out.

## HEALTH

A scientist hoping to understand something looks for the most fully realized examples of it. In geriatrics, that means patients who best conform to our very particular social notions of "old." Much of geriatric care and research focuses on the needs of the sickest, frailest, and most aged old people, rather than on elderhood in its entirety. Additionally, as is typical of medical specialties, most of our work is aimed at treating established problems instead of preventing them. Here is a common view:

> I believe our main emphasis today should be oriented to the so-called "geriatric patient" and to frail older individuals. We must convey a key message to patients, colleagues, and society: defining a geriatric patient is not only a matter of age . . . but besides they must have chronic diseases . . . polypharmacy, functional limitations . . . and social problems.

The main argument for this approach is that, since there are not enough geriatricians, we old-age specialists need to focus on the people who need us most. This view is ethically sound, practical, and popular within the field. But if the goal is to have a medical system that provides high-quality care for all Americans across the life span or a life-stage-based specialty, it doesn't work.

It's counterproductive in several other ways as well. Associating geriatric care with the oldest, frailest elders reinforces misconceptions and partial stories about old age. This makes geriatric care less an analogue to pediatrics and internal medicine and more akin to a subspecialty. It also makes it less appealing to many of the people who would benefit from age-tailored care throughout their decades of old age, which simultaneously reduces demand for it and keeps the specialty so small that it can't even adequately care for all the people in its narrowed purview. As is always the case, circular logic leads nowhere.

Since geriatricians are notoriously happy, the people harmed by this approach are patients whose medical care doesn't take their elderhood into consideration. By ignoring younger and fitter old people, geriatrics increases the conceptual distance between young and old and the chances that younger and healthier old people will become sick or frail sooner than they would have with proactive geriatric care. The circumscribed approach to geriatrics in favor these last forty to fifty years has meant most American elders get care from doctors who know little about aging bodies, late-life development, and old age. By reinforcing the conflation of the large category of "old" with its extremes, it has made it harder for people to see connections between their present and future, themselves and others, and easier for them to fill those gaps with prejudices. Surely, if a strategy has failed for nearly half a century, it's time to try something new.

Like many geriatricians, I chose my specialty because I found working with very old, frail people endlessly interesting and deeply fulfilling. Yes, dementia, debility, and death make me, my patients, and their families sad. But they are also among life's most defining events. If they are not as celebrated as new babies, graduations, weddings, and retirement, they are no less significant or meaningful. A job that allows me, year after year, to do something significant and meaningful with and for other human beings has made me a fortunate, happy person. But to give a comprehensive, accurate view of old age for this book, I had to draw from other books, the media, my family, and friends. We geriatricians can't claim to be aging specialists if we don't study and practice with patients in all the substages of old age. We also can't narrow our scope of work and then complain when others see our field as small and limited.

The solution is simple. Geriatrics means care of old people. All old people, in all settings. If there aren't enough of us and we are helpful, patients and families will make demands. To meet those demands, politicians and health system leaders will have to remove the structural and financial disincentives to a career in geriatrics—by removing barriers to all comprehensive, whole-person focused specialties. Medicine needs to stop letting diseases develop and organs fail and then providing subspecialists and costly, high-tech care to tend to the parts that broke down while it looked the other way. We will never have Population Health until that happens.

If the baby boomer generation's reputation is to be believed, few will accept a clinical team without a quarterback, or with a quarterback whose primary sport is basketball or tennis. Most have already seen what that approach did to their parents, and it's not what they want for themselves. Because a long life includes childhood, adulthood, and elderhood, a person should have a specialist for each of these major life phases: first a pediatrician, next an internist, and then a geriatrician.

### PERSPECTIVE

In response to all the media attention on the UK's aging population, the writer Ceridwen Dovey tried to write a novel from the perspective of a man in his late eighties. In describing this experience, she wrote, "I'm in my mid-thirties, but felt confident that I could imagine my way into old age. How hard could it be, really?" Her protagonist was grouchy, computer illiterate, miserably caring for his dementia-addled wife until he met a magenta-turban-wearing radical and fell in love again. After reading the first draft, an editor asked, "But what else are they, other than old?" In making her characters old, Dovey had not thought it necessary to also make them human. Instead, she created variants of two common stereotypes, the frail old depressive whose life is miserable and meaningless, and the wise eccentric who doesn't act her age.

In *Ways of Seeing*, John Berger shows that what we usually accept as objective reality changes depending on how it's presented to us. He notes that how we see things is affected by what we know and what we believe, as well as by the information we are given and the context of our viewing. A landscape of wheat fields with birds flying overhead appears charmingly bucolic until you learn it was Vincent van Gogh's last painting before he killed himself.

People who are told the same image is either a work of art or a record of everyday events evaluate it using mostly divergent criteria. With different background music, a painting of a group of men talking over dinner takes on very different tones; it can be playful or sinister, affectionate or angry. We come to disparate conclusions depending on what we are told: Is that shrunken, bent old person an escapee from the local nursing home or the author of the Supreme Court's latest erudite and transformative ruling?

What we see depends on more than what we're looking at. Even when we are trying to be objective, what we consider "fact" or "reality" depends on what precedes, follows, surrounds, and accompanies it, who we are and what we already know and believe, where we are when we see it, and whether we are shown the whole or just one small part of the picture. The same object, idea, or person, approached in different ways, can seem to mean very different things.

A friend asked me what she could do about her mother's "old lady smell." Even as I write those words, as I surround them with quotation marks, I want to protest, yet I knew exactly what my friend meant. She didn't just say that her particular mother had a surprising, noxious odor but that her mother had acquired something sufficiently common that it had its own phrase, one with the inescapable ring of truth, if also with the clang of stereotype and the grate of insult. A clean older person smells like any other clean person. But people's olfactory sense declines with age, and washing becomes more physically challenging or exhausting. Because of waning sex hormones, old people generate less odor than younger people. Frequent showers and clothes laundering begin to seem only occasionally worth the effort; the differences between recently cleaned and cleaned a few days prior are often undetectable to aged noses and eyes. Unwashed hair and skin and clothing take on a sour mustiness they don't notice.

The smell of an unwashed old person is different from the odors of an unwashed teenager or adult. At different life stages and by virtue of hormones and eating habits, our bodies contain different distributions of cells and bacteria, oils and chemicals. Tell an old person that they smell, and most are mortified—I would be. They didn't realize, and why should they? If we mention old age odor at all, we mostly ascribe it to old age itself, not to the behaviors and logic behind those behaviors. Contrast that with our approach to adult odor for which we have gym showers and deodorant and foot, jock, and feminine sprays. We offer no equivalent triggers or aides for "old person smell." Those same things would help but often aren't primarily what is needed. Adults need to mask the stronger odors they produce in the course of a regular day; very old people usually just need a world that makes it easier for them to wash more regularly.

Emphasizing the declines of aging and pathologizing life's normal progression while ignoring the essential roles played by our perceptions and physical and social environments creates disabilities where there might be only differences.

As a doctor, I find the hardest part of helping people (of any age) with advanced illness comes from knowing I can't fix the widespread cancer or end-stage lung disease, her failing brain or his permanently paralyzed left side. These feelings are, I suspect, one of the main reasons so many people (and doctors) avoid ill, debilitated, or bereft old people: the sense of one's own apparent inutility as a helper. But in indulging those discomforts, we make the ideal the enemy of the right, the kind, and the needed.

Imagine aging in a world where we spent less energy lamenting what is gone and more supporting what is present. Imagine doctors (and people generally) able to tolerate and talk about uncertainty. Imagine a society that accepted the facts of every life throughout history: we are born, we die, and in between, the lucky live by developing, changing, and aging. With this existential skill set—accessible to anyone, for free—we can be much more practically useful than we are now to people of all ages. Equally important, we will accept that sometimes we won't be at all practically useful, and that the missing pragmatics need not equate with inutility unless we consider kindness and human connection useless.

Some days when I was doing housecalls, I suspected the most important thing I did—or at least that which was most appreciated by some of my patients—was to act as a friendly visitor. I might be their only visitor for days or weeks, or one of few, or the only one who really talked to or touched them. I liked my patients, and they knew it. We laughed. If it seemed appropriate, I rested my hand on their arm. I almost always lay my left hand on a patient's shoulder when listening to their hearts or lungs. Sometimes my housecall patients clutched and squeezed my hand. Sometimes they hugged or kissed me. Sometimes they commented that they couldn't recall the last time they touched another human being.

My patients didn't do those things because they were old, although the desexualizing and relative powerlessness of old age make hugs and kisses acceptable in situations where they otherwise might be considered inappropriate, or even sexual harassment. They were starved for basic human contact, a need that transcends culture and age. That need is not a biological imperative of aging; it's the result of choices we make as individuals and as a society. We let people vanish, treating them as less than human. We tell ourselves stories of how grotesque older skin is, but hush the cultural messages inside your head, and you'll find that old skin is soft and warm and a pleasure to touch.

Consider all the public figures and neighbors and relatives you have who are visibly and undeniably old. Maybe they move slowly or maybe they don't, but you know they are in their eighth or ninth decade or beyond. Some are frail and dependent, and most are not. Yet until recently, when we heard the word *old*, we thought disdainfully of the people in the first group and pretended all those others were not old.

That's starting to change. The writer-activist Ashton Applewhite, author of *This Chair Rocks*, tells the story of an East Coast performance festival organizer who chose aging as the festival's theme in 2012. The organizer's friends warned she would lose all her subscribers. Instead, festival subscriptions tripled.

A few years later, the same thing happened to me and two colleagues when we were invited to speak about "optimizing aging" at a salon-style forum in the Napa Valley. The organizers kept warning us that attendance varied a lot, depending on the topic. It became obvious they thought our topic, the very topic that interested them and inspired them to invite us, might be off-putting to others. The evening of the event, it was standing room only, and we had to cut off the questions so people's dinner wouldn't get cold.


In 1995 Isabella Rossellini had been "the face" of Lancôme cosmetics for fifteen years when they dismissed her. She was forty-two years old. The company said women bought cosmetics to fulfill their dreams of youthful beauty, and she was too old.

It's probably worth stating the obvious: in her forties, Rossellini was more beautiful than most of us are at any age. Ditto in her sixties, but I'm getting ahead of the story . . .

Fast-forward twenty-three years. Rossellini, by then sixty-five, was told that Lancôme wanted to hire her again. She thought it only right to let them know that she hadn't gotten any younger in the interim, and if she was too old in her early forties to represent women's dreams, she didn't see how the new arrangement could possibly work. She insisted on an in-person meeting. She wanted them to see her face in its seventh decade.

At the meeting, the company's newish female CEO explained that many women felt excluded and rejected by the endless parade of only young models. They wanted to define beauty not as youth alone but as something different and more inclusive. Perhaps they wanted to hew more faithfully to the dictionary definition: "a quality of a person or thing that gives pleasure to the senses or pleasurably exalts the mind or spirit."

Describing the experience with a grin, Rossellini certainly fit the bill. "So probably women's dreams changed, did they?"

# 13. AGED

One fall, we asked our vet how we would know when it was time to put down Byron, our elderly dog. He was fourteen, half-blind, partly deaf, with dementia, arthritis, and an enlarged prostate. He occasionally walked into walls or stood staring vacantly with his tail down. He had begun wandering and whining for reasons we couldn't always decipher.

Byron had many age-related afflictions, but it was also true that he often toddled along happily on his daily walks. He sniffed bushes and stained storefronts with the measured attentiveness of a research scientist, flirted with passersby, and on occasion raised his ears and tail, marked a spot, then kicked his hind legs while growling, barking, and asserting his dominance over some generally long-gone canine competition. Since Byron was an elderly eight-pound Yorkshire terrier, this invariably provoked fond smiles in passing strangers.

Attentive to Byron's needs, we softened his food with water and sprinkled it with meat; we cuddled him when he whimpered and took him outside to relieve himself four, five, even eight times a night. We couldn't take a vacation because we couldn't imagine asking anyone, friend or dogsitter, to do what we were doing. Nor could we fully trust anyone to provide the care we thought Byron required.

When asked whether it was time to put Byron "to sleep," our vet said he used the 50 percent rule: Were at least half of Byron's days good ones? Or was it one good day for every bad, or two bad days for every good? When you get to the latter, he explained, it's time.

This conversation gave me pause for two reasons. First, what did Byron want? Was 50 percent good enough for him? There was no way to know.

Which brought me to my second reason for pause: my patients were the oldest, frailest, and sickest of old people, yet many were quite satisfied with their lives.

This isn't true for everyone at the far chronologic reaches of life. Some people are eager to say they've had enough after they find themselves bedbound or dependent, unable to do any of the things they once valued so dearly. Still others cannot express their wishes or needs but lie in bed or sit propped in chairs, frowning and grimacing despite attentive care and trials of antidepressants and pain medications.

"Why don't God want me?" Mabel asked just before her ninetieth birthday and four years after a big stroke left her bedbound and fed through a tube.

"Can't you do something?" begged an eighty-nine-year-old with advanced Parkinson's disease and incontinence who would have killed himself if only he still could.

If we had a 50 percent rule for humans, they would have welcomed the opportunity to end their lives. As it was, they had lived full lives, knew those lives were over and not coming back, but lingered. Yet others, even those with similar or equal disabilities, feel just as strongly that they want to preserve their lives at any cost.

Of course, we can't have a 50 percent rule for humans. Because who decides? These are vulnerable people, and while the world is full of dedicated, self-sacrificing caregivers, it also contains far too many people who stand to gain from death (through inheritance) or from ongoing life (in the form of Social Security checks or cheap housing).

At the same time, even if not everyone feels the despair those two patients of mine did, what if millions or tens of millions of others do? Are we going to ignore that fact, especially when we are responsible for that reality people find not worth living? Is there a difference, practically and morally, between grave illness in advanced old age and at early stages of life?

Over Byron's last year, he'd had a number of health problems, and we had intended to take a palliative approach: doing only treatments that lessened his suffering and avoiding tests and stressful vet visits. But just after we made that decision, when he was slow and slept more but seemed otherwise fairly content, his paw hurt, so we took him in. Other medical issues followed. A few months later, Byron was short of breath. We thought that was the end, but the vets disagreed. They said he needed nothing more than an X-ray to determine it was pneumonia, then oxygen and antibiotics. Without explicitly saying it, they implied that not treating such a treatable condition was dog murder. Each time he had to go to the vet, Byron shook, panted, climbed up our bodies, and tugged on his leash, his tiny body straining for the door.

Suddenly, I fully understood something I had observed at work: how it was possible to love a frail loved one, prioritize his comfort and well-being, yet repeatedly find oneself doing things that felt awful to everyone.

The situation was made worse by both a lack of consistent consensus within our family about what was the right thing to do for Byron and the well-meaning veterinary doctors. It's hard and morally unsettling to discuss a comfort-only approach with health professionals advocating for an "easy" treatment for a fixable problem. The same thing happens with humans for logical if not ideal reasons: a focus on diseases as individual entities, rather than the person's larger and more complex situation.

Eventually we realized we'd passed some no-going-back landmark in Byron's apparent well-being and made an appointment with a hospice vet. When I returned home from work on the designated night, the humans of our family were cradling Byron and looking sad. He came to me, wiggling his tail and dancing around as best he could. He hadn't eaten all day. I thawed chicken, and he gobbled it down. Someone said, "You can't kill him."

Then he followed me to the bathroom and vomited the chicken onto the floor at my feet. He stood, tail down, facing the wall.

Byron died in my arms that night.

Both before and since Byron's death, I worried that we waited too long. We counted the time he spent sleeping as contentment, tipping the scale above the 50 percent mark, when I know in elderly humans sleep is more often a sign of chronic exhaustion, depression, and avoidance of pain. In dealing with the guilt brought on by our mixed feelings—we love him; he's ruining our lives—we may have overcompensated to his detriment.

With dying humans, similar situations arise every day: hospital stays that fix the acute problem and worsen the chronic ones; emergency department visits that yield diagnoses but require weeks of recovery from the waiting and testing; surgeries that are themselves minor but provoke major confusion, complications, and hated nursing home stays. But there are, too, the relatively simple problems that might be addressed by a doctor if only seeing one didn't require an ambulance for transportation, or time off work by an adult child, or more taxi fare than remains in the Social Security check, or more effort than seems worth the while.

The issue is complicated, to say the least. A few years ago, a patient of mine with fifteen major medical problems, including a form of leukemia, decided he didn't ever want to return to the hospital, do chemotherapy, or try any of other treatments we discussed. But, for weeks after that, he railed and fumed at the prospect of palliative care, because he also wanted very badly to live.

He wanted to live—just not in the hospital, with poisons in his blood. He was sick and tired of feeling sick and tired. His was a reasoned and reasonable stance.

## NATURE

When I teach what I call public medical writing, I often quote the first line of a *New Yorker* essay by the surgeon-writer Atul Gawande, "Letting Go," which reads, "Sara Thomas Monopoli was eight months pregnant with her first child when her doctors learned she was going to die." Then I ask my students, who are sometimes medical or nursing students but more often doctors, patients, writers, and caregivers of all ages, why Gawande chose to start the essay with such an atypical death.

If my question is met by silence, I offer an alternate first sentence, asking the group to consider its relative impact: "Joann Stern Smith was ninety-four years old with dementia, advanced heart disease, and failing kidneys when her doctors learned she was going to die."

Gawande picked the real Sara for his article because she wasn't supposed to be dying. Because only a hardened heart wouldn't break at the notion of a young pregnant woman dying. Because that sort of death grabs our attention.

Gawande's brilliance notwithstanding, what matters in good writing and what matters in life aren't always the same. In life, my scenario, not his, is the norm. In a moral universe, that's as it should be. It's *natural*. Joann Stern Smith had a long life, reaching closer than most to the upper age limit for our species. Where we get into trouble is when we use this natural order of things—people shouldn't die young; dying old is our best option—as a reason *not to care* and, in medicine, not to provide the best possible care for old people.

When we think, *of course she's dying*, we forgo the thought that, whatever her age, here is a human being in need of care and compassion. Someone like us. But unless that particular human being is their grandparent or parent, people often don't consider that even if she's ninety-four and very ill, even if she has advanced dementia, her suffering counts. That her death doesn't surprise us, that it seems part of the natural order, doesn't lessen its profound significance.

When we've reached old age, we may be very experienced, but we've never died. This process of dying is always new, invariably meaningful. Our words and actions as fellow human beings, as family and friends, doctors and nurses, and as a society matter not only in death but in the life and all the living leading up to that death, regardless of the age of the dying person.

There is an undeclared war taking place across the United States. It's a battle between aging and dying that quietly began toward the end of the twentieth century. Now, several decades into the conflict, reports from the field are unequivocal: dying is winning by a landslide.

Across the country, health systems, communities, and in some cases entire states have added and touted programs and policies that give people greater control over their deaths. Strategies range from promoting discussions of values and preferences at the end of life to expanding services that support death at home and passing assistance-in-dying laws. Many of the movement's leaders are people who started their careers in aging and then moved on to dying. Most medical centers now offer palliative care services, and hospitals have special rooms for dying patients that resemble the homelike birthing rooms introduced for childbirth nearly a half century ago.

It's not that we've cured dying, moving it into the history books alongside smallpox or polio. Too many people still lack access to these improved approaches, and some deaths remain hard, even painful, despite the best efforts of highly skilled care teams. Yet recent end-of-life care advances represent meaningful systematic and attitudinal responses to stories and evidence of widespread, pointless suffering at the end of life. Newer approaches to death move beyond the medicalized, institutional, uniform method that developed as medical progress prevented or delayed certain sorts of deaths. Ironically, what's old is new again. The key step underlying many of the last two decades' death "innovations" is the acknowledgment of death's inevitability. More and more often, when it becomes clear that the high-tech approach will only extend and deepen suffering, the focus shifts to optimizing comfort and the patient's and family's unique experience of dying. Many more deaths take place at home now than fifty years ago, though not nearly as many as a century ago before death became a medical, rather than a life, event.

The media often adds confusion to American death conversations by reporting deaths from what they call "natural causes." They don't mean an earthquake or hurricane. Invariably, the dead person was old, or old enough. When a younger person dies under similar circumstances—in bed overnight, say—an investigation is launched. People whisper about drugs or suicide. The word *tragedy* is used. Both biology and philosophy are in play here. Technically, it's natural to die, one of life's few universal requirements. Our assignation of *natural* to some deaths and not others is strongly connected to our notions of old age.

In the early 1500s Leonardo da Vinci decreed a natural death as one resulting from a lack of nourishment, as blood vessels thickened and closed off with age. Although not exactly how we'd describe it today, his description of advanced old age fairly accurately captures one mechanism responsible for the gradual shutting down of organs and functions known as *senescence*. Three hundred years later, the American physician Benjamin Rush recognized that often what was written off as senescence was in fact one or more specific diseases masked by the more obvious biological changes of a long life. In his 1793 *Account of the State of the Body and Mind in Old Age, with Observations on Its Diseases and Their Remedies*, he wrote that "few persons appear to die of old age. Some one of the diseases . . . generally cuts the last thread of life."

In the modern world, where getting things done is prioritized, death can seem more manageable than old age. After all, aging takes place in mundane ways over many years or decades, while death usually has a horizon of days to months. I suspect that's why people are often more comfortable with death than aging. Death is a sprint and aging a marathon. Certainly, that attitude is common among many in medicine, where increasing numbers of trainees and clinicians of all stripes have enthusiastically embraced palliative care. While this may seem a small issue within one profession, medical trends usually reflect larger cultural tendencies. Palliative care has transformed medicine by creating a group of professionals whose primary skill set is the management of physical and existential suffering.

But it has also allowed other doctors to abdicate those territories, as if all clinicians in specialties with patient contact should not be proficient in such fundamental skills. How can it be that we have a medical system where most doctors are allowed to outsource to colleagues common, critical tasks such as having difficult conversations, relieving pain, and supporting dying patients? The answer is that as medical knowledge has expanded, we have parsed sickness not only into organs and diseases but into their subcategories. Doctors specialize not just in the heart but in rhythm disturbances, not just in the gastrointestinal tract but in hepatitis, not just in ophthalmology but in the retina.

In many ways, this makes sense. It's easier both practically and psychologically to focus on one thing, and to understand it well, than to manage not only that but also someone's hip replacement, diabetes, low vision, and heart disease. It's also the antithesis of what the health system claims to be focused on in this moment in history: "patient-centered care." When Paula, who had early dementia, chronic obstructive lung disease, and a leg ulcer, fell and hit her head, in addition to her lung doctor and skin doctor and vascular surgeon, she was told she needed one neurologist for her dementia, another for her traumatic brain injury, and a third to manage her seizures.

Palliative care not only divorces death from the diseases that cause it, it divorces dying from aging, as if those conditions are not inextricably intertwined. Most people who die are old, yet at my top medical center and elsewhere, the leading palliative care specialists unabashedly distance their work from aging and old age. Before we die, we live, and since most of us will live not just *to* old age but *in* it for decades, living there comfortably, meaningfully, and with as much ability to do useful things for ourselves and others as possible matters too. Dying as well as possible at any age requires care that takes into account a person's concerns, physiology, and context, all of which varies significantly with age. That so many palliative care doctors for adults claim their work has as much to do with pediatrics as geriatrics speaks to the depth of ageism in medical culture and to the self-defeating tendency of tribes—think Sunnis and Shiites or Tutsis and Hutus—with more in common than not to wage battle against each other instead of against the larger forces orchestrating their competition.

Ask people how they'd like to die, and most will say they hope to not wake up on the morning of the day on which a medical catastrophe would force them over the cliff from a fulfilling life into a barren gorge dominated by illness and grave disability. There are two problems with that wish. The first is that it's almost always impossible to see the cliff edge until you're already falling off it. The second is that many people who fall off terrifying-looking cliffs find lives well worth living.

Francisco Gomes was seventy-nine when he began tripping over his own feet and bumping into furniture. His daughter accused him of being drunk when she brought her family to visit. He had been an alcoholic in her childhood, and she couldn't believe he'd fallen off the wagon after twenty years of sobriety. It took him an hour to convince her he hadn't been drinking, at which point she dropped her kids with a friend and drove him to the emergency department, where a CAT scan showed a brain tumor. Three months later, the tumor was out, and Francisco took up residence in a hospital bed in his daughter's living room. He couldn't walk, but his arms and mind were fine. He could get out of bed only with the help of a lift device, and sitting in a wheelchair wore him out.

Three years later Francisco was still there, living not only with his daughter's family but holding court from a bed in the living room. In the intervening years, their apartment had become the center of the neighborhood. Francisco read to kids from buildings up and down the block and helped them with their homework after school. He taught the mailman, an immigrant from China, better English, and their families became friends, throwing Sunday parties featuring both tortillas and rice.

When she was diagnosed with esophageal cancer, Maggie Gillespie was still running the shop that had been in her family for decades, as well as volunteering in her grandson's fourth-grade class. For years, she'd made clear that if she had a dire prognosis, she wanted comfort care only. The problem was that although her tumor was extensive, it was localized, and there was a chance that with removal of most of her esophagus and local radiation, she might be cured, but she'd never be able to swallow or eat again. She agreed to a feeding tube as long as she retained the right to have it removed if things looked bleak. The surgery and early radiation treatments left her so weak and ill that she moved to the nursing home. That was where I met her seven months later. Since she wasn't my patient, our first meeting took place on her day of discharge, a Saturday when I was the only covering physician. When Maggie approached me and introduced herself, I thought she was a patient's daughter.

She laughed at my confusion and lifted up her blouse to show me her new, permanent feeding tube. "I never thought I'd want one of these," she said, "but I also always thought if I needed one I'd be totally out of it instead of just the same old me who can do everything but eat."

Sometimes we can't imagine or predict what we will be able to put up with as we move through life. For example, a 2004 study of healthy people found that most said they would rather not have medical interventions to prolong a low-quality life. However, dying people who were experiencing low quality of life almost unanimously told researchers they would use any available medical interventions to prolong their lives, even if just by a few days.

Among the frail octogenarians, nonagenarians, and centenarians I have cared for, sources of life meaning vary widely. While I could argue that there are as many types of meaning as unique individuals, it's also true that those of us who do this work have noted common themes that transcend culture and social class and can frequently be boiled down to comfort, function, and relationships.

Almost always, by the time those three things are gone, or become too difficult to access, so is a patient's ability—physical, cognitive, or both—to control their lives and communicate their preferences. Also often lost at that stage is a physician's ability to determine with sufficient certainty that death is what the patient truly does or doesn't want, that there is no coercion by family or friends either toward or away from death, and that the patient's sources of meaning haven't shifted.

Those caveats give me pause. Yet my years of geriatrics practice tell me that once most physical and sensory abilities are lost, whether the brain is failing too or simply trapped, unable to access other people, books, food, even television and most everything else, more often than not people are hoping for death, even as that prospect may still scare them. Like most things, death in old age is both similar to and different from death earlier in life.

If we return to the notion that we tell some stories more often and accurately than others, there seems to be another reason for the current popularity of death compared with aging in public programs and discussions. The challenges and opportunities of death have been featured in films, bestselling books, TED talks, newspapers, blogs, and websites. Aging is finally getting more attention, too, but until recently it got much less, and too much of the sort that's better described as catastrophic than transformative. Death, with its abbreviated trajectory, finiteness, and, depending on one's beliefs, mystical or religious associations, lends itself well to romance, while aging, its longer and messier cousin, tends more toward realism. In literature, romance refers to extraordinary exploits that take place in mysterious and exotic settings and require honorable, dutiful actions to help those in distress. By contrast, realism offers a faithful portrait of life. Given a choice between romance and realism, many people choose the former. For me, among the great joys of a career in geriatrics, one of the few fields that doesn't outsource our patients to palliative care as death nears, is that I get both.

## HUMAN

Thomas Kuhn's landmark treatise, *The Structure of Scientific Revolutions*, was one of the most influential books of the twentieth century. Its scholarly citations put Kuhn's influence well ahead of the century's other famous thinkers, including Michel Foucault and Sigmund Freud. Although the book is about science, in the decades since its publication, Kuhn's notions of paradigms and paradigm shifts have become foundational to how we see and assess the world in all sectors of life.

According to Kuhn, progress is not gradual and cumulative but occurs in revolutionary fits and starts. A paradigm, or widely accepted framework for understanding an important problem—a problem like health care—is primed for shift or overturn by periods of upheaval, uncertainty, and angst. As these crises worsen, revealing more and more flaws in the standard approach, people begin exploring different ways of thinking about the problem. Revolution occurs when enough people accept that the current paradigm is inadequate and reject it in favor of a new one.

Maybe some people are happy with the twentieth century's "normal science," the science-and-technology-are-the-best-answer-to-every-problem medical paradigm. Certainly there are many people in many parts of the world who have it far worse than most Americans do. But that doesn't mean that we don't have serious problems. And it doesn't mean that it isn't time for radical transformation. Our current medical paradigm's science-first approach has reaped huge benefits for individuals and society, but it has also had disturbing unintended consequences. We have costs no country can manage as a result of this paradigm's payment, care, education, and research systems that favor novelty and discovery over implementation of the proven and dissemination of the useful, and high-tech procedural interventions and fields over preventative, social, and relational solutions. We have astronomical rates of patient bankruptcy and dehumanization, a distribution of specialists out of line with societal needs, a demoralized workforce, and epidemics of health disparities and illness caused by our current approach to medical care.

If we need wellness centers, then "health care" is only addressing sickness. If we need programs, clinics, and special funding lines for women's health, to name just one example, then the system is not set up to care for over half the population. If our professional schools need special courses and deans to address issues of diversity and disparities, our core curricula are not adequately addressing those issues and patients of all backgrounds. If we feel the need to use catchphrases like "patient-centered care," what exactly is medicine? Shouldn't patients always be the focus of health care? Something is missing in the current system and its underlying paradigm. Something important.

The writer Jenny Diski, who died of cancer in 2016, described the problem from a patient's perspective in her final book, *In Gratitude*. Of making treatment decisions, she says: "Everything is presented to me statistically, as probabilities. I can't find the right question to break through that, to talk about the cancer that is me and mine, what it is, how it is, how it and I are with each other. Something that pans in on the singularity." And of her radiation treatment, Diski says, "I didn't doubt their ability to get me into position and to run the programme. But other things about the radiotherapy—such as my experience of it—seemed less skilfully thought-through . . . My dignity was left at the door of the treatment room each day, not because my breasts were revealed, but because as soon as I entered I became a loose component, a part the machine lacked, that had to be slotted into place to enable it to perform its function."

This is what medical practice is like now too. Everything we do—indeed, our meaning and value to our institutions and to the health care system itself—amounts to numbers: from statistics reflecting productivity or guideline adherence to billing and costs—numbers signifying value, as if what matters in health and life can be numerically expressed.

Medical centers and medical education break people down into their components: bones on floor three, joints on floor eight, hearts in this course, prostates in that one. The scientific approach requires control, and to gain control you break things down until they become manageable, and probably also because if we parse the body and diseases into categories, it makes our lives easier. Humans are complex and messy. Dealing with a whole one is slow, sometimes fraught, unpredictable, and often uncertain. It's easier not to, which is what we teach medical trainees. This "hidden curriculum" is to medicine what side effects are to drugs: it's built into the structure.

You can't separate the benefits from the harms without rethinking your entire approach.

Not long ago, I sat in on an much-touted "case-based learning" session at a medical school I was visiting, an institution rapidly acquiring a reputation for educational innovation. In a small workshop room equipped with a communal table, whiteboard, and video monitor to which one student's computer could be attached so all could see what she wrote on behalf of the group, second-year students asked smart questions about three clinical cases related to their coursework. They refined insightful queries about what was going on with the relevant organ systems, how certain drugs worked, and which symptoms had clinical import.

But in two hours of case discussions, only one student murmured a comment in response to the pathos of a patient's situation. After only the first year of what would be at minimum a seven-year process, these medical students had learned to ignore the evident suffering described in their hypothetical cases—a young boy's fear as he gasped for breath during an asthma attack, a healthy middle-aged man's sudden loss of limb and livelihood, and an older woman's repeated vomiting as a result of food poisoning.

After the session, I commented on this total focus on the pathophysiology and pharmacology to the course director, who had been lauded by my hosts as their best and most creative teacher. He said the curriculum was designed to encourage focus. It wasn't possible to teach pathophysiology and clinical care simultaneously, he said, adding that such an approach was too confusing and overwhelming for the students. They needed these fundamentals first. The patient stuff, he said, was addressed elsewhere in the curriculum. He relayed all of this with evident thoughtfulness, commitment to his learners and to medicine, and without irony.

Walking down the hallway to my next appointment, I thought about how quickly people absorb the messages we don't even realize we're sending, much like the teenager whose mother tells him to always stop at stop signs but rolls through them herself when in a hurry. It's been well documented for years that we teach our learners how and when not to care for patients via a similar hidden curriculum.

It's easier in many ways to teach medical science without knowing much about the patient as a unique human being and without expectations of feelings for them. The patients in case discussions work well as abstractions or generics, more or less interchangeable vessels for the pathophysiology new doctors must master. We can focus just on the lungs or the blood tests or the remarkable images that now pop instantly onto our screens. We can pretend that medicine is about diseases and organs rather than people and lives. We can divorce learning from caring.

Alternatively, we can take just a few seconds to recognize the human facts of the situation, letting our learners know with facial expressions and brief words of compassion, horror, and concern that it's natural—and, better yet, desirable—for doctors to feel sad when their patients are suffering. When we don't—when students are expected to read about a small boy who can't breathe and think only about the child's lung function—we teach them that being a doctor means *not* responding to distress in normal ways, including, I fear, not caring.

Empathy is feeling for the other. You might think it can't be faked, but in studies, medical trainees and doctors given words and gestures associated with true empathy created a pseudo-empathy that was perceived by patients as real empathy. Patients felt better when their clinicians faked it. And students who faked it became more empathetic. But mostly training makes doctors less empathetic. This makes me wonder: What if we rewarded people and health systems for putting patients first? What if we trained them to care? If you care, you'd want to be the best doctor you could be and have the best motivation for learning, whereas knowledge alone provides no intrinsic incentive to care.

Toward the end of my medical training, I stopped listening to music. I had seen so much in so few years that the world seemed to endlessly leak the sounds of human suffering, and I could not tolerate any more "noise."

There are so many types of suffering: physical, emotional, existential, financial, social, sexual, spiritual, psychological. That makes me wonder whether disease-focus is the right way to tackle suffering. But maybe relief of suffering, by care or cure, is not the intent of medicine. Maybe I'm confused. Maybe most doctors are primarily interested in disease, and I am the one who cares about suffering. I who look around and see it everywhere, who find it disturbing to a degree that is not infrequently disabling. Or maybe, far more likely in my experience, most doctors do care about suffering but are trained not to, and suppressing their normal human responses both allows them to function as clinicians in our unbalanced health care system and is leading to moral distress that manifests as burnout.

Science works well in settings where variables can be controlled—a petri dish, a laboratory, a data set—although, even there, we sometimes get into trouble. We can control some things about human lives but not all.

It's this human element—not just for patients but for everyone else, too—that makes medicine more than just science. The scientist works for knowledge, while the doctor works for the patient. This critical distinction is too often forgotten in our current health system. In medicine, the quintessentially human and not easily quantifiable, from illness experience and culture and social situation to political and economic structures, is frequently treated as of lesser or little import. These systematic biases for science over care and for medicine over health are at the root of the structural inequalities and current crisis in health care. With science at the center of medicine's paradigm, we prioritize *things*; if we put care at its center instead, our priority will shift to where it should be: *people*.

Most doctors are familiar with the last lines of Francis Weld Peabody's essay "The Care of the Patient." In fact, although written in 1927, his description of the role of the physician is no less apt today:

> Disease in man is never exactly the same as disease in an experimental animal, for in man the disease at once affects and is affected by what we call the emotional life (and, I would add, social environment). Thus, the physician who attempts to take care of a patient while he neglects this factor is as unscientific as the investigator who neglects to control all the conditions that may affect his experiment . . . One of the essential

qualities of the clinician is interest in humanity, for the secret of the care of the patient is in caring for the patient.

Caring for patients is why I became a doctor. It's what I still want to spend my time doing, both directly and indirectly. That caring or "provision of what is necessary for the health, welfare, maintenance, and protection" of our fellow citizens and each other can and should be the crux of our health services, training programs, research, and scholarship, because only then will "caring for the patient" take its rightful place at the center of health care and medicine.

A new paradigm must begin with assumptions. Here are ten I'd like to see on the list:

1. While the terms *medicine* and *health care* are often used interchangeably, they are not equivalent.
2. Health matters more to both individuals and society than medicine.
3. Medicine and medical science are not the same thing; the latter is one component of the former.
4. Science is necessary but not sufficient to ensure health or provide health care.
5. When we make data all that matters, we often count what can be counted rather than what counts (with thanks to Albert Einstein).
6. Technology creates new problems and questions even as it solves others; to be useful, it requires guiding principles and thoughtful consideration of risks and consequences as well as benefits.
7. Separating the medical from the human leads to a separation of the medical from the human.
8. History, with its inherent conservatism and tendency to conform to the self-interest of the powerful, has been science's partner in shaping our health care system.
9. As an institution, medicine should prioritize the interests of the people over its own.
10. The primary goal of medicine is optimization of patient health.

The only drawback to this or any new paradigm is that getting one requires a revolution. Yet, although our current system is failing both doctors and patients, we who are physicians and health system leaders are active contributors to this failure. Most of us are good citizens, company men and women working within the traditional structures of our profession, people who respond to tough challenges by putting our heads together and trying harder, almost always taking the individual and collective approaches that justice organizations have shown are ineffective in producing social or cultural change. Doctors take medicine largely as it comes because that's what we signed up for and what we're used to. We don't make waves. We don't take big risks. We don't rebel. We say we are evidence-based, but when the evidence says we are failing (The U.S. at thirty-seventh in international rankings! Fifty percent of doctors burned out!), most of us offer innovative interior design when what's called for is new structural engineering and architecture. That needs to change. A good first step would be to renounce medicine's twentieth-century paradigm and develop a new one better suited to human needs right now.

Science is a useful tool, but as a framework for optimizing human health, its emphasis is misplaced, with too much emphasis on knowledge, novelty, and the physical, and too little on helpfulness, the already proven, and the human. But if science is out, something else has to be in, and although alternate paradigms have been proposed for years, none have caught on. The biopsychosocial model seems to be a strong candidate, with its equal emphasis on the physical, mental, and social, but somehow its inclusiveness makes it seem diffuse. Also, its moniker has the nails-on-chalkboard effect of jargon. Humanism seeks to maximize the potential and dignity of all human beings and considers the whole person over the entire life span, but its nontheistic stance limits its widespread application.

The new paradigm needed—from terminology to focus—has been part of medicine at least since the age of Hippocrates, and it comes down to one simple, ancient concept: care.

The "care paradigm" begins with the desired outcome, rather than an approach that may or may not lead to that outcome. It not only can but must include science while the scientific paradigm makes no allowance whatso-ever for concepts like care.

Let me put that another way: you can have good medical science without care, but you cannot have good medical care without science. We very much need both—at all ages and stages of life.

## CONSEQUENCES

One crisp and sunny fall afternoon after a lecture about old age, a nurse, a social worker, and a physician—all middle-aged women who specialized in the care of older adults—began exchanging stories. The nurse went first, telling the others about a very old woman who wanted a different sort of care from what her doctors were recommending and how the nurse helped her get what she wanted. Instead of scans and surgery and even more time in the hospital, she went home and died there two months later.

"I know I did the right thing," the nurse concluded, "so I don't know why I keep feeling guilty and uncertain about it, except that I'm sure her doctors think I killed her."

The social worker and doctor nodded.

Then the social worker described the final days of a woman in her late eighties with end-stage neurological disease whose frequently articulated wishes had been followed in every detail. She developed an infection that probably would have responded to antibiotics, but the social worker reminded the doctors of the patient's wishes. They skipped the antibiotics, and the patient died the next week.

The doctor's story featured a frail elderly man with dementia and heart disease who could no longer shower unassisted, read, watch TV, or follow most conversations. He had made clear to his family that he never wanted to live that way, so when he fell at home and things got worse still, leaving him bedbound in severe pain helped only by painkillers that also danger-ously impaired his swallowing, the doctor arranged to put him on hospice.

"His primary care physician wasn't so sure about that," she said, exchanging a sympathetic glance with the nurse.

"Oh, they gave me hell," said the nurse.

"I can't believe we're having this conversation," said the social worker.

The nurse smiled. "Isn't it great? What a relief."

"We didn't kill our parents," the doctor said. "They died in old age of advanced illness."

The three of them looked at each other, then smiled and shook their heads.

I can relay this conversation because I was the doctor that day, and because there is a perspective from which one could say I killed my father.

To be clear: I did not commit murder. I broke no laws, committed no moral transgressions, and did not euthanize my father. My discomfort, like my two colleagues', came not from what we did do but from what we did not do: that is, follow the party line of American medicine that says that if a treatment exists, you should use it. The nurse's mother should have had her surgically curable tumor removed. The social worker's mother should have taken antibiotics for her bladder infection. My father should have been given a feeding tube. The problem with this party line is that while it considers the medical problem, it ignores the body and life in which the problem is taking place.

None of the three deaths in this story was extraordinary. Each was a variant of common old age end-of-life scenarios that play out every day for American families. We three, with our decades of experience working with sick old people, had advantages over the average person. We had seen the impact of what Sharon Kaufman has called "ordinary medicine" in old lives. And based on years of conversations with our respective parents, we knew their preferences and greatest fears, and could honor their end-of-life wishes when the time came.

The social worker and I knew each other because I'd been her mother's nursing home doctor years earlier. The two had been close, and the social worker had been a regular at the nursing home, visiting her mom and participating in activities. Seeing her again, I remembered how much I'd liked them both.

Her mother, a lively, funny woman, had developed a progressive and eventually gravely debilitating, undiagnosable neurological disorder. She had been to multiple specialists at both of the top-rated medical centers in our region. Over time, she lost her ability to walk, move, and feed herself. Her brain remained sharp until the last year, and her wishes were clear.

When she developed a bladder infection, the social worker said no to antibiotics and asked for morphine instead to ensure her mother's comfort. Later that week, her mother died in precisely the way she always said she wanted.

For that final gift of respect and agency and love—for letting nature take its course and honoring her mother's preferences—her devoted daughter was left feeling like she had done something wrong.

That's because we live in a world that assumes ill intent and because some families do try to accelerate an older relative's demise. For some, it's payback for past abuse. Others want to free themselves of the burden of care, or get at a significant inheritance, or avoid eldercare's potentially years-long drain of family resources. On the flip side are families who keep a relative alive in order to retain their job as caregiver, pocket the elder's benefits, keep living in their house or apartment, or avoid dealing with death and feeling orphaned or mortal themselves.

Sometimes the abuse is glaring. More often, there are hard-to-prove suspicions. Without seeing inside someone's mind, it can be hard to distinguish between a person who says they are respecting their critically ill parent's wishes from another who is seeing an opportunity for freedom or profit. Similarly, it's hard to discern whether someone is going to great lengths to keep a loved one alive out of a sense of filial or religious obligation or for secondary gain, all of which can coexist. It's especially hard to sort out such complexities if you don't really know the patient and family, and you won't know them if you are a hospitalist or emergency clinician or consultant or if you think taking a patient's social history means asking whether or not they smoke and drink.


My mother says the local hospital killed my grandfather. He was admitted and then, when doctors couldn't find anything specifically wrong, they sent him home. He died in his bed the next day. Not necessarily a bad way to go, well into your eighties with minimal suffering, but my mother resented the doctors' failure to diagnose whatever it was that was wrong. Up to that point my grandfather had been outgoing and active. He was old but basically fine.

Thirty years later something similar happened to my father, except he hadn't been outgoing, active, or basically fine for six months, or twelve, or maybe for several years, depending on what you think "basically fine" looks like. One evening, he fell in my parents' apartment. My mother and a visiting cousin were in the next room when they heard a crash. They got him up, and, though he couldn't remember what had happened, he seemed okay. They phoned me, and I asked a lot of questions and had him move various parts and decided maybe we'd gotten lucky. The next day, I visited. He wasn't quite right, nor was he exactly wrong either. Dad had spent an awful lot of time in hospitals in recent years, something he and we wanted to avoid again if at all possible. Almost exactly a year earlier, he'd had a serious fall followed by a surgery that had stripped him of much of his mobility, more of his mind, and almost all of his lifelong sense of humor and pleasure in life.

On the third day, he couldn't get out of bed. My mother called me, I called for an ambulance, and we reconvened at the medical center. They couldn't make a diagnosis in the emergency department, but everyone agreed he needed to be admitted.

It was the last week of the residency year. The senior resident had an apartment and job lined up in another state, and the intern was eager for his ten-day vacation and return to the hospital as a team leader. They were both as well trained as they were going to be that year.

Their workup found nothing. My father seemed okay, but also not, and he couldn't explain what was wrong.

"We could do more tests," the intern said. "But we'd be fishing. Nothing points anywhere in particular."

There didn't seem to be much point in random scans. There was no fracture or injury we would have treated with surgery after what had happened the previous year. He'd passed the tipping point on the scale of suffering versus rewards; pains outpaced gains.

We took him home the afternoon before the first day of the new interns, those young doctors who had been medical students just weeks earlier.

Although my father's mind had been fairly clear in the morning, by the time the afternoon's discharge process was complete, he was confused in an unusually lively and articulate way. In the twenty minutes it took us to drive home, he passed through Pittsburgh, Chicago, and Rome. "I'll be damned," he said more than once. "I haven't seen that in years."

He had become similarly delirious on each of his hospital stays for the previous decade. And as had happened each of those earlier times, once back in my parents' apartment, his mind cleared.

However, my father couldn't walk. He got a hospital bed, visiting nurses, and a visiting physical therapist. We pulled the commode out of storage. Also, the bedpan. He was uncomfortable and unhappy, frustrated and angry. When we raised or lowered the bed, he gritted his teeth and lashed out. He screamed in pain but couldn't say where it hurt. He couldn't do much physical therapy, even in bed, and nothing else helped either. We checked him, the nurse checked him, we reported our findings and impressions to his doctor. It wasn't clear what to do.

His doctor made a home visit. He said we could get an X-ray, but he didn't think there was a good reason to put my father through that. We wouldn't do surgery, and either way the pain needed to be treated.

He was started on morphine. The pain improved. But the drug brought out the swallowing trouble he'd had after a complicated heart bypass surgery eight years earlier. He'd had a feeding tube for several months while undergoing speech therapy and learning again how to eat safely. Eventually, though far from normal, his swallow was good enough, the tube came out, and he got to eat again, a great thing for a man who loved food as much as he did.

If he couldn't swallow safely, we faced a lose-lose choice: he could be in severe pain but eat, or he could be comfortable and the food would drop into his lungs instead of his stomach, causing him to choke and cough, maybe suffocate. His mind worsened by the day, and every attempt at getting him to choose for himself between those options failed. Another feeding tube also wasn't an option; he'd been clear he'd only want one temporarily, and besides, the latest studies showed that they didn't benefit people with dementia.

At first, we offered him small bites and sips. Sometimes it worked. But after a couple of days on morphine, although he was finally comfortable and happier, even the smallest sip of thickened liquid or smallest bite of food caused chaos. He coughed, choked, swore, and hit at whoever was in reach. We discussed the situation with his hospice nurse and agreed to stop all food and water. For a few days, it was clear he occasionally wanted something, though he could no longer ask. We gave him moist flavored sponges that he sucked like a baby. Was that a reemerging primitive reflex, or was he hungry or thirsty? There was no way to know. He looked comfortable, finally, and I consoled myself with studies of dying cancer patients who uniformly report that after the first day or a few days without food or water, as long as their mouths and lips are kept moist, they stop feeling hunger or thirst.

A day passed, then another, and another. He went into a coma, and a few days later he died. It was hard and sad, and I know that if I had to do it over, for his sake, I'd do the exact same thing.

Would my father or my colleagues' mothers have lived longer had we "done everything"? I suspect they would have, though the nurse's mother might have died sooner of surgical complications, given what a poor surgical candidate she was. As for my father, it would have been a life of pain, anger, frustration, boredom, and futility—everything he hated most and had told us he didn't want—until the infection, or the stroke, or whatever else.

In truth, he'd been dying for months or maybe a year, dying in that subacute, chronic, modern way created by late twentieth-century medicine. Right now, lots of money and thought goes into fixing and little goes into considering the downstream consequences of those fixes or when they might do more harm than good. The result is unnecessary suffering, people trapped in lives they don't want and can't escape.

Curing diseases is great through much of life. But it also produces an advanced—or, more precisely, terminal—old age lacking comfort, agency, meaning, purpose, and pleasure. Some people think they don't have to worry about that, since science will soon be able to stop aging. The unlikeliness of a perfect fix aside, cure aging, then what? A great expanse of shapeless, seasonless life? Greater competition for resources, jobs, partners, and everything else on this already crowded, environmentally failing planet? Or selective application of the technology? The biotech entrepreneurs and Hollywood celebrities investing in anti-aging will get it, and the rest of us won't.

Here are alternate, timely questions we'd all do well to consider: If a person is at the end of life's chronology and has had enough, must they continue? Is it fair to consider illness and debility ethically different in very old age than earlier in life? Certainly, if people are going to make the case that those with advanced dementia and similar grave impairments are "already gone" or "an empty shell," don't they also need to consider a different approach to those people's lives and deaths? And does asking these questions put us any more on an ethical slippery slope than not asking them, and then leaving people to fend for themselves? Different approaches for different groups can lead to injustice, or it can mean compassionate attention to particularity. The choice is ours.

After turning eighty in 2017, the British writer Penelope Lively wrote that she already barely recognized herself and hoped she'd be dead by 2030, "though I can't quite count on it. I come from a horribly long-lived family. My mother died at 93; her brother made it to 100; their mother reached 97. I look grimly at these figures; I do not wish to compete." If she's already had a full life and has a clear sense of what the future holds, should she get to decide? And if so, do we allow what might be called "passive decisions," not availing oneself of treatment options that might prolong life, or "active ones," allowing people near the end of life, chronologically and medically, to choose to die on their own terms.

Many European countries permit assisted suicide, as do increasing numbers of American states. The person has to be dying and not depressed to qualify and be able to take the medications on their own to qualify. Those requirements make sense. But they also mean the laws don't apply to old people with significant disability or dementia, and some people will end their lives sooner than they might have chosen, simply to ensure that they can. More often, they will be deprived of a right afforded younger citizens, and the privileged will have work-arounds not available to most people. The 104-year-old Australian scientist David Goodall, who in the spring of 2018 sustained a fall that further eroded his remaining quality of life, flew with three of his grandchildren to Switzerland, where he could end his life. He was in a wheelchair by then and had trouble seeing and hearing. He would have preferred to die at home, he said, but was forced by Australian law to undertake a transcontinental mission made financially feasible for him only after a web-based fund-raising campaign.

In response to Goodall's decision, the president of the Australian Medical Association said, "I think it's very sad that someone feels this way." I looked that doctor up. He's an obstetrician-gynecologist. Perhaps he's never taken care of a centenarian. I have, many times. To be sure, the Australian Medical Association president may be saying: *Isn't it sad that we have a world in which someone feels this way because we can't give his life comfort and meaning?* Or maybe he was saying it's never okay to die even if you're ancient and ready to go.

But elderhood differs from childhood and adulthood in ways that should be included in discussions of death. Treatment of the same aggressive disease has very different risks and benefits for a child, an adult, and an elder. At the end of life, we need options that recognize the different situations people find themselves in at different life stages: all old people need to be allowed to fully live, and dying old people need to be allowed to die. Policies and practices that do those two things will make life better for people of all ages.

Some people are against chosen death for religious reasons, because of a belief in the sanctity of life and the fact of human suffering. That argument is compelling. It also was formulated thousands of years ago, before science and technology interfered with the natural order of human lives. If progress can make lives longer and better, surely it can also help us make death shorter and better at the natural end of life? Even current right-to-die legislation hasn't tackled that question. Formulated largely for younger adults with terminal diseases, its requirements mean it is not available to many of the sorts of very old people who regularly ask me and my colleagues, *Why am I still here?*

Huge concepts such as past, future, and death have very different implications in very old age than in youth or middle age or early old age. Parts wear out. Options wither. Even the simplest acts become an ordeal. Here is Donald Hall, whose body didn't hold out as long as Goodall's (variation being a key trait of old age):

> In your eighties it gets hard to walk. Nearing ninety it's exhausting to pull your nightshirt on . . . You are old when mashed potatoes are

difficult to chew, or when you guess it's Sunday because the mail doesn't come. It might be Christmas. In your eighties you take two naps à day. Nearing ninety you don't count the number of naps. In your eighties you don't eat much. Nearing ninety, you remember to eat.

If you guess the date based on the postman, and sleep most of the time, you are spending your days in a quiet abyss of loneliness, not hearing other voices, alone both practically and existentially. You are in what has been called the waiting room for death.

Suffering people may arrive at a place where their days are made up solely of discomforts, waiting, and attending to diseases and basic bodily functions, a place the vast majority of humans of the past never got to until recent medicine kept other diseases from killing them when younger.

This situation is unprecedented in human history. An unprecedented situation requires an unprecedented solution.

ACCEPTANCE

Something rumbled on my bedside table. Reaching for my pager, I looked at the ceiling, where our projection clock told me it was three fourteen A.M. On the pager's rectangular green display screen the words read "labored" and "breathing."

Our call group covered two practices—the housecalls clinic for frail, homebound elderly patients, and the geriatrics clinic with patients who might be anywhere from healthy to critically ill, and from young-old to ancient.

This text said the patient John was born in 1926, and the caller's name was Gwen. Grabbing my glasses, robe, and phone, I wondered whether it was Gwen or the page operator who had used the word *labored*. Closing the bedroom door behind me, another part of my brain began considering the problems that can take breathing from automatic to hard work. In medicine, such lists are known as the differential diagnosis, and doctors' minds are full of them. A good differential contains multiple possible causes of a particular symptom. Diagnoses are sorted from most to least likely, based on the patient's story, history, exam, and lab tests.

John's daughter Gwen answered on the first ring. In geriatrics, a daughter can be anywhere between forty and eighty years old, and from the sound of Gwen's voice, I guessed she was in the middle range.

"He's struggling," she explained, "and his pajamas are soaked in sweat. It's happened every night this week, but this is worse." Gwen told me that her father had advanced lung disease but usually breathed fine when in bed. He'd had a stroke in the past year and now had trouble swallowing. He had lost sixty pounds. He did not want to go to the hospital.

"There's another problem," she said after a pause. "Three months ago I moved him down the peninsula with us. We haven't been able to get him back to San Francisco since then. We can't get him out of bed, much less out of the house. My husband has a bad back. I just had surgery. And I can't find anyone down here who will see him, so I'm calling you. I didn't know who else to call. I'm so sorry."

I told her not to worry. After asking a few more questions about her father's breathing, I googled the distance from me to John and Gwen. It was 49.7 miles. Too far.

I asked Gwen whether she and her father had discussed what they would do if he was very sick and didn't go to the hospital.

"I hate this," she said. "We have: hospice. It's time. We both know it."

That answer made hers an easier call than many. Still, sometimes people's preferences change as they move from fairly healthy to chronically ill to dying. I wanted to make sure they understood the benefits and risks of both home and hospital, and that even though I was speaking to Gwen, we were doing what John wanted, not what we wanted for him.

These can be long, difficult conversations, but we didn't have time for that. I could hear John breathing. I counted his gasps. They were not only strained but fast, his body trying to get enough oxygen by breathing at one and a half times the normal speed. Gwen and I would have to sort things out at an accelerated pace too.

I told her that I was fairly sure I knew why John couldn't breathe and that we would be even more confident once a nurse or doctor had been to the house to examine him. I also admitted that in the home we could not be as definite about his diagnoses as we could in the hospital, where machines could see inside his heart and lungs, but that at some point many people became more concerned with feeling better than with knowing precisely what was wrong.

"That's what he wants," Gwen said. "There are so many things wrong, but if he could just not suffer so much . . ."

Given John's symptoms, I was reasonably certain that I could make him comfortable in their home. But first I had to make sure they understood the larger picture. There was a good chance John would not get better. He would die.

Gwen said her father had been hospitalized many times, and it hadn't been clear that the tests made much difference, so he'd stopped going. For nearly two years, that had worked. Each time, he'd recovered and remained out of the hospital.

Keeping people healthy and out of the hospital is among the main goals of geriatrics and why housecalls are so important. Often old and frail people do far better in a setting where they're allowed to remain people first, rather than having their personhood subsumed into the patient role, and their unique humanity and priorities replaced by protocols focused on diseases and treatments, as happened the second they crossed the thresholds of our hospitals and clinics. At home, there is less disorientation and more of the things like sleeping in a comfortable bed and eating favorite foods needed to restore health.

Much more than most people imagine can be done in the home: almost every part of the physical examination, blood draws, X-rays, joint injections, gynecologic tests, IV infusions, minor surgeries, and much more. Add to that the many, considerable dangers of hospitals that people avoid by staying home, and it becomes clear why studies and a large federal demonstration program have shown that housecalls lead to better care and better lives for chronically ill older adults like John.

But John wasn't just sick, he was terminally ill. I gently reminded Gwen that her father was eighty-eight years old and his heart, lungs, liver, and kidneys weren't working well. For some people in John's situation, living longer is the main goal, while others prioritize staying home and being comfortable. I also said that there was no right answer, only the right answer for John and his family.

"He knows he's dying," she said. "He says he just wants to feel less awful. And to stay here, with us. I know he's right. I just don't know what we can do for him at four in the morning."

Her use of the D word reassured me. Most people, doctors included, avoid it, and it's clear from studies across populations and educational backgrounds that when doctors don't use it, people are more surprised and angry when their loved one dies. Not using it also reinforces the delusion, unique to this time and place in human history, that with the right medical care death is optional. Using it, by contrast, provides people with the time and power to get used to something they may not like but cannot avoid and opportunities to do and say things before it's too late.

I got lucky that night. Both John and Gwen were able to use the D word, and they were unified in their clear preferences about how to proceed with his care.

I asked what drugs they had in the house, hoping for at least two types that would ease John's breathing. Morphine and its chemical cousins mute the air hunger of struggling or drowning lungs, and antianxiety medicines help with the natural distress that occurs when a person tries to breathe and can't get enough air.

"Oh, God," Gwen said. "We don't have anything like that. He didn't need it the last time he saw a doctor."

I hesitated, then asked what medications Gwen had been given after her own recent surgery.

"Oh," she said in a way that made clear she understood what I was thinking. "Hold on, I'll get them."

Now wide-awake, I turned on my computer and wrapped a blanket around my shoulders and bare feet. I could practically see the heaves and drops of John's chest, his sweaty brow, and the catch of light on his open mouth. I imagined, too, the minutes and hours that would follow this phone call: Gwen rearranging John's blankets and pillows, forcing herself to smile and make small talk, touching him here and there, whether necessary or not, as if to say: *I'm here, and so far, so are you.* And although I'd never met or so much as spoken to John, I had known enough fathers to see one more part of this scene: his efforts to pretend things weren't so bad in order to reassure the daughter he still wanted to protect, even now, long after the reversal of their original roles, though they both knew that very soon he'd have to abandon even that most fundamental piece of himself.

One of the most interesting things about being a doctor is how we are trained to keep personal feelings at bay while continuing to perform necessary, professional tasks. I felt a familiar tug, a tension gathering in my cells as if they were under the sway of a giant magnet pulling me south down the peninsula to that one lit room in a dark house on a darker street. Since I, too, had recently been the responsible daughter of a dying, elderly father, I imagined I knew how Gwen felt—the sadness and need to make things better, the fatigue and anxiety, the love and anticipation of an imminent, permanent transformation of her life. I noted my feelings, recognized them as projections, then squelched them and continued doing my job.

"Doctor?" Gwen read me the names on each of her pill bottles. *Bingo*, I thought when she stumbled over a particular chemical name. Next, I advised something that, along with some of his own medications, would relieve John's distress, something families do often but that doctors are not supposed to recommend. This combination would see him through until daylight, when we could get hospice and the right medicines into their house.

"I can't believe I didn't think of this," Gwen said. "What a relief!"

We made a plan for that night and one for the morning. Then I made Gwen promise to call again if John wasn't comfortable within the next hour.

She thanked me. Although she was appropriately serious and sad, there was also an energy to her voice that hadn't been there at the start of the call. Hanging up, I thought, not for the first time, how wrong people were when they said geriatrics was depressing or that having a patient die meant failure for the doctor. I felt deeply sad for Gwen and John, but that's not the same as depression, which suggests hopelessness and meaninglessness. These moments were hard for John and Gwen, likely among the hardest of their lives, but they were also profound, important, and meaningful.

\* \* \*

Recently, when I sent a condolence note to a friend about her stepfather's death, I received a long e-mail reply that included this paragraph:

> One of the many mysterious takeaway's from J's death and gigantic legacy is how it has made me feel terrifically alive and urgent to get more shit done, but also to pause and take time for those who matter and I don't get to see . . . In those last days . . . we all struggled with the protocols and systems around seeing an old man breathe his last breaths with dignity in the midst of [a] Shakespearean drama . . . Super weird and sad and comical and intense. Luckily my whole family circled the wagons . . . We all camped out in my Mom's apartment for the week to help manage the chaos and hold my mother up. So of course there's that other mystery, which is that it's been a lot of fun with loads of laughs. When else do I get so much prolonged time with my family without anyone feeling like there's another place to be, other responsibilities to maintain? We were all just there. Sitting. Eating. Answering the door. Loading and unloading the dishwasher . . .

In life, different people and families value different things; in death, they tend to value the same few fundamentals, and one of the surprises of an expected and mostly comfortable death at life's natural end is the license it gives everyone to put those fundamentals first.

John didn't die that night or that week, though he did die a few months later, in hospice.

# DEATH

*If we had the courage to think and reflect about life and death, we would raise our children differently . . . we would make death and dying a part of life again.*
—Elisabeth Kübler-Ross

# 14. STORIES

In an essay titled "On Sixty-Five," Emily Fox Gordon said she'd really begun to feel her age. But in the next paragraph, she wrote: "I hasten to add that though my muscles may be weakening and my joints stiffening, I'm not infirm. I'm as vigorous as I ever was, and reasonably healthy." A young person reading that passage might logically think: Hold on, now, you can't have it both ways: either you're weak and stiff or you're vigorous. Which is it? Fox Gordon offered similar contradictions about her cognition. "Mentally I'm quite intact, though my memory, always bad, grows worse." The point of the essay was that her body and life had changed in significant ways, and also, she seemed to lack many of what she took to be the defining manifestations of old age. Her acquaintances agreed with that assessment: "People tell me I seem younger than my years." By which, they presumably meant she still seemed like a "normal" human being.

Here are the facts: One, Fox Gordon was over halfway through her seventh decade, an "old person" by accepted definitions throughout most of human history and legally in the United States—she qualified for retirement, Social Security, and Medicare. Two, her body and mind had changed with age, mostly for the worse. Three, in her estimation and in the opinions of people who called her young-looking, being old wasn't half bad. The only logical conclusion one can draw from these facts is that there's a disconnect between the reality of old age and our beliefs about it—at least for the young-old.

People acknowledge their transition from adult to elder at different ages. Approaching her eighth decade, Doris Grumbach wrote: "This is different. The month at seventy seems disastrous, so without redeeming moments." The British book editor Diana Athill, looking back at her younger-old self from ninety, had a similar reaction: "All through my sixties I felt

I was still within hailing distance of middle age, not safe on its shores, perhaps, but navigating its coastal waters . . . Being 'over seventy' is being old: suddenly I was aground on that fact and saw that the time had come to size it up." By the summer of 2018, both Athill and Grumbach were one hundred years old. Both had published books in their nineties and essays in their hundredth year. If this qualifies them for the "exceptional elder" mantle, it also proves that seventy is not, by definition, an unmitigated disaster.

It is different, however. All ages are. At eighty, Penelope Lively described her aged self as almost becoming a new person:

> This someone else, this alter ego who has arrived, is less adventurous, more risk-averse, costive with her time . . . There is the matter of the spirit and the flesh, and that is the crux of it: the spirit is still game for experience, anything on offer, but the body most definitely is not, and unfortunately calls the shots.

The body is also what most people respond to, whether looking at someone else or at ourselves. Twenty-one years before she died at the age of ninety-four, Doris Lessing also referenced the growing distance between her body and self: "The great secret that all old people share is that you really haven't changed in seventy or eighty years. Your body changes, but you don't change at all. And that, of course, causes great confusion." Comments like these, common as they are among both great writers and my patients, make me wonder whether the greatest challenge of elderhood is overcoming our tendency to look at old age and see only bodily decline, forgetting that inside the body is a fellow human being.

At eighty-two, May Sarton wrote: "I have begun this journal at a time of difficult transition because I am now entering real old age. At seventy-five, I felt much more able than I do now . . . forgetting so much makes me feel disoriented sometimes and also slows me up. How to deal with continual frustration about small things like trying to button my shirt, and big things like how to try for a few more poems. That is my problem." Reading this, I picture a small, white-haired woman moving slowly. But also present in that passage are emotions and experiences I share: I, too, was more able seven years ago, in my forties; I, too, now forget things I once would have remembered; I, too, have things I'd like "to try for" in the remainder of my life. Look closely, and we are more similar than different.

By age ninety, Diana Athill lamented that "dwindling energy is one of the most boring things about being old. From time to time you get a day when it seems to be restored, and you can't help feeling that you are 'back to normal,' but it never lasts. You just have to resign yourself to doing less—or rather, taking more breaks than you used to in whatever you are doing." Even here, there is universality. Although old age is a particular state, replace *being old* in the first sentence with *being pregnant* or *being injured* or *being overworked* and the rest of Athill's words could describe any of us. Old age doesn't change our normal human responses.

Still, elderhood is different, and not just because of changes in the body and brain. "I'm ninety-three," wrote Roger Angell, "and I'm feeling great." There was, however, also this: "It shouldn't surprise me if at this time next week I'm surrounded by family, gathered on short notice to help decide, after what's happened, what's to be done with me now." Illness and death loom more prominently in elderhood than in earlier life stages. The tragedy of old age, wrote the Pulitzer Prize–winning geriatrician Robert Butler nearly fifty years ago, is "not the fact that each of us must grow old and die, but that the process of doing so has been made unnecessarily and at times excruciatingly painful, humiliating, debilitating, and isolating."

For one month in 2018, I conducted a thought experiment. Everywhere I went, I imagined the people I saw without hair dye or implants or comb-overs. The more I looked, the more I found—after all, men's first gray hairs generally appear at thirty, and women get their first, on average, by thirty-five. People from all ethnic groups. People who looked rich and people who looked poor. People who were adults, middle-aged, senior, old, elderly, and aged. Everywhere I looked (including in the mirror), I saw people pretending to be something other than what they were. How can it be that we have created a society where a majority of adults and elders feel ashamed of their basic identity? And if we are pretending to be something we are not, how can we be surprised or disappointed when others disparage what we are?

Imagine if everyone who was middle-aged or old looked middle-aged or old. Imagine if when we looked at our bus drivers, nurses, world leaders, teachers, rock stars, investment bankers, caregivers, cops, doctors, tech executives, grocery clerks, real estate brokers, lawyers, manicurists, and favorite actors, we saw what they really look like, who they really are. Imagine gray, white, and absent hair signaling the completion of youth and the ascent of maturity. Imagine if all those gray-, white-, and absent-haired people did all the things they already do. Imagine we liked, loved, respected, admired, and were inspired by them as we already are, and when they got older still and needed some help from us, we offered them a world and a worldview that said: *We still see you, and we still like, love, respect, admire, and are inspired by you, both for who you were and for who you are, a person completing the full arc of a human life.* Imagine old people seeming less "other" and more "us."

Most people want to look good, but when we define *good* as young, we set ourselves up for failure. We tell just one of the many stories of old age. Life offers just two possibilities: die young or grow old. The latter is the better option for most people, but it's not nearly as good an option as it could be. As go our hair color and health care dollars, so go our lives. If we pander to prejudice, we should not be surprised to find ourselves invisible, overlooked, or discarded.

# CODA

*It was my intention to write with a polemic voice.*
—Terese Marie Mailhot

# OPPORTUNITY

I have devoted as much of this book to history, literature, philosophy, anthropology, sociology, and stories as to science. The position that science will solve our species' greatest sources of anxiety and anguish already has vocal, powerful advocates. I wanted to add another perspective, to show that when we take a single approach to a complex challenge, we sacrifice not only accuracy and truth but opportunities to make life more of what we hope for and need and less of what we fear and dread.

A good life, like a good story, requires a beginning, a progression, and an ending. Without those defining elements, it feels partial, even tragic; it lacks shape, purpose, and meaning. The end may be hard and sad, but even when we don't want a story to end, the best ones leave us with a sense of completion and satisfaction.

The left-brain fixers among us offer only instruments. Sometimes these are lifesaving or life enhancing; other times, their unintended consequences overshadow any benefits. Without due diligence about who chooses the questions and tools, who benefits, and who might be gravely harmed, what appears to be progress can be anything but. Science and technology can only ask and answer certain sorts of questions. Those instruments, although now considered synonymous with progress in both medicine and life generally, will become socially and morally responsible only when they are paired at the outset with equal consideration of their origins, intent, and impact on people of all ages and backgrounds.

Events are judged not on their entirety but on their moments of peak intensity and on their endings. And what is life but a long, messy, awful, wonderful event? Elderhood is life's third and final act; what it looks like is up to us.

# ACKNOWLEDGMENTS

I owe a huge debt to:

The many writers and scholars quoted herein, not only those who have done so much for old age, but also those whose brilliant brave work taught me about writing, thinking, difference, and life. Particular thanks to Claudia Rankine, Ursula K. Le Guin, Andrew Solomon, Mary Beard, Matthew Desmond, and Maggie Nelson for showing me what was possible.

Victoria Sweet, for that September phone call when she gave me the advice that changed my approach to this book and helped me make it so much more of what I wanted it to be.

The medical institutions that made me the doctor I am: Harvard and, especially, UCSF. As two of the best in the country, they know their strengths. If in these pages I sometimes point out their opportunities for improvement, it's only because I know they can lead the nation to a better, more just, inclusive, and effective medical system.

My writing group—Catherine Alden, Natalie Baszile, Susi Jensen, Kathryn Ma, Edward Porter, Bora Reed, and Suzanne Wilsey—for the enduring pleasure of their friendship, good food, wise advice, and gracious indulgence of my deviation from fiction into writing the real.

The MacDowell Colony, where a years-old mess of documents and files was miraculously and almost instantaneously transformed into the first real draft of this book.

Bill Hall, whose remarkable achievements in medicine, unique erudition, widely learned lectures, and endless support have meant more to me than he appreciates.

David Shields, who told me the "weird" stuff I wanted to do in my writing was interesting and important.

Katy Butler and Sunita Puri, fellow travelers whose support always cheers me.

The editors who published parts of this book (before I knew that's what they were) in the following publications: the *New York Times*, the *New England Journal of Medicine*, the *Lancet*, *Health Affairs*, the *Washington Post*, *Academic Medicine*, and *New England Review*.

My patients, past, present, and future. The word *doctor* comes from the Latin *docere*, but any physician who has practiced medicine knows we learn as much from patients as they do from us. I cannot thank mine enough for entrusting me with their care.

My agent, Emma Patterson, and my editor, Nancy Miller, for their unwavering confidence and patience over the many years this book didn't get started, then the couple of years it didn't get finished, and their help once it was on its way.

My father, who taught me so much, directly and indirectly, and whom I miss.

My mother, always my biggest fan, whose elderhood I aspire to emulate and fear I won't.

Jane, especially and always.

# NOTES

**Conception**

xi **"never just a body"** Featherstone, M., & Wernick, A. (1995). *Images of aging: cultural representations of later life*. London, UK: Routledge.

**1. Life**

5 **over 40 percent of hospitalized adults** AHRQ Reports: Healthcare Costs and Utilization Project. (2010). *Overview statistics for inpatient hospital stays*.

**3. Toddler**

**History**

24 **"the book for the transformation of an old man into a youth"** Magner, L. N. (1992). *A history of medicine*. (35). New York, NY: Marcel Dekker.

24 **variability of old age** Plato, Grube, G. M. A., & Reeve, C. D. C. (1992). *Republic*. Indianapolis: Hackett Pub. Co.

24 **"end aging forever"** Buhr, S. (September 15, 2014). The $1 million race for the cure to end aging. *TechCrunch*; De Grey, A., & Rae, M. (2007). *Ending aging: The rejuvenation breakthroughs that could reverse human aging in our lifetime*. New York, NY: St. Martin's Press; McNicoll, A. (October 3, 2013). How Google's Calico aims to fight aging and "solve death." CNN; National Academy of Medicine. (October 19, 2015). *Special session: innovation in aging and longevity*. Special session of the Symposium on Aging at the NAM Annual Meeting, Washington, DC.

25 **similar stipulations for older adults** Span, P. (April 13, 2018). The clinical trial is open: the elderly need not apply. *New York Times*.

25 **exercise, diet, sleep, and management of constipation** Mulley, G. (2012). A history of geriatrics and gerontology. *European Geriatric Medicine*. 3(4), 225–227.

26 **"Apostle of Senescence"** Birren, J. E. (2007). History of gerontology. In Birren, J. E. (Ed.), *Encyclopedia of Gerontology* (2nd edition). San Diego: Academic Press (Elsevier); Peterson, M., & Rose, C. L. (1982). Historical antecedents of normative vs. pathological perspectives in aging. *Journal of the American Geriatrics Society*. (30)4, 292.

26 **moderation and personal responsibility** Walker, W. B. (1954). Luigi Cornaro, a renaissance writer on personal hygiene. *Bulletin of the History of Medicine*. 28(6), 525–534.

26 **Francis Bacon studied long-lived people** Peterson, M., & Rose, C. L. (1982). Historical antecedents of normative vs. pathological perspectives in aging. *Journal of the American Geriatrics Society*. (30)4, 292.

26 **he was right on all counts** Carp, F. (1977). Impact of improved living environment on health and life expectancy. *Gerontologist*. 17(3), 242–249; Fontana, L., & Partridge, L. (2015). Promoting health and longevity through diet: from model organisms to humans. *Cell*. 161(1), 10–118; Gravina, S., & Vijg, J. (2010). Epigenetic factors in aging and longevity. *Pflügers Archiv—European Journal of Physiology*. (459)2, 247–258; Terracciano, A., Löckenhoff, C. E.,

Zonderman, A. B., Ferrucci, L., & Costa, P. T. (2008). Personality predictors of longevity: activity, emotional stability, and conscientiousness. *Psychosomatic Medicine*. 70(6), 621–627.

26 **Discourse of the Preservation of the Sight** Susan, A. G., & Williams, M. E. (1994). A brief history of the development of geriatric medicine. *JAGS*. 42, 335–340.

27 **Struldbruggs** Swift, J. (1953). Chapter 10. *Gulliver's travels, book 3*. (234–249). London/Glasgow, UK: Collins.

27 **"progressive hardening of all fibres of the body"** Schafer, D. (2002). "That senescence itself is an illness": a transitional medical concept of age and ageing in the eighteenth century. *Medical History*. 46, 525–548.

27 **"old-age infirmity is no illness"** Parker, S. (2013). *Kill or cure: an illustrated history of medicine*. New York, NY: DK Publishing.

28 **"creating respectable cowards"** Cole, T. (1992). *The journey of life: a cultural history of aging in America*. Cambridge, UK: Cambridge University Press. (191).

28 **descriptions of dementia** Day, G. E. (1849). *Practical treatise on the domestic management and most important diseases of advanced life*. Philadelphia, PA: Lea and Blanchard.

28 **impact of early life habits** Fothergill, J. M. (1885). *The diseases of sedentary and advanced life: a work for medical and lay readers*. New York, NY: D. Appleton & Co.

28 **multimorbidity** Maclachlan, D. (1863). A *practical treatise on the diseases and infirmities of advanced age*. London, UK: John Churchill & Sons.

29 **"the mother of British geriatrics"** Kong, T. K. (2000). Marjory Warren: the mother of geriatrics. *Journal of the Hong Kong Geriatrics Society*. 10(2), 102–105.

29 **physical rehabilitation of the sick elderly** Matthews, D. A. (1984). Dr. Marjory Warren and the origin of British geriatrics. *Journal of the American Geriatrics Society*. 32(4), 253–258.

29 **radically different in function** Nevins, M. (2012). Chapter 9. *More meanderings in medical history*. (122). Bloomington, IN: iUniverse.

29 **"so-called 'incurable' cases"** Warren, M. W. (1943). Care of chronic sick. *British Medical Journal*. 2(4329), 822–823; Warren, M. W. (1946). Care of the chronic aged sick. *Lancet*. (247)6406, 841–843.

30 **approaches currently touted as innovative or transformational** Both who is doing the work and who is most likely to benefit from it have now, as they always have, a lot to do with money and power. See Friend, T. (2017). Silicon valley's quest to live forever. *New Yorker*.

39 **"not cooperating"** Span, P. (July 21, 2017). Another possible indignity of age: arrest. *New York Times*.

39 **taking care of older patients is the only necessary qualification** Diachun, L., Van Bussel, L., Hansen, K. T., Charise, A., & Rieder, M. J. (2010). "But I see old people everywhere": dispelling the myth that eldercare is learned in nongeriatric clerkships. *Academic Medicine*. 85(7), 1221–1228.

40 **many police departments . . . increasingly recognize the unintended harms** Brown, R. T., Ahalt, C., Steinman, M. A., Kruger, K., & Williams, B. A. (2014). Police on the front line of community geriatric healthcare: challenges and opportunities. *Journal of the American Geriatrics Society*. 62(11), 2191–2198; Brown, R. T., Ahalt, C., Rivera, J., Cenzer, I. S., Wilhelm, A., & Williams, B. A. (2017). Good cop, better cop: evaluation of a geriatrics training program for police. *Journal of the American Geriatrics Society*. 65(8), 1842–1847.

## 4. Child

### Houses

41 **would be called ethnic literature** Gilman, S. L. (1998) Introduction: ethnicity-ethnicities-literature-literatures. *PMLA*. 113(1), 19–27; Le, N. (2006). Love and honour and pity and pride and compassion and sacrifice. *Zoetrope: All Story*. 10(2); Lee, K. (February 23, 2012). Should we still be using the term "ethnic literature"? Huffington Post.

43 **a better job when treating bodies** Macapagal, K., Bhatia, R., & Greene, G. J. (2016). Differences in healthcare access, use, and experiences within a community sample of racially

diverse lesbian, gay, bisexual, transgender, and questioning emerging adults. *LGBT Health*. 3(6), 434–442; Rahman, M., Li, D. H., & Moskowitz, D. A. (2018). Comparing the healthcare utilization and engagement in a sample of transgender and cisgender bisexual+ persons. *Archives of Sexual Behavior.*

44 **bestselling medical novel** Shem, S. (2010). The house of God. New York, NY: Berkley Books.

### Resurrection

48 **"prescribing cascade"** Rochon, P. A., & Gurwitz, J. H. (1997). Optimising drug treatment for elderly people: the prescribing cascade. *British Medical Journal*. 315, 1096–1099.

### Confusion

51 **"barely noticeable until everything around has disappeared"** Bayley, J. (1999). Chapter 7. *Elegy for iris*. (115). New York, NY: Picador.

52 **"against invisible threats"** Ernaux, A. (1987). *A woman's story*. New York, NY: Seven Stories Press. (71–72).

52 **Americans fear dementia** (September 12, 2017) Why are we so afraid of dementia? *Conversation.*

52 **only about half the people with dementia have been diagnosed** Bradford, A., Kunik, M. E., Schulz, P., William, S. P., & Singh, H. (2009). Missed and delayed diagnosis of dementia in primary care: Prevalence and contributing factors. *Alzheimer's Disease and Associated Disorders*. 23(4), 306–314.

53 **significant variability among ethnic group subtypes** Mayeda, E. R., Glymour, M. M., Quesenberry, C. P., & Whitmer, R. A. (2016). Inequalities in dementia incidence between six racial and ethnic groups over fourteen years. *Alzheimer's & Dementia: The Journal of the Alzheimer's Association* 12(3), 216–224.

53 **doctors frequently miss the diagnosis of dementia** Valcour, V. G., Masaki, K. H., Curb, J. D., & Blanchette, P. L. (2000). The detection of dementia in the primary care setting. *Archives of Internal Medicine*. 160(19), 2964–2968; Callahan, C. M., Hendrie, H. C., & Tierney, W. M. (1995). Documentation and evaluation of cognitive impairment in elderly primary care patients. *Annals of Internal Medicine*. 122(6), 422–429; Lin, J. S., O'Connor, E., Rossom, R. C., Perdue, L. A., Eckstrom, E. (2013). Screening for cognitive impairment in older adults: a systematic review for the U.S. preventive services task force. *Annals of Internal Medicine*. 159(9), 601–612.

53 **3 percent of patients over age sixty-five were documented in 2018 as having some kind of cognitive impairment** Park, A. (March 24, 2015). Many doctors don't tell patients they have Alzheimer's. *Time*; Alzheimer's Association. (2015). 2015 Alzheimer's disease facts and figures. *Alzheimer's and Dementia*. 11(3), 332–384.

### Standards

57 **"I would have to watch this torture"** Gabow, P. (2015). The fall: aligning the best care with standards of care at the end of life. *Health Affairs*. 34(5), 871–874.

58 **treats *diseases* rather than attending to *illness*** Kleinman, A. (1988). *Illness narratives*. New York, NY: Basic Books.

58–59 **cause significant suffering** Jecker, N. S. (2017). Doing what we shouldn't: medical futility and moral distress. *American Journal of Bioethics*. 17(2), 41–43; Derse, A. R. (2017). "Erring on the side of life" is sometimes an error: physicians have the primary responsibility to correct this. *American Journal of Bioethics*. 17(2), 39–41.

### Other

62 **"a list of the things that were wrong"** Gross, T., & Brown, M. M. (August 4, 2017). Poet imagines life inside a 1910 building that eugenics built. Fresh Air: *NPR*. 31:18—31:44, 32:15–33:48, 34:01–34:06.

62 **"shared meaning and coherence"** Cole, T. (1992). *The journey of life: a cultural history of aging in America.* (230). Cambridge, MA: Cambridge University Press.

62 **"less than" compared with youth** Haraven, T. K. (1976). The last stage: historical adulthood and old age. *American Civilization: New Perspectives.* 105(4), 13–27.

### 5. Tween
#### Normal

64 **history of Western medicine** Much of what I cite as history in this book is in fact merely the history of Europe and the North American continent. Written in English, that literature is more accessible to me, and because the book's focus is the United States, it's often also most relevant to American beliefs and institutions.

64 **more soldiers if fewer children died** Brosco, J. P. (2012). Navigating the future through the past: the enduring historical legacy of federal children's health programs in the United States. *American Journal of Public Health.* 102(10), 1849–1857.

67 **entirely absent from current AAMC surveys** Association of American Medical Colleges. (2018). Medical school graduation questionnaire.

67 **"hidden curriculum"** Hafferty, F. W. (1998). Beyond curriculum reform: confronting medicine's hidden curriculum. *Academic Medicine.* 73(4), 403–407.

68 **taken-for-granted aspects in the clinical setting** Esteghamati, A., Baradaran, H., Monajemi, A., Khankeh, H. R., & Geranmayeh, M. (2016). Core components of clinical education: a qualitative study with attending physicians and their residents. *Journal of Advances in Medical Education & Professionalism.* 4(2), 64–71.

68 **the maroon 1987 edition** Bickley, L. S. (2003). *Bates' guide to physical examination and history taking.* Philadelphia: Lippincott Williams & Wilkins.

#### Different

69 **"on the road to eliminating them"** Allport, G. W. (1954). *The nature of prejudice.* Cambridge, MA: Addison-Wesley Pub. Co.

70 **"because they are old"** Butler, R. N. (1975). *Why survive?: Being old in America.* Baltimore, MD: Johns Hopkins University Press.

70 **"time preceding death"** Butler, R. N. (1975). *Why survive?: Being old in America.* Baltimore, MD: Johns Hopkins University Press.

70 **"older people as different"** Butler, R. N. (1975). *Why survive?: Being old in America.* Baltimore, MD: Johns Hopkins University Press.

72 **"the child of ignorance"** Hazlitt, W. On prejudice. In *Sketches and essays.* London, UK: Richards.

72 **"frailty and error"** Voltaire. (1984). Tolerance. In T. Besterman (Ed.), Philosophical dictionary. London, UK: Penguin Classics.

72 **"resistant to all evidence"** Allport, G. W. (1954). *The nature of prejudice.* Cambridge, MA: Addison-Wesley Publishing Co.

### 6. Teen
#### Evolution

79 **Similar sentiments** Goldman, D. P., Chen, C., Zissimopoulos, J., Rowe, J. W., & the Research Network on an Aging Society. (2018). Opinion: measuring how countries adapt to societal aging. *Proceedings of the National Academy of Sciences of the United States of America.* 115(3), 435–437.

80 **didn't expect to grow old** Thane, P. (2003). Social histories of old age and aging. *Journal of Social History.* 37(1), 93–111.

81 **"divine and ancestral sources"** Falkner, T. M., & De Luce, J. (Eds.). Homeric heroism, older age and the end of the *Odyssey* in *Old age in Greek and Latin literature* (25). Albany, NY: State University of New York Press.

81 **one-line short story** Davis, L. (July 10, 2017). Fear of ageing. *New York Tyrant.*

**Perversions**

85 **more harm than good** Finlayson, E. (2015). Surgery in the elderly: aligning patient goals with expected outcomes. [PowerPoint slides]; Suskind, A., Jin, C., Cooperberg, M. R., Finlayson, E., Boscardin, W. J., Sen, S., & Walter, L. C. (2016). Preoperative frailty is associated with discharge to skilled or assisted living facilities after urologic procedures of varying complexity. *Urology.* 97, 25–32.

**Rejuvenation**

87 **They offer the hope** Featherstone, M., & Hepworth, M. (1995). Images of positive aging: a case study of Retirement Choice magazine. In M. Featherstone, & A. Wernick (Eds.) *Images of aging: cultural representations of later life.* (29–48). London, UK: Routledge.

88 **"geroscience hypothesis"** Austad, S. (2016). The geroscience hypothesis: is it possible to change the rate of aging? In F. Sierra, & R. Kohanski (Eds.). *Advances in Geroscience.* (1–36). Bethesda, MD: Springer International Publishing.

88 **interrupting the aging process** Cristofalo, V. J., Gerhard, G. S., & Pignolo, R. J. (1994). Molecular biology of aging. *Surgical Clinics of North America.* 74(1), 1–21; Pignolo, R. J. (n.d.). The biology of aging: an overview. [PowerPoint slides]. Retrieved from https://www.med.upenn.edu/gec/user_documents/Pignolo-BiologyofAging2012GGRFINAL.pdf.

88 **lived to 120 years old** Herodotus. (1920). Book III in A. D. Godley (Ed.) *The Histories.* (23). Cambridge, UK: Harvard University Press.

89 **hormone injections popular** Gruman, G. J. (1961). The rise and fall of prolongevity hygiene, 1558–1873. *Bulletin of the History of Medicine.* 35, 221–225.

89 **caloric restriction** Weindruch, R., & Sohal, R. S. (1997). Caloric intake and aging. *New England Journal of Medicine.* 337(14), 986–994.

89 **positive hormonal changes** Roth, G. S., Mattison, J. A., Ottinger, M. A., Chachich, M. E., Lane, M. A., & Ingram, D. K. (2004). Aging in rhesus monkeys: relevance to human health interventions. *Science.* 305(5689), 1423–1426.

90 **resveratrol . . . activates sirtuins** Baur, J. A., Pearson, K. J., Price, N. L., Jamieson, H. A., Lerin, C., Kalra, A., et al. (2006). Resveratrol improves health and survival of mice on a high-calorie diet. *Nature.* 444(7117), 337–342.

90 **"looking for drug targets"** Buck Institute for Research on Aging. (September 5, 2017). Ketogenic diet improves healthspan and memory in aging mice. *Eurekalert!*

90 **"senolytics"** Kirland, J. L., Tchkonia, T., Zhu, Y., Niedernhofer, L. J., & Robbins, P. D. (2017). The clinical potential of senolytic drugs. *Journal of American Geriatrics Society.* 65(10), 2297–2301.

90 **certain aging-associated markers** Baker, D. J., Wijshake, T., Tchkonia, T., LeBrasseur, N. K., Childs, B. G., van de Sluis, B., et al. (2011). Clearance of p16$^{Ink}$4$^a$—positive senescent cells delays ageing-associated disorders. *Nature.* 479(7372), 232–236.

91 **prolong life in flies** Bitto, A., Ito, T. K., Pineda, V. V., LeTexier, N. J., Huang, H. Z., Sutlief, E., et al. (2016). Transient rapamycin treatment can increase lifespan and healthspan in middle-aged mice. *eLife.* 5, 16351; Bjedov, I., Toivonen, J. M., Kerr, F., Slack, C., Jacobson, J., Foley, A., & Partridge, L. (2010). Mechanisms of life span extension by rapamycin in the fruit fly *Drosophila melanogaster. Cell Metabolism.* 11(1), 35–46; Blagosklonny, M. V. (2013). Rapamycin extends life- and health span because it slows aging. *Aging (Albany NY).* 5(8), 592–598; Ehningher, D., Neff, F., & Xie, K. (2014). Longevity, aging, and rapamycin. *Cellular and Molecular Life Sciences.* 71(22), 4325–4346.

91 **Stem cells** Barber, G. (March 27, 2018). The Science behind the pursuit of youth. Wired.

91 **use of hormones** Perls, T. T., Reisman, N. R., & Olshansky, S. J. (2005). Provision or distribution of growth hormone for "antiaging": clinical and legal issues. *JAMA.* 294(16), 2086–2090.

92 **finitude of cell divisions** Hayflick, L., and Moorhead, P. S. (1961). "The serial cultivation of human diploid cell strains." *Experimental Cell Research* 25:585–621.

92 **"they may be harmful"** Olshansky, S. J., Hayflick, L., & Carnes, B. A. (2002). Position statement on human aging. *Journals of Gerontology. Series A, Biological Sciences and Medical Sciences.* 57(8), B292–297.

### Gaps

94 **top four drugs** O'Connor, A. (November 23, 2011). Four drugs cause most hospitalizations in older adults. *New York Times.*

95 **There were no requirements to include them** National Institutes of Health (May 25, 2018). *Inclusion Across the Lifespan—Policy Implementation.*

95 **what happens in the real world** Hughes, L. D., McMurdo, M. E., & Guthrie, B. (2013). Guidelines for people not for diseases: the challenges of applying UK clinical guidelines to people with multimorbidity. *Age Ageing.* 42(1), 62–69.

96 **conditions that commonly coexist** Boyd, C. M., Darer, J., Boult, C., Fried, L. P., Boult, L., & Wu, A. W. (2005). Clinical practice guidelines and quality of care for older patients with multiple comorbid diseases: implications for pay for performance. *JAMA.* 294(6), 716–724.

96 **The exclusion of old people from studies** Shenoy, P., & Harugeri, A. (2015). Elderly patients' participation in clinical trials. *Perspectives in Clinical Research.* 6(4), 184–198.

96 **a disease of old people** Brauer, C. A., Coca-Perraillon, M., Cutler, D. M., & Rosen, A. B. (2009). Incidence and mortality of hip fractures in the United States. *JAMA.* 302(14), 1573–1579.

96 **Cochrane Library Database** McCarvey, C., Coughlan, T., & O'Neill, D. (2017). Ageism in studies on the management of osteoporosis. *Journal of the American Geriatrics Society.* 65(7), 1566–1568.

97 **cancer screening** Walter, L. C., & Covinsky, K. E. (2001). Cancer screening in elderly patients: a framework for individualized decision making. *JAMA.* 285(21), 2750–2756.

97 **to surgery** Suskind, A. M., Zhao, S., Walter, L. C., Boscardin, W. J., & Finlayson, E. (2018). Mortality and functional outcomes after minor urological surgery in nursing home residents: a national study. *Journal of the American Geriatrics Society.* 66(5), 909–915.

98 **homebound old people** American Academy of Home Care Physicians. (n.d.). The case for home care medicine: access, quality, cost.

99 **cost of one emergency visit** Ornstein, K., Wajnberg, A., Wajnberg, A., Kaye-Kauderer, H., Winkel, G., DeCherrie, L., et al. (2013). Reduction in symptoms for homebound patients receiving home-based primary and palliative care. *Journal of Palliative Medicine.* 16(9), 1048–1054; Totten, A. M., White-Chu, E. F., Wasson, N., Morgan, E., Kansagara, D., Davis-O'Reilly, C., & Goodlin, S. (2016). Home-based primary care interventions. *Comparative Effectiveness Reviews, No. 164.*

### Adulthood

103 **"well-meaning and competent"** Mount, B. M. (1976). The problem of caring for the dying in a general hospital; the palliative care unit as a possible solution. *Canadian Medical Association Journal.* 115.

### 7. Young Adult
### Modern

110 **little interest to most doctors** Vaughan, C. P., Fowler, R., Goodman, R. A., Graves, T. R., Flacker, J. M., & Johnson, T. M. (2014). Identifying landmark articles for advancing the practice of geriatrics. *Journal of American Geriatrics Society.* 62(11), 2159–6162.

110 **languishing in a no-man's-land** Friedman, S. M., Shah, K., & Hall, W. J. (2015). Failing to focus on healthy aging: a frailty of our discipline? *Journal of American Geriatrics Society.* 63(7), 1459–1562.

110 **paucity of geriatrics-trained nurses** Morley, J. E. A brief history of geriatrics. *Journals of Gerontology. Series A Biological Sciences and Medical Sciences* 2004;59:1132–1152.

110 **"unmet need among the elderly"** Bynum, W. F., & Porter, R. (Eds.). (1993). *Companion encyclopedia of the history of medicine.* (1107). New York, NY: Routledge.

111 **not supporting big health means not getting reelected** Rosenthal, E. (2017). *An American sickness: how healthcare became big business and how you can take it back.* New York: Penguin Press.

### Mistakes

119 **doctors who apologize** Robbennolt, J. K. (2009). Apologies and medical error. *Clinical Orthopaedics and Related Research.* 467(2), 376–382.

120 ***normal* is defined as** Peterson, M., & Rose, C. L. (1982). Historical antecedents of normative vs. pathological perspectives in aging. *Journal of the American Geriatrics Society.* 30(4), 289–294.

120 **"the fevers of old men are less acute"** Gunnarsson, B. L. (2011). *Languages of science in the eighteenth century.* Berlin, DE: Walter de Gruyter GmbH & Co. (273).

120 **increased vulnerability to disease** Ritch, A. (2012). History of geriatric medicine: from Hippocrates to Marjory Warren. *Journal for the Royal College of Physicians of Edinburgh.* 42(4), 368–374.

120 **several diseases simultaneously** Banerjee, S. (2014). Multimorbidity-older adults need health care that can count past one. *Lancet.* 385(9968), 587–589; Wolff, J. L., Starfield, B, & Anderson, G. (2002). Prevalence, expenditures, and complications of multiple chronic conditions in the elderly. *Archives of Internal Medicine.* 162(20), 2269–2276.

120 **"special characteristics"** Charcot, J. M. (1881). *Clinical lectures on the diseases of old age.* New York, NY: William Wood & Co.; Charcot, J. M. (1889). *Clinical lectures on diseases of the nervous system.* London, UK: The New Sydenham Society.

### Competence

124 ***competence . . . capacity*** American Bar Association Commission on Law and Aging, & American Psychological Association. (2008). *Assessment of older adults with diminished capacity: a handbook for psychologists.* American Bar Association Commission on Law and Aging & American Psychological Association. (12); Leo, R. J. (1999). Competency and capacity to make treatment decisions: a primer for primary care physicians. *The Primary Care Companion to the Journal of Clinical Psychiatry.* 1(5), 131–141; Moye, J., & Marson, D. C. (2007). Assessment of decision-making capacity in older adults: an emerging area of practice and research. *Journals of Gerontology: Series B.* 62(1), 3–11; Silberfeld, M., Stevens, D., Lieff, S., Checkland, D., & Madigan, K. (1992). Legal standards and threshold of competence. *Advocates' Quarterly.* 14, 482.

124 **against their well-being** Moye, J., Marson, D. C., Edelstein, B. (2013). Assessment of capacity in an aging society. *American Psychologist.* 68(3), 158–171.

124 **mildly disabling hearing loss** Cruickshanks, K. J., Tweed, T. S., & Wiley, T. L. (2003). The five-year incidence of progression of hearing loss: the epidemiology of hearing loss study. *JAMA Otolaryngology—Head & Neck Surgery.* 129(10), 1041–1046.

### Bias

129 ***The White Album*** Didion, J. (1979). *The white album.* New York, NY: Noonday.

130 **demographic groups express distress in different ways** Lewis-Fernandez, R., & Díaz, N. (2002). The cultural formulation: a method for assessing cultural factors affecting the clinical

encounter. *Psychiatric Quarterly*. 73(4), 271–295; Myers, H. F., Lesser, I., Rodriguez, N., Mira, C. B., Hwang, W. C., Camp, C., et al. (2002). Ethnic differences in clinical presentation of depression in adult women. *Cultural Diversity and Ethnic Minority Psychology*, 8(2), 138–156; Takeuchi, D. T., Chun, C. A., Gong, F., & Shen, H. (2002). Cultural expressions of distress. *Health: An Interdisciplinary Journal for the Social Study of Health, Illness and Medicine*. 6(2).

131 **"the Negro in America"** Baldwin, J., & Peck, R. (Writers) & Peck, R. (Director). (2016). *I am not your negro*. United States: Magnolia Pictures.

132 **altered mental status was delirium** Oh, E. S., Fong, T. G., Hshieh, T. T., & Inouye, S. K. (2017). Delirium in older persons: advances in diagnosis and treatment. *JAMA* 318(12), 1161–1174.

133 **research on biases in medicine** FitzGerald, C., & Hurst, S. (2017). Implicit bias in healthcare professionals: a systematic review. *BMC Medical Ethics*, 18(1), 19; Shaband, H. (August 29, 2014). How racism creeps into medicine. *Atlantic*.

133 **wouldn't want to be old** Levy, B. R. (2003). Mind matters: cognitive and physical effects of aging self-stereotypes. *Journals of Gerontology: Series B*. 58(4): 203–211.

133 **the importance of *intersectionality*** Crenshaw, K., Gotanda, N., Peller, G., & Thomas, K. (1995). *Critical race theory: the key writings that formed the movement* (6th edition). New York, NY: New Press; hooks, b. (1990). *Yearning: race, gender, and cultural politics*. Boston, MA: South End; Crenshaw, K. (September 24, 2015). Why intersectionality can't wait. *Washington Post*.

134 **scientifically sound and morally distressing data** Goddu, P., O'Conor, K. J., Lanzkron, S., Saheed, M. O., Peek, M. E., Haywood, C., & Beach, M. C. (2018). Do words matter? Stigmatizing language and the transmission of bias in the medical record. *Journal of General Internal Medicine*. 33(5), 685–691; Haider, A. H., Sexton, J., Sriram, N., Cooper L. A., Efron, D. T., Swoboda, S., et al. (2011). Association of unconscious race and social class bias with vignette-based clinical assessments by medical students. *JAMA*. 306(9), 942–951; Hall, W. J., Chapman, M. V., Lee, K. M., Merino, Y. M., Thomas, T. W., Payne, K., et al. (2015). Implicit racial/ethnic bias among health care professionals and its influence on health care outcomes: a systematic review. *American Journal of Public Health*. 105(12), e60–e76; Hamberg, K. (2008). Gender bias in medicine. *Women's Health*. 4(3), 237–243; Jackson, C. L., Agénor, M., Johnson, D. A., Austin, S. B., & Kawachi, I. (2016). Sexual orientation identity disparities in health behaviors, outcomes, and services use among men and women in the United States: a cross-sectional study. *BMC Public Health*. 16, 807; Scheck, A. (2004). Race, gender, and age affect medical care, so why does bias persist? *Emergency Medical News*. 26(5), 18–21.

134 **two patients of the same age and grooming and class** Kaul, P., Armstrong, P. W., Sookram, S., Leung, B. K., Brass, N., & Welsh, R. (2011). Temporal trends in patient and treatment delay among men and women presenting with ST-elevation myocardial infarction. *American Heart Journal*. 161(1), 91–97; Liakos, M., & Parikh, P. B. (2018). Gender disparities in presentation, management, and outcomes of acute myocardial infarction. *Current Cardiology Reports*. 20, 64; Vaccarino, V., Rathore, S. S., Wenger, N. K., Frederick, P. D., Abramson, J. L., Barron, H. V., et al. (2005). Sex and racial differences in the management of acute myocardial infarction, 1994 through 2002. *New England Journal of Medicine*. 353, 671–682.

134 **primary language is English** Nguyen, M., Ugarte, C., Fuller, I., Haas, G., & Portenoy, R. K. (2005). Access to care for chronic pain: racial and ethnic differences. *Journal of Pain*. 6(5), 301–314; Campbell, C. M., & Edwards, R. R. (2012). Ethnic differences in pain and pain management. *Pain Management*. 2(3), 219–230.

136 **when they began dialysis** Grubbs, V. (2017). *Hundreds of interlaced fingers: a kidney doctor's search for the perfect match*. United States: Amistad.

NOTES // 415

## 8. Adult

### Oblivious

137 **The Unknown Profession** Campbell, J. Y., Durso, S. C., Brandt, L. E., Finucane, T. E., & Abadir, P. M. (2013). The unknown profession: a geriatrician. *Journal of American Geriatrics Society.* 61(3), 447–449.

139 **Calling an older person cute** Whitbourne, S. K., & Sneed, J. R. (2004). Chapter 8: The paradox of well-being, identity processes, and stereotype threat: ageism and its potential relationships to the self in later life. In T. D. Nelson (Ed.), *Ageism: stereotyping and prejudice against older persons.* (247). Cambridge, MA: MIT Press.

139 **"does not fit the speaker's stereotypes about old"** The Old Women's Project. (n.d.). *Real-life examples of ageist comments.*

### Language

141 **"If I'm ninety and believe I'm forty-five"** Le Guin, U. K. (2017). *No time to spare: thinking about what matters.* (193). Boston, MA: Houghton Mifflin.

141 **"Old age is for"** Le Guin, U. K. (2017). *No time to spare: thinking about what matters.* (201). Boston, MA: Houghton Mifflin.

141 **"to tell me I don't exist"** Le Guin, U. K. (2017). *No time to spare: thinking about what matters.* (243). Boston, MA: Houghton Mifflin.

142 **a metaphor for happiness** Sontag, S. (1972). The double standard of aging. *Saturday Review.* 29–38.

142 **"'Old' means you're past your prime"** Morris, W. (July 19, 2017). Jay-Z and the politics of rapping in middle age. *New York Times.*

143 **illness metaphors** Sontag, S. (1979). *Illness as metaphor.* (3). New York, NY: Vintage Press.

### Vocation

145 **Dr. Ken Brummel-Smith's** Kemp, B., Brummel-Smith, K., & Ramsdell, J. (Eds.). (1990) *Geriatric rehabilitation.* Austin, TX: Pro-Ed Press.

146 **medical training doesn't just erode doctors' empathy** Dyrbye, L. N., Thomas, M. R., & Shanafelt, T. D. (2005). Medical student distress: causes, consequences, and proposed solutions. *Mayo Clinic Proceedings.* 80(12), 1613–1622; West, C. P., Huschka, M. M., Novotny, P. J., Sloan, J. A., Kolars, J. C., Haberman, T. M., & Shanafelt, T. D. (2006). Association of perceived medical errors with resident distress and empathy: a prospective longitudinal study. *JAMA.* 296, 1071–1078.

146 **Greek words for old age physician** Nascher, I. L. (1909). Geriatrics. *New York Medical Journal.* 90(17), 358–359; Nascher, I. L. (1914). *Geriatrics: the diseases of old age and their treatment.* Philadelphia, PA: P. Blakiston's Son & Co.

146 **"senility and its diseases apart from maturity"** Nascher, I. L. (1909). Longevity and rejuvenescence. *New York Medical Journal.* 89(16), 794–800.

146 **the state of being old** Dodd, Mead, & Co. (1916). *The new international encyclopaedia.* (703). New York, NY: Dodd, Mead and Co.; Ozarin, L. (2008). I. L. Nascher, MD (1863–1944): the first American geriatrician. *Psychiatric News.* https://doi.org/10.1176/pn.43.22.0024.

146 **"have never been numerous or powerful"** Thane, P. (1993). Chapter 46: Geriatrics. In W. F. Bynum & R. Porter (Ed.), *Companion Encyclopedia of the History of Medicine* (1092). London, UK; New York, NY: Routledge.

146 **"The conservation of old people . . . has been neglected"** Freeman, J. T. (1950). François Ranchin contributor of an early chapter in geriatrics. *Journal of the History of Medicine and Allied Sciences.* 5(4), 422–431; Thane, P. (2005). *A history of old age.* Oxford, UK: Oxford University Press.

147 **gérocomie** (Greek: *geron*—old man; *komeo*—to take care of it) Bynum, W. F., & Porter, R. (Eds.). (1993). *Companion encyclopedia of the history of medicine: volume 2.* (1095). London, UK; New York, NY: Routledge.

147 **the lack of lectures about old patients** Freeman, J. T. (1961). Nascher: excerpts from his life, letters, and works. *Gerontologist*, 1, 17–26.

148 **the first geriatrics lecture** Burstein, S. R. (1946). Gerontology: a modern science with a long history. *Postgraduate Medical Journal*.

148 **"a reaction against the belief"** Howell, T. H. (1975). *Old age: some practical points in geriatrics* (3rd edition). London, UK: H. K. Lewis. (101).

148 **medical care harms and kills** Gabow, P. A., Hutt, D. M., Baker, S., Craig, S. R., Gordon, J. B., & Lezotte, D. C. (1985). Comparison of hospitalization between nursing homes and community residents. *Journal of the American Geriatrics Society*. 33(8), 524–529; Graham, J. (December 8, 2016). You're not just "growing old" if this happens to you. *Kaiser Health News*; Piers, R. D., Van den Eynde, M., Steeman, E., Vlerick, P., Benoit, D. D., & Van Den Noortgate, N. J. (2012). End-of-life of the geriatric patient and nurses' moral distress. *Journal of the American Medical Directors Association*. 13(1), 7–13; Pijl-Zier, E., Armstrong-Esther, C., Hall, B., Akins, L., & Stingl, M. (2008). Moral distress: an emerging problem for nurses in long-term care? *Quality in Ageing and Older Adults*. 9(2), 29–48; Span, P. (June 22, 2018). Breathing tubes fail to save many older patients. *New York Times*; Tedeschi, B. (March 28, 2018). With the help of a loved one, a family finds what is essential in the end. *STAT*.

**Distance**

155 **"an old person in a nursing home"** Lynn, J. (2008). *Aging America: a reform agenda for living well and dying well*. Hastings Center Bioethics Agenda 08: America Ages.

**Values**

155 **physician career satisfaction** Leigh, J. L., Kravitz, R. L, Schembi, M., Samuels, S. J., & Mobley, S. (2002). Physician career satisfaction across specialties. *Archives of Internal Medicine*. 162(14), 1577–1584; Leigh, J. P., Tancredi, D. J., & Kravitz, R. L. (2009). Physician career satisfaction within specialties. *Biomedical Central Health Services Research*. (9, 166); Siu, A. L., & Beck, J. C. (1990). Physician satisfaction with career choices in geriatrics. *The Gerontologist*. 30(4), 529–534.

156 **elder-friendly hospitals** American Geriatrics Society Expert Panel on the Care of Older Adult with Multimorbidity. (2012). *Journal of American Geriatrics Society*. 60(10), E1–E25; Capezuit, E. A. (2015). *Geriatrics models of care: bringing "best practice" to an aging America*. New York, NY: Springer; Coleman, E. A., & Boult, C. (2003). Improving the quality of transitional care for persons with complex care needs. *Journal of the American Geriatrics Society*. 51(4), 556–557; Counsell, S. R., Holder, C. M., Libenauer, L. L., Palmer, R. M., Fortinsky, R. H., Kresivic, D. M., et al. (2000). Effects of multicomponent intervention on functional outcomes and process of care in hospitalized older patients: a randomized controlled trial of Acute Care for Elders (ACE) in a community hospital. *Journal of the American Geriatrics Society*. 48(12), 1572–1581; Fulmer, T., & Berman, A. (November 3, 2016). Age-friendly health systems: how do we get there? *Health Affairs*; Meier, D. E., & Gaisman, C. (2007). Palliative care is the job of every hospital. *Medscape General Medicine*. 9(3), 6.

156 **to what they are** Sandberg, S. (2013). *Lean in: women, work, and the will to lead*. New York, NY: Alfred A. Knopf; Mody, L., Boustani, M., Braun, U. K., & Sarkisian, C. (2017). Evolution of geriatric medicine: midcareer faculty continuing the dialogue. *Journal of the American Geriatrics Society*. 65(7), 1389–1391.

156 **"not equally been extended"** Nascher, I. L. (1914). *Geriatrics: the diseases of old age and their treatment*. (XV) Philadelphia, PA: P. Blakiston's Son & Co.

156 **"The cause of this neglect"** Nascher, I. L. (1914). *Geriatrics: the diseases of old age and their treatment*. (V) Philadelphia, PA: P. Blakiston's Son & Co.

156–57 **"treatment of diseases in senility"** Nascher I. L. (1909). Longevity and rejuvenescence. *New York Medical Journal*.

157 **"those who are economically worthless"** Nascher, I. L. (1914). *Geriatrics: the diseases of old age and their treatment*. (VI). Philadelphia, PA: P. Blakiston's Son & Co.

159 **"a ton of problems"** Higashi, R. T., Tilack, A. A., Steinman, M., Harper, M., & Johnson, C. B. (2012). Elder care as "frustrating" and "boring": understanding the persistence of negative attitudes toward older patients among physicians-in-training. *Journal of Aging Studies*. 26(4), 476–483.

### Truth

170 **interact with other parts** Steel, N., Abdelhamid, A., Stokes, T., Edwards, H., Fleetcroft, R., Howe, A., & Qureshi, N. (2014). A review of clinical practice guidelines found that they were often based on evidence of uncertain relevance to primary care patients. *Journal of Clinical Epidemiology*, 67(11), 1251–1257; Jansen, J., McKinn, S., Bonner, C., Irwig, L., Doust, J., Glasziou, P., et al. (2015). Systematic review of clinical practice guidelines recommendations about primary cardiovascular disease prevention for older adults. *BMC Family Practice*, 16, 104; Upshur, R. E. G. (2014). Do clinical guidelines still make sense? No. *Annals of Family Medicine*, 12(3), 202–203.

170 **clinicians struggle to personalize** Bodenheimer, T., Lo, B., & Casalino, L. (1999). Primary care physicians should be coordinators, not gatekeepers. *JAMA*. 281(21), 2045–2049; Wenrich, M. D., Curtis, J. R., Ambrozy, D. A., Carline, J. D., Shannon, S. E., & Ramsey, P. G. (2003). *Journal of Pain and Symptom Management*. 25(3), 236–246.

170 **social services that might improve their lives** Bradley, E. H., Canavan, M., Rogan, E., Talbert-Slagle, K., Ndumele, C., Taylor, L., Curry, L. A. (2016). Variation in health outcomes: the role of spending on social services, public health, and health care, 200–209. *Health Affairs*. 35(5), 760–768; Schneider, E. C., & Squires, D. (2017). From last to first—could the U.S. health care system become the best in the world? *New England Journal of Medicine*. 377, 901–904.

170–71 **falls have innumerable causes** Delbaere, K., Close, J. C., Brodaty, H., Sachdev, P, & Lord, S. R. (2010). Determinants of disparities between perceived and physiological risk of falling among elderly people: cohort study. *British Medical Journal*. 341, 4165.

### Biology

173 **seven stages** Shakespeare, W. (1963). *As you like it*. H. H. Furness (Ed.). New York, NY: Dover Publications.

173 **losing the ability to self-regulate** Cristofalo, V. J., Allen, R. G., Pignolo, R. J., Martin, B. G., & Beck, J. C. (1998). Relationship between donor age and the replicative lifespan of human cells in culture: a reevaluation. *Proceedings of the National Academy of Sciences of the United States of America*. 95(18), 10614–10619; Cristofalo, V. J., Gerhard, G. S., Pignolo, R. J. (1994). Molecular biology of aging. *Surgical Clinics of North America*. 74(1), 1–21; Cristofalo, V. J., Lorenzini, A., Allen, R. G., Torres, C., & Tresini, M. (2004). Replicative senescence: a critical review. *Mechanisms of Ageing and Development*. 125(10–11), 827–848.

174 **autolysis** Morales, A. (2016). *The girls in my town*. (92). Albuquerque, NM: University of New Mexico Press.

174 **single-celled populations are immortal** Masoro, E. J. (Ed.). (1995). *Handbook of physiology Sect 11: Aging*. (3–21). Oxford, UK: Oxford University Press.

174 **gradually deteriorate from maturation** Finch, C. E. (1990). *Longevity, senescence, and the genome*. Chicago, IL: University of Chicago Press.

174 **human body as it ages** Benetos, A., Okuda, K., Lajemi, M., Kimura, M., Thomas, F., Skurnick, J., et al. (2018). Telomere length as an indicator of biological aging. *Hypertension*. 37, 381–385; Epel, E. S., Blackburn, E. H., Lin, J., Dhabhar, F. S., Adler, N. E, Morrow, J. D., & Cawthon, R. M. (2004). Accelerated telomere shortening in response to life stress. *Proceedings of the National Academy of Sciences of the United States of America*. 101(49),

17312–17315; Harley, C. B., Futcher, A. B., & Greider, C. W. (1990). Telomeres shorten during ageing of human fibroblasts. *Nature.* 345(6274), 458–460; Marniciak, R., & Guarente, L. (2001). Human genetics: testing telomerase. *Nature.* 413(6854), 370–371, 373; Rudolph, K. L., Chang, S., Lee, H. W., Blasco, M., Gottlieb, G. J., Greider, C., & DePinho, R. A. (1999). Longevity, stress response, and cancer in aging telomerase-deficient mice. *Cell.* 96(5), 701–712.

175 **Evolutionary theories** Bowles, P. J. (1986). *Theories of human evolution: a century of debate, 1844–1944.* Baltimore, MD: Johns Hopkins University Press.

176 **life expectancy is nearly ninety years** Central Intelligence Agency. (2017). Country comparison: Life expectancy at birth. *World Factbook*; The US Burden of Disease Collaborators. (2018). The state of US health, 1990–2016: Burden of diseases, injuries, and risk factor among US states. *JAMA.* 319(14), 1444–1472

177 **"it's a massacre"** Roth, P. (2006). *Everyman.* New York, NY: Houghton Mifflin.

178 **communities also support healthy options** Ehrenreich, B. (March 31, 2018). Why are the poor blamed and shamed for their deaths? *Guardian.*

179 **"This is what 40 looks like"** Savan, S. (2006). *Slam dunks and no-brainers: Pop language in your life, the media, business, politics, and like, whatever.* New York, NY: Vintage.

## Outsourced

183 **living meaningful lives** American Geriatrics Society Geriatrics Healthcare Professionals. (2017). AGS extends hip fracture co-management program that sees geriatrics mending more than bones; Friedman, S. M., Mendelson, D. A., Kates, S. L., & McCann, R. M. (2008). Geriatric co-management of proximal femur fractures: total quality management and protocol-driven care result in better outcomes for a frail patient population. *Journal of American Geriatrics Society.* 56(7), 1349–1356.

184 **transfers to nursing homes** Burke, R. E., Lawrence, E., Ladebue, Ayele, R., Lippman, B., Cumbler, E., Allyn, R., & Jones, J. (2017). How hospital clinicians select patients for skilled nursing facilities. *Journal of American Geriatrics Society.* 65(11), 2466–2472.

184 **"I'll jump out the window"** Ernaux, A. (1996). *A woman's story.* New York, NY: Seven Stories Press. (73).

184 **"no longer a place for her"** Ernaux, A. (1996). *A woman's story.* New York, NY: Seven Stories Press. (74).

184 **she kept trying to escape** Ernaux, A. (1996). *A woman's story.* New York, NY: Seven Stories Press. (78).

184 **"she lost her self-respect"** Ernaux, A. (1996). *A woman's story.* New York, NY: Seven Stories Press. (80–81).

186 **beginning in Constantinople** Clarfield, A. M. (1990). Dr. Ignatz Nascher and the birth of geriatrics. *Canadian Medical Association Journal.* 143(9), 944.

186 **Not until the Poor Laws** Kelly, M., & Ó Gráda, C. (2011). The poor law of Old England: institutional innovation and demographic regimes. *Journal of Interdisciplinary History.* 41(3), 339–366.

188 **unsafe living conditions** San Francisco Ombudsman program, personal communication, 2018.

188 **"deprivatization of experience"** Gubrium, J. F., & Holstein, J. A. (1999). The nursing home as a discursive anchor for the ageing body. *Ageing & Society.* 19(5), 519–538.

188 **"nothing to do but sit"** Nevins, M. (2012). Chapter 9: *More meanderings in medical history* (119). Bloomington, IN: iUniverse.

189 **comfortable and meaningful lives** Warren, M. W. (1946). Care of the chronic aged sick. *Lancet.* 1, 841–843.

189 **"old 'master and inmate' relationship"** Gilleard, C., & Higgs, P. (2010). Aging without agency: theorizing the fourth age. *Aging & Mental Health.* 14(2), 121–128.

189 **aging homeless population** Knight, H. (March 5, 2016). Fast-aging homeless population may lead to public health crisis. *San Francisco Chronicle*; Sabatini, J. (April 11, 2016). Report: SF needs to adapt services for an aging homeless population. *San Francisco Examiner*.

189 **"taking care of the failing"** *Here and Now*. (September 14, 2017). Florida nursing home under investigation after at least eight die. NPR.

### Zealot

191 **"upsetting those responsible for their care"** Mount, B. M. (1976). The problem of caring for the dying in a general hospital; the palliative care unit as a possible solution. *Canadian Medical Association Journal*. 115, 119–121.

191 **even when they are unlikely to benefit a patient** Polite, B., Conti, R. M., & Ward, J. C. (June 2, 2015). Reform of the buy-and-bill system for outpatient chemotherapy care is inevitable: perspectives from an economist, a realpolitik, and an oncologist. *2015 ASCO Annual Meeting*; Wynne, B. (2016). For Medicare's new approach to physician payment, big questions remain. *Health Affairs*. 35(9).

### 9. Middle-aged
### Stages

192 **three, four, six, or twelve** Thane, P. (1993). Chapter 46: Geriatrics. In *Companion encyclopedia of the history of medicine, volume 1*. W. F. Bynum, & R. Porter (Eds.). (1093). New York, NY: Routledge.

192 **growth, stasis, and decline** Higgs, P., & Gilleard, C. (2015). *Rethinking old age: theorising the fourth age*. London, UK: Palgrave Macmillan.

192 **seven age groups** Thane, P. (1993). Chapter 46: Geriatrics. In *Companion encyclopedia of the history of medicine, volume 1*. W. F. Bynum, & R. Porter (Eds.). (1093). New York, NY: Routledge.

192 **"legislation is passed and agencies are created"** Hareven, T. K. (1976). The last stage: historical adulthood and old age. *American Civilization: New Perspectives*. 105(4), 13–27.

193 **a late-life analogue of adolescence** Hall, G. S. (1922). *Senescence, the last half of life*. New York, NY: D. Appleton and Co.

193 **"a real wisdom that only age can teach"** Hall, G. S. (1922). *Senescence, the last half of life*. (366). New York, NY: D. Appleton and Co.

193 **Bernice Neugarten** Neugarten, B. (1974). Age groups in American society and the rise of the young-old. *Annals of the American Academy of Political and Social Science*. 415, 187–198.

193 **increasing numbers of people over age eighty-five** Suzman, R., & Riley, M. W. (1985). Introducing the "oldest old." *Milbank Memorial Fund Quarterly, Health and Society*. 63(2), 175–186.

193 **go-go, go-slow, and no-go** Palmore, E. (1999). *Ageism: negative and positive* (2nd edition). (55). New York, NY: Springer Publishing.

193 **healthy, chronically ill, frail, and dying** Carey, E. C., Covinksy, K. E., Lui, L., Eng, C., Sands, L. P., & Walter, L. C. (2008). Prediction of mortality in community-living frail elderly people with long-term care needs. *Journal of the American Geriatrics Society*. 56, 68–75; Lunney, J. R., Lynn, J., & Hogan, C. (2002). Profiles of older Medicare decedents. *Journal of the American Geriatrics Society*. 50(6), 1108–1112.

194 **"progressive, not retrogressive"** Nascher, I. L. (1916). *Geriatrics; the diseases of old age and their treatment: including physiological old age, home and institutional care, and medicolegal relations*. (1). Philadelphia, PA: P. Blakiston's Son & Co.

194 **"take a similar view of senility"** Nascher, I. L. (1916). *Geriatrics; the diseases of old age and their treatment: including physiological old age, home and institutional care, and medicolegal relations*. (11). Philadelphia, PA: P. Blakiston's Son & Co.

194 **"a period of life rather than as a bodily condition"** Martin, L. J. (1930). *Salvaging old age*. London, UK: Macmillan Co.

### Help

197 **worse than death** Rubin, E. B., Buehler, A. E., & Halpern S. D. (2016). States worse than death among hospitalized patients with serious illness. *JAMA Internal Medicine.* 176(10), 1557–1559.

200 **correct doses** Fiatarone, M. A., Marks, E. C., Ryan, N. D., Meredith, C. N., Lipsitz, L. A., & Evans, W. J. (1990). High-intensity strength training in nonagenarians: effects on skeletal muscle. *JAMA.* 263(22), 3029–34; Reid, D. F., Callahan, D. M., Carabello, R. J., Philips, E. M., Frontera, W. R., & Fielding, R. A. (2008). Lower extremity power training in elderly subjects with mobility limitations: a randomized controlled trial. *Aging Clinical and Experimental Research.* 20(4), 337–343.

200 **purpose, meaning, and relevant options** McKnight, P. E., & Kashdan, T. B. (2009). Purpose in life as a system that creates and sustains health and well-being: an integrative, testable theory. *Review of General Psychology.* 13(3), 242–251; Stoyles, G., Chadwick, A., & Caputi, P. (2015). Purpose in life and well-being: the relationship between purpose in life, hope, coping, and inward sensitivity among first-year university students. *Journal of Spirituality in Mental Health.* 17(2), 119–134; Reker, G. T., Peacock, E. J., & Wong, P. T. P. (1987). Meaning and purpose in life and well-being: a life-span perspective. *Journal of Gerontology.* 42(1), 44–49.

203 **"the Fourth Age"** Gilleard, C., & Higgs, P. (2010). Aging without agency: theorizing the fourth age. *Aging & Mental Health.* 14(2), 121–128.

### Prestige

205 **physicians' annual income by specialty** Kane, L. (April 11, 2018). Medscape physician compensation report 2018. *Medscape.*

205 **ranked thirty-seventh among nations** Schneider, E. C., Sarnak, D. O., Squires, D., Shah, A., & Doty, M. M. (2017). Mirror, mirror, 2017: international comparison reflects flaws and opportunities for better U.S. health care. *Commonwealth Fund.*

205 **procedural and majority male** Vassar, L. (February 18, 2015). How medical specialties vary by gender. *AMA Wire.*

207 **women . . . are going into surgery** Farber, O. N. (August 6, 2018). Women survive a heart attack more often when their doctor is female, study finds. *STAT.*

207 **half with a man's name, half with a woman's** Moss-Racusin, C. A., Dovidio, J. F., Brescoll, V. L., Graham, M. J., & Handelsman, J. (2012). Science faculty's subtle gender biases favor male students. *Proceedings of the National Academy of Sciences of the United States of America.*

### Complexity

209 **people don't designate a proxy** Span, P. (January 19, 2018). One day your mind may fade: at least you'll have a plan. *New York Times*; Givens, J. L., Sudore, R. L., Marshall, G. A., Dufour, A. B., Kopits, I., & Mitchell, S. L. (2018). Advance care planning in community-dwelling patients with dementia. *Journal of Pain and Symptom Management.* 55(4), 1105–1112.

209 **does not actually include "everything"** Committee on Approaching Death: addressing key end of life issues; Institute of Medicine. (2015). *Dying in America: improving quality and honoring individual preference near the end of life.* Washington, DC: National Academies Press; Huffman, J. C., & Stern, T. A. (2003). Compassionate care of the terminally ill. *The Primary Care Companion to the Journal of Clinical Psychiatry.* 5(3), 131–136.

### Sexy

222 **link sexuality with youth** Freeman, J. T. (1979) *Aging, its history and literature.* New York, NY: Human Sciences Press.

223 **buff, and beautiful version of sexual attractiveness** G. Herdt & B. deVries. (Eds.) (2004). Gay and lesbian aging: Research and future directions. New York: Springer. Fredriksen-Goldsen K. I., Cook-Daniels L., Kim H.-J., Erosheva E. A., Emlet C. A., Hoy-Ellis, C. P, et al. (2014). Physical and mental health of transgender older adults: An at-risk and underserved

population. *Gerontologist*, 54, 488–500; Choi, S., & Meyer, I. H. (2016). *LGBT Aging: A Review of Research Findings, Needs, and Policy Implications.* Los Angeles: Williams Institute.

223 **in his nineties, put it this way** Angell, R. (February 17 and 24, 2014). This old man. *The New Yorker.*

224 **"a new sort of freedom"** Athill, D. (2008). *Somewhere towards the end.* New York, NY: W. W. Norton & Co.

224 **"Talk to me, not my daughter!"** Hawthorne, F. (May 9, 2012). Talk to me, not my daughter. *New York Times.*

226 **Thirteen million Americans are incontinent** Gorina, Y., Schappert, S., Bercovitz, A., Elgaddal, N., & Kramarow, E. (2014). Prevalence of incontinence among older Americans. *Vital and Health Statistics:* Series 3. 36, 1–33.

226 **haven't asked about incontinence** Cochran, A. (2000). Don't ask, don't tell: the incontinence conspiracy. *Managed Care Quarterly.* 8(1), 44–52; Hahn, S. R., Bradt, P., Hewett, K. A., & Ng, D. B. (2017). Physician-patient communication about overactive bladder: results of an observational sociolinguistic study. *Public Library of Science One.* 12(11).

227 **our present notions of male and female speech and power** Beard, M. (2017). *Women and power: a manifesto.* New York, NY: Liveright Publishing.

228 **"difficult and unappealingly limited"** Gawande, A. (2014). *Being mortal: medicine and what matters in the end.* New York, NY: Metropolitan Books.

## Disillusionment

230–31 **too anxious to leave his office** Shaw, B. (2015). *Last night in the OR: a transplant surgeon's odyssey.* New York, NY: Plume.

231 **because of the constant tension** Rush, T., & Shannon, D. (2018). Why I left medicine: a young doctor's views on burnout and non-clinical transitions. *ReachMD.*

231 **"it meant I fell behind"** Shannon, D. (December 2, 2015). Physician burnout: it's bad and getting worse, survey finds. *WBUR.*

231 **"There is no escape and no relief"** Personal e-mail communication, 2015.

231 **experiencing burnout** Shanafelt, T. D., Hasan, O., Dyrbye, L. N., Sinsky, C., Satele, D., Sloan, J., & West, C. P. (2015). Changes in burnout and satisfaction with work-life balance in physicians and the general US working population between 2011 and 2014. *Mayo Clinic Proceedings.* 90(12), 1600–1613.

231 **similar education and work hours** Huynh, C., Bowles, D., Yen, M.S., Phillips, A., Waller, R., Hall, L., & Tu, S. P. (2018). Change implementation: the association of adaptive reserve and burnout among inpatient medicine physicians and nurses. *Journal of Interprofessional Care.*

231 **"quality of the health care delivery system"** Shanafelt, T. D., Hasan, O., Dyrbye, L. N., Sinsky, C., Satele, D., Sloan, J., & West, C. P. (2015). Changes in burnout and satisfaction with work-life balance in physicians and the general US working population between 2011 and 2014. *Mayo Clinic Proceedings.* 90(12), 1600–1613.

231 **a shortage of forty-five thousand to ninety thousand physicians** Association of American Medical Colleges. (2015). *The complexities of physician supply and demand: projections from 2013 to 2025.* Washington, DC: Association of American Medical Colleges.

232 **poignant essays about burnout** Hill, A. B. (March 23, 2017). Breaking the stigma—a physician's perspective on self-care and recovery. *New England Journal of Medicine.* 376, 1103–1105; Humikowski, C. A. (July 2018). Beyond burnout. *JAMA.* 320(4), 343–344; Métraux, E. (March 20, 2108). I experienced trauma working in Iraq: I see it now among America's doctors. *STAT*; Talbot, S. G., & Dean, W. (July 26, 2018). Physicians aren't "burning out." They're suffering from moral injury. *STAT*; Xu, R. (May 11, 2018). The burnout crisis in American medicine. *The Atlantic.*

**Priorities**

233 **her eyes strayed from me to her screen** Alkureishi, M. A., Lee, W. W., Lyons, M., Press, V. G., Imam, S., Nkansah-Amankra, A., et al. (2016). Impact of electronic medical record use on the patient-doctor relationship and communication: a systematic review. *Journal of General Internal Medicine.* 31(5), 548–560.

233 **not sequenced in the way our conversation was proceeding** Friedberg, M. W., Chen, P. G., Van Busum, K. R., Aunon, F. M., Pham, C. Caloyeras, J. P., et al. (2013). *Factors affecting physician professional satisfaction and their implications for patient care, health systems, and health policy.* Santa Monica, CA: RAND Corporation.

233 **an ever-growing list of tasks** Sinsky, C., Colligan, L., Li, L., Prgomet, M., Reynolds, S., Goeders, L., et al. (2016). Allocation of physician time in ambulatory practice: a time and motion study in four specialties. *Annals of Internal Medicine.* 165(11), 753–760; McDonald, C. J., Callaghan, F. M., Weissman, A., Goodwin, R. M., Mundkur, M., & Kuhn, T. (2014). Use of internist's free time by ambulatory care Electronic Medical Record systems. *JAMA Internal Medicine.* 174(11), 1860–1863.

233 **midlevel providers** Brown, D. F., Sullivan, A. F., Espinola, J. A., & Camargo, C. A. (2012). Continued rise in the use of mid-level providers in the US emergency departments, 1993–2009. *Internal Journal of Emergency Medicine.* 5(21); Liu, H., Robbins, M., Mehrota, A., Auerbach, D., Robinson, B. E., Cromwell, L. F., & Roblin, D. W. (2017). *Medical Care.* 55(1), 12–18.

233 **scribes** Soudi, A., & McCague, A. B. (2015). Medical scribes and electronic health records. *JAMA.* 314(5), 518–519; Yan, C., Rose, S., Rothberg, M. B., Mercer, M. B., Goodman, K., & Misra-Hebert, A. D. (2016). Physician, scribe, and patient perspectives on clinical scribes in primary care. *Journal of General Internal Medicine.* 31(9), 990–995.

235 **belies my internist's greater experience** Darves, B. (October 3, 2014). Compensation in the physician specialties: Mostly stable. *New England Journal of Medicine CareerCenter.*

235 **always expensive, and sometimes nonsensical care** Brownlee, S., Saini, V., & Cassel, C. (April 25, 2014). When less is more: issues of overuse in health care. Health Affairs Blog; Fuchs, V. R. (July 2104). Why do other rich nations spend so much less on healthcare? *The Atlantic.*

235 **"differences in access"** U.S. National Library of Medicine. (2016). *Health Disparities.* Bethesda, MD: National Institutes of Health.

236 **shown to prevent illness** Starfield, B., Shi, L., & Macinko, J. (2005). Contribution of primary care to health systems and health. *Milbank Quarterly.* 83(3), 457–302.

236 **high rates of overuse and waste** Smith, M., Saunders, R., Stuckhardt, L., & McGinnis, J. M. (Eds.). (2012). *Best care at lower cost: the path to continuously learning health care in America.* Washington, DC: National Academies Press.

237 **"embedded in the political and economic organization"** Farmer, P. E., Nizeye, B., Stulac, S., & Keshavjee, S. (2006). Structural violence and clinical medicine. *PLOS Medicine.* 3(10), e449.

237 **American health care** Stone, T. (December 6, 2016). Incremental fixes won't save the U.S. health care system. *Harvard Business Review.*

237 **far exceeded those of the other countries** Papanicolas, I., Woskie, L. R., & Jha, A. K. (March 13, 2018). Health care spending in the United States and other high-income countries. *JAMA.* 319(10), 1024–1039.

237 **a system-less system** Parente, S. T. (2018). Factors contributing to the higher health care spending in the United States compared with other high-income countries. *JAMA.* 319(10), 988–990.

237 **we fail to prioritize care that most helps patients** Yao, N., Ritchie, C., Camacho, F., & Leff, B. (2016). Geographic concentration of home-based medical care providers. *Health Affairs.* 35(8), 1404–1409; Lown, B. A., Rosen, J., & Marttila, J. (2011). An agenda for improving

compassionate care: a survey shows about half of patients say such care is missing. *Health Affairs*. 30(9), 1772–1778.

237 **harder for clinicians** Bodenheimer, T. (2006). Primary care—will it survive? *New England Journal of Medicine*. 355, 861–864; Beckman, H. (2015). The role of medical culture in the journey to resilience. *Academic Medicine*. 90(6), 710–712.

**Sympathy**

238 **found him wholly unreceptive** Weinstein, M. S. (2018). Out of the straitjacket. *New England Journal of Medicine*. 378, 793–795.

**10. Senior**

**Ages**

241 **"the idea of childhood did not exist"** Aries, P. (1965). *Centuries of childhood: a social history of family life*. (R. Baldick, Trans.). (125). New York, NY: Vintage Books. (Original work published 1960).

241 ***sentiment . . . idea*** Ulanowicz, A. (2005). *Philippe Ariès*. Representing Childhood project, University of Pittsburgh.

241 **he did not approve of this change** Acocella, J. (August 18, 2003). Little people. *New Yorker*.

242 **The human brain naturally makes categories** Thomas, B. (December 26, 2012). Meaning on the brain: how your mind organizes reality. *Scientific American*.

243 **"a term not already tarnished"** Laslett, P. (1991). *A fresh map of life: the emergence of the third age*. (3). Cambridge, MA: Harvard University Press.

243 **could not overlap with the Fourth** Laslett, P. (1991). *A fresh map of life: the emergence of the third age*. (4). Cambridge, MA: Harvard University Press.

243 **"crown of life"** Laslett, P. (1991). *A fresh map of life: the emergence of the third age*. (vii). Cambridge, MA: Harvard University Press.

244 **more attention** Gilleard, C., & Higgs, P. (2010). Aging without agency: theorizing the fourth age. *Aging & Mental Health*. 14(2), 121–128.

244 **more a set of behaviors and attitudes** Gilleard, C., & Higgs, P. (2005). *Contexts of ageing: Class, cohort, and community*. Cambridge, UK: Polity Press.

244 **inevitable decline and "ignominy"** Laslett, P. (1991). *A fresh map of life: the emergence of the third age*. (3–5). Cambridge, MA: Harvard University Press.

244 **"failure by institutional forms of care"** Gilleard, C., & Higgs, P. (2010). Aging without agency: theorizing the fourth age. *Aging & Mental Health*. 14(2), 122.

244 **"social and cultural capital that is most valued"** Gilleard, C., & Higgs, P. (2010). Aging without agency: theorizing the fourth age. *Aging & Mental Health*. 14(2), 123.

244 **"developments in health and social policy"** Gilleard, C., & Higgs, P. (2010). Aging without agency: theorizing the fourth age. *Aging & Mental Health*. 14(2), 125.

244 **"denied them their status"** Laslett, P. (1991). *A fresh map of life: the emergence of the third age*. (viii). Cambridge, MA: Harvard University Press.

**Pathology**

248 **medicalization of American aging** Estes, C. L., & Binney, E. A. (1989). The biomedicalization of aging: dangers and dilemmas. *Gerontologist*. 29(5), 587–596.

248 **advanced old age as an accomplishment** Hareven, T. R. (1976). The last stage: historical adulthood and old age. *Daedalus*. 105(4), 13–27.

248 **"paradigmatic polarity of normality and pathology"** Cole, T. (1992). *The journey of life: a cultural history of aging in America*. (202). Cambridge, UK: Cambridge University Press.

249 ***Old age itself is a disease*** H. T. Riley (Ed.). (1874). Act III, scene 1 in *The comedies of Terence: Phormio*. (George Colman, Trans.). New York, NY: Harper & Bros.

**Freedom**

253 **"I don't worry about dying"** Delany, S. L., Delany, E., & Hearth, A. H. (1994). *Having our say: the Delany sisters' first 100 years*. New York, NY: Dell Publishing.

253 **"the room it provides for rotten news"** Angell, R. (February 17 and 24, 2014). This old man. *New Yorker*.

253 **"not only one's own life, but others', too"** Sacks, O. (July 6, 2013). The joy of old age. (No kidding.) *New York Times*.

254 **"microaggressions"** Sue, D. W. (2010). *Microaggressions and marginality: manifestation, dynamics, and impact*. (229–233). Hoboken, NJ: John Wiley & Sons.

255 **lowest life satisfaction** Stone, A. A., Schwartz, J. E., Broderick, J. E., & Deaton, A. (2010). A snapshot of the age distribution of psychological well-being in the United States. *Proceedings of the National Academy of Sciences of the United States of America*. 107(22), 9985–9990.

255 **a U-shape across life** Steptoe, A., Deaton, A., & Stone, A. A. (2018). Psychological wellbeing, health, and ageing. *Lancet*. 385(9968), 640–648; Rock, L. Life gets better after 50: why age tends to work in favour of happiness. (May 5, 2018). *Guardian*.

255 **well-being comparable to those of twenty-year-olds** Blanchflower, D. G., & Oswald, A. J. (2008). Is well-being U-shaped over the life cycle? *Social Science & Medicine*. 66(8), 1733–1749.

255 **anxiety marched steadily upward** Stone, A. A., Schwartz, J. E., Broderick, J. E., & Deaton, A. (2010). A snapshot of the age distribution of psychological well-being in the United States. *Proceedings of the National Academy of Sciences*. 107 (22) 9985–9990.

255 **"wonderfully freeing"** Naimon, D., & Ruefle, M. (June 3, 2015). *Between the Covers* podcast. (00:29).

256 **"many whose feelings are quite different"** Plato. (1943). *Plato's The Republic*. New York: Books, Inc.


**Longevity**

260 **mostly better, with less poverty** Engelhardt, G. V., & Gruber, J. (2006). Social security and the evolution of elderly poverty. In *Public Policy and the Income Distribution*, A. J. Auerbach, D. Card, & J. M. Quigley (Eds.) (259–287). New York, NY: Russell Sage Foundation; DeNavas-Walt, C., Proctor, B. D., & Smith, J. C. (2014). *Income and Poverty in the United States: 2013*. Current Population Report P60-249. Washington, DC: U.S. Census Bureau.

260 **fewer years of disability** Chen, Y., & Sloan, F. A. (2015). Explaining Disability Trends in the U.S. Elderly and Near-Elderly Population. *Health Services Research*. 50(5), 1528–1549.

260 **as the numbers of older people grew** Fischer, D. H. (1978). *Growing old in America*. Oxford, UK: Oxford University Press.

260 **"a person's stage in the life cycle"** Shoven, J. B. (2007). New age thinking: alternative ways of measuring age, their relationship to labor force participation, government policies and GDP. *National Bureau of Economic Research*.

260 **"compression of morbidity"** Fries, J. F. (1980). Aging, natural death, and the compression of morbidity. *New England Journal of Medicine*. 303(3), 130–135.

260 *very old or elderly* Vernon, S. (June 29, 2017). What age is considered "old" nowadays? *Money Watch*.

261 **lives that are both longer and healthier** Fried, L. P. (2016). Investing in health to create a third demographic dividend. *Gerontologist*. 56(2), S167–S177.

262 **around one in ten** Thane, P. (2005). *A history of old age*. Oxford, UK: Oxford University Press.

262 **our species' life span hasn't changed** Gaylord, S. A., & Williams, M. E. (1994). A brief history of the development of geriatric medicine. *Journal of the American Geriatrics Society*. 42(3), 335–340.

263 **blue zones** Buettner, D. (2005). The secrets of long life. *National Geographic*.

263 **they live longer than people who aren't religious** Ducharme, J. (February 15, 2018). You asked: do religious people live longer? *Time*.

264 **human surviving past the age of 122** Deiana, L., Pes, G. M., Carru, C., Ferrucci, L., Francheschi, C., & Baggio, G. (2008). The "oldest man on the planet." *Journal of the American Geriatrics Society*. 50(12), 2098–2099; Robine, J. M., & Allard, M. (1998). The oldest human. *Science*. 279(5358), 1834–1835.

264 **"didn't stop to think if they should"** Wang, J. (January 23, 2018). Jeff Bezos gains $2.8 billion after Amazon Go's debut, reaches highest net worth ever. *Forbes*; Silverman, S. (January 24, 2018). Retrieved from https://twitter.com/SarahKSilverman/status/956166109585063937.

**Childproof**

264 *Five Flights Up* Burch, C. (Producer), & Loncraine, R. (Director). (2014). *Five flights up*. [Motion Picture]. United States: Lascaux; Latitude; Revelations.

265 **child deaths from medications** Rodgers, G. B. (2002). The effectiveness of child-resistant packaging for aspirin. *Archives of Pediatrics and Adolescent Medicine*. 156(9), 929–933.

265 **Poison Prevention Packaging Act** US Consumer Product Safety Commission. (2005). *Poison prevention packaging: a guide for healthcare professionals*. Washington, DC.

265 **were nearly cut in half** Rodgers, G. B. (1996). The safety effects of child-resistent packaging for oral prescription drugs. Two decades of experience. *JAMA*. 275(21), 1661–1665.

266 **not only on children** United States Environmental Protection Agency. (February 27, 1996). *PRN 96-2: changes to child-resistant packaging (CRP) testing requirements*.

266 **some kind of arthritis** Barbour, K. E., Helmick, C. G., Boring, M., Zhang, X., Lu, H., & Holt, J. B. (2016). Prevalence of doctor-diagnosed arthritis at state and county levels—United States 2014. *Morbidity and Mortality Weekly Report*. 65(19), 489–494.

267 **"easy open" ones** How to open a child proof pill container. (2018) *wikiHow*; Whitson, G. (January 1, 2013). Turn a childproof pill bottle in an easy-open one. *lifehacker*.

267 **those adults most likely to take pills** United States Consumer Product Safety Commission. (October 4, 2008). *Poison prevention packaging act*. (4). (Originally published December 30, 1970).

**Elderhood**

271 *"For age is opportunity no less"* Longfellow, H. W. (1866). *The poetical works of Henry Wadsworth Longfellow*. (210–314). Boston, MA: Ticknor and Fields.

**11. Old**
**Exceptional**

274 **study of successful aging** Rowe, J. W., & Kahn, R. L. (1997). Successful aging. *Gerontologist*. 37(4), 433–440.

274 *eugeria* Aristotle. (1926). Book 1, Chapter 5 in *Rhetoric*. J. H. Freese, Trans. Cambridge, UK: Harvard University Press.

**Distress**

281 **a hospital ward geared to the unique needs of older adults** Barnes, D. E., Palmer, R. M., Kresevic, D. M., Fortinsky, R. H., Kowal, J., Chren, M. M., & Landefeld, C. S. (2012). Acute care for elders units produced shorter hospital stays at lower cost while maintaining patients' functional status. *Health Affairs*. 31(6), 1227–1236; Flood, K. L., & Allen, K. R. (2013). ACE units improve complex patient management. *Today's Geriatric Medicine*. 6(5), 28; Landfeld, C. S., Palmer, R. M., Kresevic, D. M., Fortinsky, R. H., & Kowal, J. (1995). A randomized trial of care in a hospital medical unit especially designed to improve the functional outcomes of acutely ill older patients. *New England Journal of Medicine*. 332(20), 1338–1344; Palmer, R. M., Landefeld, C. S., Kresevic, D., & Kowal, J. (1994). A medical unit for the acute care of the elderly. *Journal of the American Geriatrics Society*. 42(5), 545–552.

281 **our hospital was starting one too** Clark, C. (April 25, 2013). If ACE units are so great, why aren't they everywhere? *HealthLeaders*.

286 **jargon like "age-friendly health system"** Institute for Healthcare Improvement. (2018). *Age-friendly health systems.*

286 **one that meets the needs of older people** World Health Organization. (2018). *Ageing and life-course: health systems that meet the needs of older people.*

### Worth

288 **tend to oversave** Eisenberg, R. (March 26, 2018). Are retirees spending too little? *Next Avenue*; Ghilarducci, T. (March 2, 2018). America's unusual high rates of old-age poverty and old-age work. *Forbes.*

288 **poorer by the year** National Council on Aging. (2016). Economic security for seniors facts.

288 **two years after retirement** Gallegos, D. (February 11, 2018). Why so many men die at sixty-two. *Wall Street Journal.*

288 **"unretiring"** Maestas, N., Mullen, K. J., Powell, D. von Wachter, T., & Wenger, J. B. (2017). Working conditions in the United States: results of the 2015 American working conditions survey. Rand Corporation.

288 **working population** Toosi, M., & Torpey, E. (May 2017). Older workers: labor force trends and career options. Bureau of Labor Statistics.

288 **"burden" of old people's unemployment** Jaffe, I. (March 28, 2017). Older workers find age discrimination built right into some job websites. NPR; Palmer, K. (n.d.) Ten things you should know about age discrimination. *AARP: Work Life Balance.*

289 **"even *indispensable*"** Parker, S. (2013). Medicine and care for the elderly in *Kill or cure: an illustrated history of medicine.* (279). New York, NY: Dorling Kindersley Ltd.

289 **accepted that misconception** Burstein, S. R. (1950). Lillien Jane Martin—Pioneer in old age rehabilitation. *Medicine Illustrated.* 4(2), 82–90; Burstein, S. R. (1950). Lillien Jane Martin— Pioneer in old age rehabilitation. *Medicine Illustrated.* 4(3), 153–158.

### Beloved

291 **"the positive pathologies"** Hayes, Bill. (2017). *Insomniac city: New York, Oliver, and me.* New York, NY: Bloomsbury.

### Places

294 **longest study of human happiness** Waldinger, R. (November 2015). What makes a good life? Lessons from the longest study on happiness. *TEDxBeaconStreet.*

295 **engagement . . . and meaning** May, D. R., Gilson, R. L., Harter, L. M. (2010). The psychological conditions of meaningfulness, safety, and availability and the engagement of the human spirit at work. *Journal of Occupational and Organizational Psychology.* 77(1), 11–37; Peterson, C., Park, N., & Seligman, M. E. (2005). Orientations to happiness and life satisfaction: the full life versus the empty life. *Journal of Happiness Studies.* 6(1), 25–41.

295 **not just to unhappiness** Perissinotto, C. M., Stikacic Cenzer, I., & Covinsky, K. E. (2012). Loneliness in older persons: a predictor of functional decline and death. *Archives of Internal Medicine.* 172(14), 1078–1083.

295 **fifteen cigarettes a day** Connect2affect. (n.d.). About isolation. AARP.

295 **loneliness increases mortality by 26 percent** Holt-Lunstad, J., Smith, T. B., Baker, M., Harris, T., & Stephenson, D. (2015). Loneliness and social isolation as risk factors for mortality: a meta-analytic review. *Perspectives on Psychological Science.* 10(2), 227–237.

### Comfort

300 **for millennia people died at home** Davies, D. (2005). *A brief history of death.* Malden, MA: Blackwell Publishing.

300 **five out of six deaths took place in hospitals** Institute of Medicine (US) Committee on Care at the End of Life; Field, M. J., & Cassel, C. K. (Eds.). (1997). Approaching death:

improving care at the end of life. Washington, DC: National Academies Press; 2, A profile of death and dying in America.

300 **one in three deaths occur at home** Gleckman, H. (February 6, 2013). More people are dying at home and in hospice, but they are also getting more intense hospital care. *Forbes*; Teno, J. M., Gozalo, P. L., & Bynum, J. P. (2013). Change in end-of-life care for Medicare beneficiaries: site of death, place of care, and health care transitions in 2000, 2005, and 2009. *JAMA*. 309(5), 470–477.

**Tech**

301 **jobs in need of many people** Poo, A. (2015). *The age of dignity: Preparing for the elder boom in a changing America*. New York, NY: New Press.

302 **the harms of that approach** Walton, A. G. (April 16, 2018). How too much screen time affects kids' bodies and brains. *Forbes*.

303 **the need for instant gratification** (n.d.). Health and technology. Digital Responsibility; Cook, J-R. (March 29, 2016). Technology doesn't ruin health, people do. *Zócalo Public Square*; Pew Research Center (April 2018). The Future of Well-Being in a Tech-Saturated World. *Pew Research*.

305 **"quantified self" movement** Wolf, G. (n.d.). Quantified self. *Antephase*; Wolf, G. (June 2010). The quantified self. *TED@Cannes*.

307 **large numbers of tech-using old people** Kuchler, H. (July 30, 2017). Silicon Valley ageism: "They were, like, wow, you use Twitter?" *Financial Times*.

**Meaning**

308 **would stop most medical care at age seventy-five** Emanuel, E. J. (October 2014). Why I hope to die at 75. *Atlantic*.

308 **as have so many doctors** Murray, K. (March–April 2013). How doctors die. *Saturday Evening Post*; Byock, I. (June 30, 2016). At the end of life, what would doctors do? *New York Times*; Chen, P. (2007) *Final exam: a surgeon's reflections on mortality*. New York, NY: Alfred A. Knopf.

309 **everyone has dementia by age one hundred** Remnick, D., & Emmanuel, E. (July 14, 2017). The man who would be king (of Mars), and Trumpcare revisited. *New Yorker Radio Hour*.

311 **"treated as socially useless and even invisible"** Fried, L. P. (June 1, 2014). Making aging positive. *The Atlantic*.

311 **personal goals in old age** Clark, M. (1976). The anthropology of aging, a new area for studies of culture and personality. *Gerontologist*. 7(1), 55–64; Perkinson, M. A., & Solimeo, S. L. (2014). Aging in cultural context and as narrative process: conceptual foundations of the anthropology of aging as reflected in the works of Margaret Clark and Sharon Kaufman. *Gerontologist*. 54(1), 101–107.

311 **"being themselves in old age"** Kaufman, S. (1986). The ageless self: sources of meaning in later life. (6). Madison, WI: University of Wisconsin Press.

**Imagination**

313 **second-class citizens of twenty-first-century life** Douthat, R. (August 8, 2018). Oh, the humanities! *New York Times*.

**Bodies**

317 **a majority of people who become disabled** Albrecht, G. L., & Devlieger, P. J. (1999). The disability paradox: high quality of life against all odds. *Social Science & Medicine*. 48(8), 977–988; Viemerö, V., & Krause, C. (1998). Quality of life in individuals with physical disabilities. *Psychotherapy and Psychosomatics*. 67(6), 317–322.

318 **life-space** Brown, C. J., & Flood, K. L. (2013). Mobility limitations in the older patient: a clinical review. *JAMA*.

318 **Social isolation and loneliness** Perissinotto, C. M., Cenzer, I. S., & Covinsky, K. E. (2012). Loneliness in older persons: a predictor of functional decline and death. *Archives of Internal Medicine.* 172(14), 1078–1083.

318 **a young man spent a week alone** (September 21, 2017). The Loneliness Project. *The Campaign to End Loneliness;* Worland, J. (March 18, 2015). Why loneliness may be the next big public-health issue. *Time.*

**Classification**

321 **which shots patients should get** Centers for Disease Control. (2018). *Recommended immunization schedule for adults aged 19 years or older, United States 2018.* Atlanta, GA: U.S. Department of Health & Human Services.

321 **young-old and old-old** Marcum, C. S. (2011). Age differences in daily social activities. *RAND Center for the Study of Aging.*

321 **infections most likely to sicken and kill us in old age** Aspinall, R., & Lang, P. O. (2014). Vaccine responsiveness in the elderly: best practice for the clinic. *Expert Review of Vaccines.* 7, 885–894.

322 **enhancing the aging immune system** Del Guidice, G., Weinberger, B., & Grubeck-Loebenstein, B. (2015). Vaccines for the elderly. *Gerontology.* 61, 203–210.

322 **caused functional decline and death** Suskind, A., & Cox, L. C. (May 6–10, 2016). AUA 2016: baseline functional status predicts postoperative treatment failure in nursing home residents undergoing transurethral resection of the prostate (turp)-session highlights. *UroToday.*

322 **lymphoma and breast and lung cancers** Balducci, L. (2006). Management of cancer in the elderly. *Oncology.* 20(2), 135–143.

322 **acute myeloid leukemia** American Cancer Society. (2014). *Treatment response rates for acute myeloid leukemia.* Retrieved from https://www.cancer.org/cancer/acute-myeloid-leukemia/treating/response-rates.html.

323 **The older-old have more functional impairments** Ansah, J. P., Malhotra, R., Lew, N., Chiu, C., Chan, A., Bayer, S., & Matchar, D. B. (2015). Projection of young-old and old-old with functional disability: Does accounting for the changing educational composition of the elderly population make a difference? *PLOS One.* 10(5).

323 **greater debility and shorter life expectancies** Lee, S. J., Leipzig, R. M., & Walter, L. C. (2013). "When will it help?" Incorporating lagtime to benefit into prevention decisions for older adults. *JAMA.* 310(23), 2609–2610.

323 **without living to see the benefits** Brownlee, S., Saini, V., & Cassel, C. (April 25, 2014). When less is more: issues of overuse in health care. Health Affairs. Retrieved from https://www.healthaffairs.org/do/10.1377/hblog20140425.038647/full/.

323 **hip, knee** Skinner, D., Tadros, B. J., Bray, E., Elsherbiny, M., & Stafford, G. (2016). Clinical outcome following primary total hip or knee replacement in nonagenarians. *Annals of the Royal College of Surgeons of England.* 98(4), 258–264.

323 **aortic valve** Barreto-Filho, J. A., Wang, Y., Dodson, J. A., Desai, M. M., Sugeng, L., Geirsson, A., & Krumholz, H. M. (2013). Trends in aortic valve replacement for elderly patients in the United States, 1999–2015 2011. *JAMA.* 310(19), 2078–2085.

323 **poorly equipped and organized our health care system is** Gawande, A. (January 23, 2017). The heroism of incremental care. *New Yorker.*

**12. Elderly**

**Duality**

336 **a certain sort of appearance for women** Sontag, S. (1997). Chapter 1: the double standard of aging. In *The other within us: feminist explorations of women and aging,* M. Pearsall (Ed.). New York, NY: Routledge.

### Education

341 **populations that dominated health care a century ago** Association of American Medical Colleges. (2018). *Curriculum reports*. Retrieved from https://www.aamc.org/initiatives/cir/ curriculumreports/.

342 **a specialized rotation in geriatrics** Diachun, L., Van Bussel, L., Hansen, K., Charise, A., & Rieder, M. (2010). "But I see old people everywhere": Dispelling the myth that eldercare is learned in nongeriatric clerkships. *Academic Medicine*. 85(7), 1221–1228.

343 **put health professionals off old patients** Bagri, A. S., MD, & Tiberius, R. (2010). Medical student perspectives on geriatrics and geriatric education. *Journal of American Geriatrics Society*. 58, 1994–1999.

343 **futile or harmful treatment** Butler, K. (2013). *Knocking on heaven's door: the path to a better way of death*. New York, NY: Scribner; Zitter, J. N. (2017). *Extreme measures: finding a better path to the end of life*. New York, NY: Avery.

### Resilience

345 **"death by a thousand clicks"** Eisenstein, L. (2018). To fight burnout, organize. *New England Journal of Medicine*. 379, 509–511.

347 **"the need for the need"** Cole, T. (March 21, 2012). The White-Savior Industrial Complex. *Atlantic*.

348 **"in spite of his age; in spite of his losses"** Fadiman, A. (2017). *The wine lover's daughter: a memoir*. New York, NY: Farrar, Straus and Giroux.

### Attitude

348 **"Letter from Greenwich Village"** Gornick, V. (2014). Letter from Greenwich Village. In J. J. Sullivan (Ed.), *The best American essays 2014*. (61–62). Boston, MA: Houghton Mifflin Harcourt Publishing Company.

349 **"the minimum of discomfort to self and inconvenience to others"** Athill, D. (2009). Chapter 15. *Somewhere towards the end*. (1655). Kindle ed. New York, NY: W. W. Norton & Company.

351 **marked increases in old age** Stone, A. A., Schwartz, J. E., Broderick, J. E., & Deaton, A. (2010). *Proceedings of the National Academy of Sciences of the United States of America*. (107)22, 9985–9990.

351 **marked ageism** World Health Organization. (2018). Ageing and life-course.

351 **Preventive health measures improve health** Westerhof, G. J., Miche, M., Brothers, A. F., Barrett, A. E., Diehl, M., Montepare, J. M., et al. (2014). The influence of subjective aging on health and longevity: a meta-analysis of longitudinal data. *Psychology and Aging*, 29, 793–802; Kim, E. S., Moored, K. D., Giasson, H. L., & Smith, J. (2014). Satisfaction with aging and use of preventive health services. *Preventive Medicine*, 69, 176–180.

351 **people with more positive attitudes about aging** Levy, B. R., & Myers, L. M. (2004). Preventive health behaviors influenced by self-perceptions of aging. *Preventive Medicine*. 39(3), 625–629.

351 **intervention that strengthened positive age stereotypes** Levy, B. R., Pilver, C., Chung, P. H., & Slade, M. D. (2014). Subliminal strengthening: improving older individuals' physical function over time with an implicit-age-stereotype intervention. *Psychological Science*. 25(12), 2127–2135.

351 **self-fulfilling prophesies** Sargent-Cox, K. A., Anstey, K. J., & Luszcz, M. A. (2014). Longitudinal change of self-perceptions of aging and mortality. *Journals of Gerontology, Series B: Psychological Sciences and Social Sciences*. 69, 168–173.

351 **ageism is more common than sexism or racism** Carretta, H. J., Sutin, A. R., Stephan, Y., & Terracciano, A. (2015). Perceived discrimination and physical, cognitive, and emotional health in older adulthood. *American Journal of Geriatric Psychiatry: Official Journal of the American Association for Geriatric Psychiatry*. 23(2), 171–179.

#### Design

355 **patient-centered design features** Reiling, J., Hughes, R. G., & Murphy, M. R. (2008). Chapter 28: The impact of facility design on patient safety in R. G. Hughes (Ed.) *Patient safety and quality: an evidence-based handbook for nurses.* Rockville, MD: Agency for Healthcare Research and Quality; Siddiqui, Z. K., Zuccarelli, R., Durkins, N., Wu, A. W., & Brotman, D. J. (2015). Changes in patient satisfaction related to hospital renovation: experience with a new clinical building. *Journal of Hospital Medicine.* 10(3), 165–171.

#### Health

356 **. . . and social problems** Ribera Casaro. J. M. (2012). The history of geriatric medicine. The present: problems and opportunities. *European Geriatric Medicine.* 3, 230.

#### Perspective

358 **"I could imagine my way into old age"** Dovey, C. (October 1, 2015). What old age is really like. *New Yorker.*

358 **what we usually accept as objective reality** Berger, J. (1972). *Ways of seeing.* London, UK: British Broadcast Corporation.

362 **"the face" of Lancôme** Hughes, S. (July 9, 2016). Isabella Rossellini: "There is no work between 45 and 60—you're in limbo." *Guardian.*

362 **"pleasurably exalts the mind or spirit"** Merriam-Webster. (n.d.). Definition of beauty. Retrieved from https://www.merriam-webster.com/dictionary/beauty.

#### 13. Aged
##### Nature

366 **"Sara Thomas Monopoli . . . when her doctors learned she was going to die"** Gawande, A. (August 2, 2010). Letting go. *New Yorker.*

368–69 **obvious biological changes of a long life** Ritch, A. (2012). History of geriatric medicine: from Hippocrates to Marjory Warren. *Journal of the Royal College of Physicians of Edinburgh.* 42(4), 368–374.

369 **"few persons appear to die of old age"** Rush, B. (1793). Account of the state of the body and mind in old age, with observations on its diseases and their remedies in *Medical Inquiries and Observations*, 2, Butterfield (Ed.). Edinburgh, UK: Sinclair.

369 **"patient-centered care"** What is patient-centered care? (January 1, 2017). *NEJM Catalyst.*

371 **rather not have medical interventions** Pelham, B. (April 2004). Affective forecasting: the perils of predicting future feelings. *American Psychological Association.*

##### Human

374 **catchphrases like "patient-centered care"** Bardes, C. L. (2012). Defining "patient-centered medicine." *New England Journal of Medicine.* 366, 782–783.

374 **"to enable it to perform its function"** Diski, J. (2016). *In gratitude.* New York, NY: Bloomsbury.

376 **words and gestures associated with true empathy** Newton, B. W., Savidge, M. A., Barber, L., Cleveland, E., Clardy, J., Beeman, G., & Hart, T. (2000). Differences in medical students' empathy. *Academic Medicine.* 75(12), 1215.

376 **training makes doctors less empathetic** Neumann, M., Edelhäuser, F., Tauschel, D., Fischer, M. R., Wirtz, M., Woopen, C., et al. (2011). Empathy decline and its reasons: a systematic review of studies with medical students and residents. *Academic Medicine.* 86(8), 996–1009.

378 **"the secret of the care of the patient is in caring for the patient"** Peabody, F. W. (1927). The care of the patient. *JAMA.* 88(12), 877–882.

379 **individual and collective approaches** For a good example of this, see the work of *Race Forward* or read this article: Murphy, T. (2017). A new way to look at race. *Brown Alumni Magazine.*

**Consequences**

381 **"ordinary medicine" in old lives** Kaufman, S. R. (2015). *Ordinary medicine: extraordinary treatments, longer lives, and where to draw the line.* Durham, NC: Duke University Press.

384 **Another feeding tube also wasn't an option** Finucane, T. E., Christmas, C., & Leff, B. A. (2007). Tube feeding in dementia: how incentives undermine health care quality and patient safety. *Journal of American Medical Directors Association.* 8(4), 205–208; Dzeng, E., Colaianni, A., Roland, M., Levine, D., Kelly, M. P., Barclay, S., & Smith, T. J. (2016). Moral distress amongst American physician trainees regarding futile treatments at the end of life: a qualitative study. *Journal of General Internal Medicine.* 31(1), 93–99.

385 **the rest of us won't** Friend, T. (April 3, 2017). Silicon Valley's quest to live forever. *New Yorker.*

386 **"I do not wish to compete"** Lively, P. (October 5, 2013). So this is old age. *Guardian.*

386 **where he could end his life** Westcott, B. (May 3, 2018). 104-year-old Australian scientist to fly to Switzerland to end life. CNN.

388 **"don't count the number of naps"** Hall, D. (2018). Notes nearing ninety. *Narrative Magazine.*

**Acceptance**

390 **housecalls lead to better care** Leff, B., Carlson, C. M., Saliba, D., & Ritchie, C. (2015). The invisible homebound: setting quality-of-care standards for home-based primary and palliative care. *Health Affairs.* 34(1), 21–29.

390 **only the right answer for John and his family** Sudore, R. L. (2009). A piece of my mind. Can we agree to disagree? *JAMA.* 302(15), 1629–1630.

**Death**

395 **"a part of life again"** Kübler-Ross, E. (1970). On death and dying. New York, NY: Collier Books/Macmillan Publishing Co.

**14. Stories**

397 **"On Sixty-Five"** Fox Gordon, E. On sixty-five. (2014). In Sullivan, J. J. and Atwan, R. (Ed.). *Best American essays 2014.* New York, NY: Houghton-Mifflin Harcourt.

397 **"so without redeeming moments"** Grumbach, D. (1991). *Coming into the end zone: a memoir.* New York, NY: W. W. Norton & Co.

398 **"the time had come to size it up"** Athill, D. (2008). *Somewhere towards the end.* New York, NY: W. W. Norton & Co.

398 **"and unfortunately calls the shots"** Lively, P. (October 5, 2013). So this is old age. *Guardian.*

398 **"And that, of course, causes great confusion"** Lessing, D. (May 10, 1992). *Sunday Times.*

398 **"That is my problem"** Sarton, M. (1997). *At eighty-two: a journal.* New York, NY: W. W. Norton & Co.

399 **"in whatever you are doing"** Athill, D. (2008). *Somewhere towards the end.* New York, NY: W. W. Norton & Co.

399 **"and I'm feeling great"** Angell, R. (2015). *This old man: all in pieces.* New York, NY: Anchor Books.

399 **"humiliating, debilitating, and isolating"** Butler, R. N. (1975). *Why survive?: Being old in America.* Baltimore, MD: Johns Hopkins University Press.

**Coda**

401 **"a polemic voice"** Mailhot, T. M. (2018). *Heart berries: a memoir*. Berkeley, CA: Counterpoint.

**Opportunity**

403 **moments of peak intensity** Frederickson, B. L., & Kanheman, D. (1993). Duration neglect in retrospective evaluations of affective episodes. *Journal of Personality and Social Psychology*. 65(1), 45–55; Kahneman, D. (2000). Evaluation by moments, past and future. In *Choices, values, and frames*, D. Kahneman, & A. Tversky (Eds.). (693). Cambridge, UK: Cambridge University Press.

# BIBLIOGRAPHY

Adichie, C. N. (2009). The danger of the single story. *TEDGlobal*. Retrieved from https://www.ted
.com/talks/chimamanda_adichie_the_danger_of_a_single_story/transcript?language=en.

Angell, R. (2015). *This old man: all in pieces*. New York: Anchor Books.

Applewhite, A. (2016). *This chair rocks: a manifesto against ageism*. New York: Networked Books.

Aries, P. (1982). *The hour of our death: the classic history of western attitudes toward death over the last
one thousand years*. New York: Vintage Books.

Athill, D. (2008). *Somewhere towards the end*. New York: W. W. Norton & Co.

Barnes, J. (2008). *Nothing to be frightened of*. New York: Random House.

Bayley, J. (1998). *Elegy for Iris: a memoir of Iris Murdoch*. London: Duckworth Overlook.

Beard, M. (2017). *Women & power: a manifesto*. New York: Liveright Publishing.

Berger, J. (1972). *Ways of seeing*. London: Penguin Books.

Blythe, R. (1979). *The view in winter: reflections on old age*. London: Penguin Books.

Booth, W. C. (1992). *The art of growing older: writers on living and aging*. Chicago: University of
Chicago Press.

Brownlee, S. (2007). *Overtreated: why too much medicine is making us sicker and poorer*. New York:
Bloomsbury.

Buettner, D. (2008). *The blue zones: nine lessons for living longer from the people who've lived the
longest*. Washington, DC: National Geographic Society.

Butler, K. (2013). *Knocking on heaven's door: the path to a better way of death*. New York: Scribner.

Butler, R. N. (1975). *Why survive?: being old in America*. Baltimore: Johns Hopkins University Press.

Carstensen, L. (2011). *A long bright future*. New York: PublicAffairs.

Chast, R. (2014). *Can't we talk about something more pleasant?: a memoir*. New York: Bloomsbury.

Cicero, M. T. (1927). *De senectute, de amicitia, de divinatione*. London: W. Heinemann,
G. P. Putnam's Sons.

Cole, T. (1992). *The journey of life*. Cambridge, UK: Cambridge University Press.

Cole, T. R., & Winkler, M. G. (Eds.). (1995). *The oxford book of aging: reflexions on the journey of life*.
Oxford, UK: Oxford University Press.

Crenshaw, K., Gotanda, N., Peller, G., & Thomas, K. (Eds.). (1995). *Critical race theory: the key
writings that formed the movement*. New York: New Press.

de Beauvoir, S. (1996). *The coming of age*. (P. O'Brian, Trans.). New York: W. W. Norton & Co.
(Original work published 1970).

Desmond, M. (2016). *Evicted: poverty and profit in the American city*. New York: Crown Publishers.

Didion, J. (2005). *The year of magical thinking*. New York: Alfred A. Knopf.

Ehrenreich, B. (2018). *Natural causes: an epidemic of wellness, the certainty of dying, and killing
ourselves to live longer*. New York: Hachette Book Group.

Ernaux, A. (1991). *A woman's story*. (T. Leslie, Trans.). New York: Seven Stories Press. (Original work
published 1988).

Fischer, D. H. (1978). *Growing old in America*. Oxford, UK: Oxford University Press.

Foucault, M. (1994). *The birth of the clinic: an archaeology of medical perception*. (A. Sheridan, Trans.). New York: Vintage Books. (Original work published 1963).

Friedan, B. (1993). *The fountain of age*. New York: Simon & Schuster.

Gawande, A. (2015). *Being mortal: medicine and what matters in the end*. New York: Picador.

Gillick, M. R. (2017). *Old and sick in America: the journey through the health care system*. Chapel Hill, NC: University of North Carolina Press.

Groopman, J. (2007). *How doctors think*. New York: Houghton Mifflin Co.

Grumbach, D. (2014). *Coming into the end zone: a memoir*. New York: Open Road.

Hall, D. (2014). *Essays after eighty*. New York: Houghton Mifflin Harcourt.

Hall, D. (2018). *A carnival of losses: notes nearing ninety*. New York: Houghton Mifflin Harcourt.

Heilbrun, C. (1997). *The last gift of time: life beyond sixty*. New York: Ballantine Books.

Hemingway, E. (1952). *The old man and the sea*. New York: Scribner.

Kaufman, S. R. (1986). *The ageless self: sources of meaning in late life*. Madison: University of Wisconsin Press.

Kaufman, S. R. (2015). *Ordinary medicine: extraordinary treatments, longer lives, and where to draw the line*. Durham, NC: Duke University Press.

Kidder, T. (1993). *Old friends*. New York: Houghton Mifflin Company.

Kleinman, A. (1988). *The illness narratives: suffering, healing, and the human condition*. New York: Basic Books.

Kohn, M., Donley, C. C., & Wear, D. (Eds.). (1992). *Literature and aging: an anthology*. Kent, OH: Kent State University Press.

Kozol, J. (2015). *The theft of memory: losing my father, one day at a time*. New York: Random House.

Le Guin, U. K. (2017). *No time to spare: thinking about what matters*. New York: Houghton Mifflin Harcourt.

Leland, J. (2018). *Happiness is a choice you make: lessons from a year among the oldest old*. New York: Farrar, Straus and Giroux.

McPhee, J. (1984). *Heirs of general practice*. New York: Farrar, Straus and Giroux.

Mendelsohn, D. (2017). *An odyssey: a father, a son, and an epic*. New York: Alfred A. Knopf.

Mukherjee, S. (2011). *The emperor of all maladies: a biography of cancer*. New York: Scribner.

Nuland, S. B. (1994). *How we die: reflections on life's final chapter*. New York: Vintage Books.

O'Neil, M., & Haydon, A. (2015). *Aging, agency, and attribution of responsibility: shifting public discourse about older adults*. Washington, DC: FrameWorks Institute.

Pipher, M. (1999). *Another country: navigating the emotional terrain of our elders*. New York: Riverhead Books.

Poo, A. (2015). *The age of dignity: preparing for the elder boom in a changing America*. New York: New Press.

Rankine, C. (2014). *Citizen: an American lyric*. Minneapolis: Graywolf Press.

Rosenthal, E. (2017). *An American sickness: how healthcare became big business and how you can take it back*. New York: Penguin Books.

Sarton, M. (1995). *Encore: a journal of the eightieth year*. New York: W. W. Norton.

Segal, L. (2013). *Out of time: the pleasures and the perils of ageing*. Brooklyn, NY: Verso.

Shem, S. (1978). *The house of God*. New York: Bantam Dell.

Shenk, D. (2003). *The forgetting: Alzheimer's: portrait of an epidemic*. New York: Anchor Books.

Skloot, R. (2011). *The immortal life of Henrietta Lacks*. Portland, OR: Broadway Books.

Sloan, J. (2009). *A bitter pill: how the medical system is failing the elderly*. Vancouver, CA: Greystone Books.

Solomon, A. (2012). *Far from the tree: parents, children, and the search for identity*. New York: Scribner.

Sontag, S. (1979). *Illness as metaphor*. New York: Vintage Books.

Span, P. (2009). *When the time comes: families with aging parents share their struggles and solutions.* New York: Hachette Book Group.

Sweet, V. (2017). *Slow medicine: the way to healing.* New York: Riverhead Books.

Thane, P. (2005). *A history of old age.* Oxford, UK: Oxford University Press.

Thomas, W. H. (1996). *Life worth living: how someone you love can still enjoy life in a nursing home: the Eden Alternative in action.* Acton, MA: VanderWyk & Burnham.

Weil, A. (2005). *Healthy aging: a lifelong guide to your physical and spiritual well-being.* New York: Alfred A. Knopf.

Winakur, J. (2008). *Memory lessons: a doctor's story.* New York: Hyperion.

# INDEX

AAMC (Association of American Medical Colleges), 66–67

AARP, 268

abuse, elder neglect and, 188, 303–4, 382

accessibility, 352–56

accomplishment, reduced, 221

accountable care organization approach, 212

*Account of the State of the Body and Mind in Old Age* (Rush), 27–28, 369

active dying, 300

Acute Care for Elders (ACE), 280–87, 354

acute myeloid leukemia, 322

adaptability, 311

adulthood and revised life cycle, 270. *See also* young adulthood

Adult Protective Services (APS), 151, 306

advance directives, 122, 151–52

advanced old age
 age-related mortality in, 264
 contrasted with earlier stages, 76, 81
 da Vinci's description of, 368
 dread of, 197, 203, 245–47, 317
 as Fourth Age, 203, 243–46, 282
 gender imbalance in, 335–37
 history of, 185–86, 248
 immune system in, 322
 social stance in, 349–51
 suffering and unhappiness in, 195–204

advocacy, 179–82

African Americans, 129–34, 136

age blindness, 136

age-friendly health system, 286

ageism, 69–74, 156, 164, 261, 351, 352, 370

aging
 benefits of, 78–79, 253–56, 351
 bias against, 73 (*See also* ageism)
 biology and, 90, 173–79, 194, 321–23, 350–51
 *vs.* dying, 367–72

evolution through stages of, 75–81

history of ideas about, 24–30, 76, 81, 88–89, 261–62

increased interest in topic of, 361–62

nurture and, 176–77

pathological, 28, 30, 120, 147, 148, 247–49

scientific strategies to affect, 90–91, 92

successful, 140, 273–78

aging-in-place homes, 355

aging projects in companies, 228

AIDS, 126–29, 223

airport security, 273

Albert, 190

alcoholism, 15, 122

Algizar, 25

Allan, 149–50

Allport, Gordon, 69–70, 72

Alzheimer, Alois, 28

Alzheimer's disease, 49, 50, 51, 52, 210, 251. *See also* dementia

American Academy of Anti-Aging Medicine, 92

American College of Physicians, 144

American Medical Association, 231

American Medical Group Management Association (AMGA), 235

Americans with Disabilities Act, 353

Angell, Roger, 223, 225, 253, 399

anti-aging products and therapies, 86–93

antianxiety medications, 391

antidepressants, 20–21, 23, 37–38, 196

anti-inflammatory drugs, 48

antioxidant supplementation, 90

anxiety, 53, 217, 230–31, 255

apologies, 119, 121

appendix, ruptured, 30–34, 113

Applewhite, Ashton, 361

APS (Adult Protective Services), 151, 306

Arabia, 25

Ariès, Philippe, 241–42

Aristotle, 8, 24, 80, 120, 192, 274
arthritis, 26, 172, 226, 266
arthritis medications, 19
Arturo, 97–99
Asian Americans, 176–77
aspirin, 93–94, 122
assisted dying laws, 203–4, 386–87
assisted living, 150, 169, 188, 190, 196,
    200–203, 293–94. *See also* old-age
    institutions
Association of American Medical Colleges
    (AAMC), 66–67
assumptions, incorrect, 34–40
*As You Like It* (Shakespeare), 173
Athill, Diana, 224, 349, 397–98, 399
atrial fibrillation, 94–95
attitude, 277–78, 348–51
Australia, 386–87
Australian Medical Association, 387
autism, blaming mothers for, 65
autonomy, loss of, 254, 305–8
Avicenna, 25

baby boomer blip, 263
Babylon, 88
Bacon, Francis, 26–27
Bacon, Roger, 25–26, 88
Baldwin, James, 1, 131
Bayley, John, 51
Beard, Mary, 227
Beauvoir, Simone de, 60, 223, 268
Beers Criteria, 46
behavior and aging
    exceptional seniors and, 274, 275, 276
    history of ideas about, 24, 25, 26, 28, 29, 88
    psychosocial theories and, 175
beloved, death of, 291–93
Berger, John, 102, 358
beta-hydroxybutyricacid (BHB), 90
Bezos, Jeff, 264
bias
    age blindness, 136
    against aging, 73 (*See also* ageism)
    medicine and, 65–66, 69–74, 118, 129–36,
        204, 207, 235–36
Biohub, 278–79
biology and aging, 90, 173–79, 194, 321–23,
    350–51
biopsychosocial model, 379
bladder infections, 330, 382

blindness. *See* vision loss
blood infections, 330
blood pressure, 19, 68, 135, 172, 179–80
blood pressure medications, 23, 48, 66
blood replacement, 91
blood sodium levels, 22–23
blood sugar levels, 325–26, 329, 331–32
blood thinners, 94, 125, 180
blue zones, 263
bodies, aging, 13, 14, 317–20
body as machine, 62
body weight, 90, 263. *See also* obesity
brain tumors, 370
breast cancer, 153, 322
Britain, 26, 186. *See also* England; United
    Kingdom
Brown, Molly McCully, 61–62
Brown-Séquard, Charles-Édouard, 89
Brummel-Smith, Ken, 145–46
burden, 290
burnout, physician, 214–21, 229–32, 238–40,
    305, 345–47, 377
Butler, Robert, 70, 399
Byrne, Steve, 291–92
Byron, 363–65

Calderon, Maria, 120–21
caloric restriction, 89–90, 263
cancer. *See also* chemotherapy; radiation
    treatment
    age differences in, 322–23
    breast, 153, 322
    colon, 97
    dementia and, 50, 53, 56
    esophageal, 371
    home care and, 151–54
    lung, 322
    old age compared to, 59
    pain and, 284–85
    progression of, 298
    treatment for, 68, 82–86, 92, 374
*The Canon of Medicine* (Avicenna), 25
capacity, 124
care coordination, 168, 171, 211–12
caregiving
    difficulty of, 18–19, 20, 51, 98, 209, 247,
        301–2
    distance and, 150–55
    low wages for, 327, 334, 336–37
    meaningfulness of, 247

caregiving (*continued*)
  physicians and support for, 21, 55, 172–73
  RAISE Act, 24
  by robots, 301–5
  by undocumented workers, 326–35
"The Care of the Patient " (Peabody), 377–78
care paradigm, 379–80
care *vs.* treatment, 343
caring for patients, 337–41, 375–80
Carl, 150–51
case-based learning sessions, 375
Cathy, 298–300
Cavaglieri, Cookie, 198–202
Cavaglieri, Frank, 195–204
Centers for Disease Control (CDC), 49–51,
  266, 321–22, 323
*Centuries of Childhood* (Ariès), 241
cerebral palsy, 61
Chad, 176
Chan, Priscilla, 278–79
Chan Zuckerberg Initiative, 278–80
Charcot, Jean-Martin, 120
chemotherapy, 82–86, 114, 153, 189–90,
  322–23, 366
Cher, 61
chest tube insertion, 106–8
child development, 42, 44, 77
childhood, 241–42, 270, 277
childhood memories. *See* memories, childhood
child labor laws, 64
child-resistant bottles, 264–68
China, ancient, 88
Chinese writers, 242
Christianity, 25, 88, 186, 274
chronic diseases, 27, 69, 79, 260, 278, 318
Cicero, 24, 25
Clark, Margaret, 311
clinical pathways, 56–58
clothing and fashion, 227–28
Cochrane Library Database, 96
coding, 32–33
cognitive impairment, 53, 54, 55, 68, 135, 307.
  *See also* dementia
Cole, Teju, 347
Cole, Thomas, 248
college experiences, 41–42
colon cancer, 97
colonoscopy, 83–85, 219
*The Coming of Age* (Beauvoir), 268
commencement speech, 312–17

communication
  dementia and, 249–53, 330–31, 337–40
  with families of geriatric patients, 34–39,
    46–48, 94–95, 180–82
  primary care and, 21–22
  value of, 109
companies, aging projects in, 228
compassion, 109
competence, 122–25
complaining, 157–58, 288
compression of morbidity, 260, 261
Condorcet, Marquis de, 27
confusion. *See also* delirium; dementia
  as condition worse than death, 197
  feeding tubes and, 84
  hospitalization and, 98
  medications and, 95, 99
  paramedics and, 38–39
  urinary tract infections and, 330
conscience, 116
constipation, 25, 226
Consumer Product Safety Commission, 266
contractures, 87
Cornaro, Luigi, 26
courage, 348
*The Cure of Old Age and the Preservation of
  Youth* (Bacon), 25–26
cures, late effects of, 92–93

Dalai Lama, 312–13
dating, 15–16
daughters, 150–55
da Vinci, Leonardo, 368
Davis, Lydia, 81
death
  acceptance of, 388–92
  aging *vs.*, 366–72
  of a beloved, 291–93
  CDC top ten causes of, 49–51
  comfort with, 298–300
  conditions identified as worse than, 197
  language of, 141–42
  medical education and, 68
  medicalization of, 191, 300
  neglect of old age preceding, 70–71
  polypharmacy and, 168
  stress and risk of, 79
  in traditional societies, 81
Deborah, 190
DeGeneres, Ellen, 312–13

deinstitutionalization, 187
Delany, Sadie, and sister Bessie, 253
delirium
    definition in medicine, 36
    emergency departments and, 131–33
    hip fracture surgeries and, 182, 183
    hospitalization and, 251, 384
    medical education and, 67
    medications and, 95
    paramedics and, 36–37
Dell School of Medicine, 342
dementia
    Alzheimer's disease, 49, 50, 51, 52, 210, 251
    American approach to old age and, 56
    assumptions of, 124–25
    author as expert on, 143–44
    CDC top ten causes of death and, 49–51
    communication and, 209–10, 249–53,
        330–31, 337–40
    delirium and, 36
    diabetes and, 325–26
    early research on, 28
    families and, 51, 55, 149–50
    feeding tubes and, 384
    hearing loss and, 135
    housecalls and, 208–12
    informed consent and, 97
    institutions for people with, 111
    medical education and, 68
    medications and, 45–49, 53, 150
    misunderstandings about, 39
    post-hospitalization, 97
    progression of, 51–53
    quality of life and, 246, 309
    robot caregivers and, 303
    science of, vs. patient care, 54–55
    screening for, 123
    types of, 210
De Niro, Robert, 222
Denver Health, 56–57
Department of Health and Human Services,
    231
depersonalization, 220
depression, 20–23, 26, 29, 53, 216–17, 255
Descartes, René, 26–27
De sedibus, et causis morborum (Morgagni), 27
de Senectute (Cicero), 24
design, elder-friendly, 352–56
DHEA, 89
diabetes, 210, 325–26, 329

dialysis, 136, 284
diapers, 152–53
Dickens, Charles, 237
Didion, Joan, 129–31, 134
diet, 24, 25, 26, 56, 275, 277, 351
differential diagnosis, 130–31, 134, 388
difficult patients and families, 43, 173, 181–82,
        185, 245, 288–89
disability, living with, 317–18
discharge planning, 282, 283
Discorsi della vita sobria (Cornaro), 26
Discourse of the Preservation of the Sight; of
        Melancholic Diseases; of Rheumes and of
        Old Age (Laurens), 26
disease eradication, 278–80
disillusionment, 229–32
Diski, Jenny, 374
dizziness, 121
doctor-patient relationship, 217–20, 305
dogs and 50% rule, 363–65
Do Not Resuscitate (DNR), 168
Dot, 301, 304–5
"The Double Standard of Aging" (Sontag), 142
Dovey, Ceridwen, 358
driving, giving up, 275
drusen, 68
dual eligibility, 153

Economist, 290
Edward and Carmen, 267
Egypt, ancient, 24, 80
Einstein, Albert, 313, 317, 378
elder-friendly design, 352–56
elder-friendly hospitals, 156, 282–83
elderhood. See also advanced old age; aging; old
        age; old-old and oldest old people;
        young-old people
    geriatrics and, 356–58
    life cycle, revised version of, and, 270
    reclamation of, 268–70
    as third act, 8–9, 323, 403
elder neglect and abuse, 188, 303–4, 382
elder vs. old, 4–7
electronic medical records (EMRs)
    doctor-patient relationship and, 217, 219, 305
    limitations to using, 35, 37, 171, 218–19, 233
    physician burnout and, 217–20
    physician work schedules and, 217, 231
    surprises in, 93–94
    vision difficulties and, 229, 285

*Elegy for Iris* (Bayley), 51
Elenoa, 328–35
Elizabeth, Queen, 275, 276
Emanuel, Zeke, 308–10
emergency rooms, 122–23, 249–51
Emile and Lilly, and daughter Karen, 293–94, 295–96
emotional exhaustion, 216
empathy, 115–17, 146, 376
EMRs. *See* electronic medical records (EMRs)
encore careers, 288
end-of-life care, 68, 189–91, 367–68, 380–93. *See also* hospice care; palliative care
end-of-life wishes and planning
   advance directives, 122, 151–52
   importance of establishing, 58, 168–69, 209–10
   reluctance to follow, 190, 380–81
   speaking to patients and families about, 47, 55, 154
energy efficiency, 90
England, 64, 88, 186–87, 243. *See also* Britain; United Kingdom
Ernaux, Annie, 52, 184–85
erosion of doctor-patient relationship, 217–20
esophageal cancer, 371
Estes, Carroll, 248
Esther, 312
*eugeria*, 274
eukaryotes, 174
Europe
   childhood as life stage and, 64
   history of medicine and ideas about aging in, 25–27, 88, 110, 146–47
   history of old-age institutions in, 185–87
   medical and social care combined in, 111
   Middle Ages and Renaissance in, 242
   social companion robot designed in, 302
   well-being in, 255
Eva, 163–73
evolutionary theories, 175
evolution through stages of aging, 75–81
exceptional seniors, 140, 273–78, 282, 350, 398
exercise
   apps for, 307
   attitude and, 351
   dementia and, 56
   elderly widows in the past and, 14
   fitness in old age and, 25, 86–87, 275

ketogenesis and, 90
   lack of access to, 7
expressions used to talk about aging, 140–41

faces, 319, 320
Fadiman, Anne, 348
Fadiman, Clifton, 348
Fall in Eden, 88, 274
falls
   in assisted living facilities, 196
   dementia and, 210
   hospitalization following, 383–84
   medical education and, 67
   medications and, 96, 168
   Parkinson's disease and, 121
   research and, 110
   social isolation and, 226
   strokes compared to, 170–71
   thinning bones and, 177
   urinary tract infections and, 330
families of geriatric patients
   blame for bad outcomes and, 74, 182–83
   communicating and working with, 34–39, 46–48, 94–95, 139, 180–82
   dementia and, 51, 55, 149–50
   digital technology and, 305–6, 307, 308
   distance and, 150–55
   end-of-life care and, 380–82, 388–93
family medicine, 102
*The Faraway Nearby* (Solnit), 116
Farber, Sidney, 314
Farmer, Paul, 237
fear, 256–58
feeding tubes, 83–84, 371, 384
*Five Flights Up* (film), 264–65
flu vaccines, 321–22
Fonda, Jane, 221
forgetfulness, 25. *See also* dementia
*A Fortunate Man* (Berger), 102
*4:44* (Jay-Z), 142
Fourth Age, 203, 243–46, 282. *See also* advanced old age
Fox Gordon, Emily, 397
fragmented care, 167–68
France, 89, 120, 146–47, 186–87, 243
Frankel, Mark, 193
freedom in aging, 253–56
Freeman, Morgan, 264–65
Freudenberger, Herbert J., 231
Fried, Linda, 310–11

frontotemporal dementia, 210
function and environment, 178

Gabow, Patricia, 56–59
Galen and Galenic tradition, 24, 25, 27, 88–89
Gallagher, Betty, 324–35
Gallup World Poll, 255
Gates Foundation, 279
Gawande, Atul, 366–67
gay males, 221, 223–24. *See also* LGBT health; LGBTQ elders
gender and longevity, 276, 335–37
genetics, 26, 28, 175, 276
George, and wife Bessie, 249–51, 253
Georgia, 284
geriatric medicine and geriatricians
    ACE units, 280–87, 354
    aim and goal of, 157
    dementia and, 53
    elder-friendly design and, 282–83, 354
    elderhood and, 356–58
    gaps in, 9
    geriatrics as term, 73, 146
    history of, 29–30, 70, 110–11, 146–48
    lessons in, 16–23
    lower status of, as specialty, 44–45, 69, 137–38, 147–48, 155–56, 205, 228–29, 343
    medical education and, 6, 66–68
    on-call duty and, 34, 162
    oncology and, 86
    pediatrics compared to, 44, 146, 148
    struggles in, 7
    Third and Fourth Ages and, 244
    values and, 155–63
    as vocation, 143–48, 155, 158–63, 372
geriatric patients, 4, 5–6, 7, 28–29, 138–40. *See also* families of geriatric patients
*Geriatrics* (Nascher), 156
geriatrics education and training, 39–40
"Geriatrics Year in Review" lecture, 54–55
Germany, 28, 89
*gerocomeia*, 186
*gérocomie*, 147
*Gerontocomia* (Zerbi), 26
gerontology, 44, 203
geroscience hypothesis, 87–88
Gilgamesh, 88
Gilleard, Chris, 244, 246
Gillespie, Maggie, 371

glandular grafts, 89
glasses, 111
glaucoma, 99
Golden Age or Place, 88
gomers, 44
Gomes, Francisco, 370–71
Goodall, David, 386–87
Google, 24
Gornick, Vivian, 348–51
gout, 48
*Grace and Frankie* (TV show), 221–22
grandparents, 13–16, 42
gray hair, 173, 175–76, 178–79, 399–400
Gray Panthers, 16, 261
greatest generation, 263
Greece, ancient, 24, 25, 80, 227, 256
Greek writers, 242
grief, 20
Grimm, Brothers, 324
Grumbach, Doris, 397, 398
*Gulliver's Travels* (Swift), 27
gynecologists, 205, 336

Hall, Donald, 60, 224, 225, 387–88
Hall, G. Stanley, 193
Hareven, Tamara, 192
Harvard Medical School, 64–65, 148, 342
Harvard Medical School Alumni Council, 236
Hayes, Bill, 291–93
Hayflick, Leonard, 92
Hayflick limit, 92
Hazlitt, William, 72
headaches, 38–39
health and health care *vs.* medicine, 378
health care system, U.S.
    care coordination and home care and, 211–12
    change needed in approach to, 7–8, 373–80
    dementia and, 53–54
    division between medical and social care, 111, 170–72, 200–201, 209–10
    EMRs and, 218–19
    history and, 378
    perversion of brutal treatments and, 86
    physician burnout and, 232
    priorities in, 22, 29, 235–36
    spending by, 237
    standards of care and, 56–59
    sympathy lacking in, 240
    time spent talking to patients and families and, 182

health span, 88, 90

hearing aids, 111, 124–25, 135, 190

hearing loss, 124–25, 135, 190, 202, 226, 354–55

heart, aging's effects on, 177

heart attacks, 66, 68, 92, 122–23, 136, 267

heartburn, 48

heart disease, 43, 50, 53, 56, 59, 68. *See also* heart attacks; strokes

*Heirs of General Practice* (McPhee), 102

Helena, 312

helplessness, 29, 197

Hemoglobin A1c test, 331–32

Henry VIII, King, 186

*Here and Now* (Young), 189

heredity. *See* genetics

Herodotus, 88

Herz-Sommer, Alice, 277

hidden curriculum, 67–68

Higgs, Paul, 244, 246

hip fractures, 182–83

Hippocrates, 24, 99, 120, 379

Hippocratic oath, 158

Hoffman, Veronica, and mother Lynne, 34–40

Hollywood, 222, 265

homebound people, 98–99

home health care, 156, 211–14, 353. *See also* housecalls

Homeland Security, 273

homelessness, 79

homeostasis, loss of, 177

homosexuality. *See* gay males; LGBT health; LGBTQ elders; sexual orientation

hormone injections, 89

hospice care, 154, 182, 190, 203, 284, 298–300, 389

hospices, 147, 186–87

hospitalists, 124–25, 205, 284, 285, 337–40

hospitalization

    adverse events/complications during, 149, 282, 283

    confusion and, 98

    delirium and, 251, 384

    dementia following, 97

    following falls, 383–84

    harm caused by, 171

    home care and prevention of, 169, 211–12, 390–92

    polypharmacy and, 168

    trauma of, 211

    unhappiness with, 199

Hospital Readmissions Reduction Program (2012), 211

housecalls. *See also* home health care

    appearance of patients and, 324–26

    benefits of, 98–99

    for dementia patients, 208–12

    emergencies discovered during, 122–23

    geriatrics practices and, 169, 172, 220, 258

    human connection and, 301, 360–61

*The House of God* (Shem), 44

Howell, Trevor, 148

humanism, 379

humoralism, 27, 88–89, 91, 336

Hutter, Jakob, 27

*Hygiene* (Galen), 25

illness metaphors, 143

*The Illness Narratives* (Kleinman), 58

imagination, 312–17, 348

immortality, 26, 27, 88

immune system, 89, 90–91, 175, 321–22

immunizations, 321–22, 323

immunosenescence, 322

incarceration, 79

Inclusion Across the Lifespan Policy, 95

incontinence, 67, 172, 197, 226, 364

indoctrination, 112–17

Inez and Esteban, 337–41

infantilization, 306

infections

    blood, 330

    cures for, 68

    dementia and, 53, 210

    novel strategies for prevention of, 322

    survival of, 92

    susceptibility to, 321

    urinary tract, 330, 382

    wound, 182

inferiority, 291

inflammation, 90, 175

*In Gratitude* (Diski), 374

insomnia, 25, 226

*Insomniac City* (Hayes), 291–93

insulin, 89, 329, 333–35

*The Intern* (film), 222

internal bleeding, 180–81

internal medicine and internists, 102, 205, 216–17, 232–33, 235

intersectionality, 133

invisibility, 224–26, 255, 310–11

Iranian writers, 242
Irina (nurse), 45–46, 48
isolation, 318–19. *See also* loneliness
Italy, 26, 147, 263

Jacobi, Abraham, 156
Japan, 111, 263, 302, 303, 309
Jay-Z, 142
Jobs, Steve, 312–13, 314
John, and daughter Gwen, 388–92, 393
Johns Hopkins, 137
*Journal of the American Medical Association*, 96
*The Journey of Life* (Cole), 248
"The Joy of Old Age. (No Kidding.)" (Sacks),
    253
Juan, 189–90

Kahn, Robert L., 274
Kaiser emergency department, 129–31, 134
Kaufman, Sharon, 311–12, 381
ketogenic diet, 90
ketone bodies, 90
Kid, 93–94
kidney failure, 98–99
kidney transplants, 136
Kleinman, Arthur, 58
Knausgaard, Karl Ove, 171
Kraepelin, Emil, 28
Kübler-Ross, Elisabeth, 395
Kuhn, Thomas, 373

Lancôme cosmetics, 362
language of aging and death, 140–43
Laslett, Peter, 243–45
Latinos, 136
Laurens, André du, 26, 288
*Lean In* (Sandberg), 156
learned helplessness, 29
Le Guin, Ursula K., 141
Lessing, Doris, 398
lessons in geriatric medicine, 16–23
Les Universités du Troisième Age, 243
"Letter from Greenwich Village" (Gornick),
    348–51
"Letting Go" (Gawande), 366–67
leukemia, 314, 322, 366
Lewy body dementia, 210
LGBT health, 67
LGBTQ elders, 223–24, 352
life cycle, revised version of, 270

life expectancy in U.S., 176–77, 260, 262, 264.
    *See also* life span; longevity
life-space, 318
life span. *See also* life expectancy in U.S.;
    longevity
    behavior and, 88
    calorie restriction and, 89
    changes throughout, 77–78
    Christianity and, 274
    consistency of, 262, 264
    disease manifestation at both ends of, 36
    historically, 8
    longer, consequences of, 80–81, 93, 279
    resveratrol and, 90
life stages, 192–95, 241–47, 270
Lincoln, Abraham, 245
Liszt, Franz, 277
Lively, Penelope, 386, 398
Living Well, Dying Well, 155
Loma Linda, California, 263
loneliness, 24, 318–19, 388
Loneliness Project, 318–19
longevity. *See also* life expectancy in U.S.;
        life span
    anti-aging medicine and, 91–92
    doubling of, 8
    failure of body and mind and, 197–98
    gender and, 276, 335–37
    historical ideas about, 25, 26, 88–89
    immunosenescence and, 322
    increased, causes and consequences of,
        260–64, 279
    research on, 89–91
    retirement age and, 76
    silver tsunami and, 16
*Longevity and Rejuvenescence* (Nascher), 146
*Longevity in Man* (Thoms), 26
Longevity Prize, 71
Longfellow, Henry Wadsworth, 271
lumbar punctures, 127–28
lung cancer, 322
lymphoma, 322
Lynn, Joanne, 11, 155
Lynne, 34–40

Mabel, 131–33, 364
MacArthur Foundation study (1997), 274
Maclachlan, Daniel, 120
macular degeneration, 68
Mailhot, Terese Marie, 401

malnutrition, 182
Malthus, Thomas, 27
mammograms, 207
Manguso, Sarah, 60–61
Marc, 314–15
marriage, 28
Martin, Lillien J., 194, 289
Maslow's hierarchy of needs, 318
Matthew 12:25, 245
Mayo Clinic, 231
McFarlane, Arthur E., 92
McPhee, John, 102
meaningfulness, 308–12, 371–72, 392
*médecine des vieillards*, 147
Medicaid, 111, 153, 188, 263–64, 327
medical education
    age-inclusive curriculum, 343–44
    care *vs.* treatment, 343
    case-based learning sessions, 375
    clinical rotations, 100–102, 126, 341–42, 344
    death and, 300
    geriatrics and, 66–68, 341–43
    normality and, 63–69, 120
    pediatrics and, 63–64
    science as primary focus of, 3–4, 43–44, 45
    sexual orientation and, 117–18
    topics not covered in, 18–19
    women's and minority health and, 64–66
medical internships, 118, 126
medical residencies, 16–23, 105–9, 115–16,
    117, 119–21, 125–29, 143–44
medical students
    childhood memories and, 32, 33
    debt and, 236
    empathy and, 116–17
    exercise with, 4–6
    housecalls and, 325
    observations of, 138–39, 140, 340–41
    perspectives on older patients, 159, 160, 342,
        343
Medicare, 153
medications. *See also specific medication names
        and types*
    adjustment of, 172, 200
    attitude and, 351
    Beers Criteria, 46
    child-resistant containers for, 264–68
    delirium and, 37–38
    dementia and, 45–49, 53, 150
    polypharmacy, 168

prescribing cascades, 45–49
    reviewing, 332–33
    risks and side effects of, 19–23, 48, 93–99,
        149, 168
    stopping, 203
medicine
    bias and, 65–66, 69–74, 118, 129–36, 204,
        207, 235–36
    history of, 24–30
    imagination and, 313–17
    paradigm shift needed in, 373, 378–80
    prestige and salaries in, 204–8, 235–36
    priorities in, 232–37
    in the twentieth and twenty-first centuries, 7,
        24–25, 29–30, 109–11, 187–88, 237, 259
    violence in, 112–17
medieval times, 88
memories, childhood, 13–16, 30–34, 41,
        256–57
memory, 90. *See also* dementia
menopause, 336
mental health, 239, 311. *See also* anxiety;
        depression
mental institutions, 187
Metchnikoff, Élie, 89
Micco, Guy, 4–7, 177
microaggressions, 254
middle age
    AARP and, 268
    dread of, 81
    hearing loss and, 354–55
    in Hollywood, 222
    life cycle, revised version of, and, 270
    packaging testing and, 266
    Shakespeare and, 173
    as stage of life, 192
    transition into, 77–78, 79
    well-being and, 254–56
Middle Ages, 242
Middle East, 25
mild cognitive impairment, 55
Millie, 122–23
minister of loneliness, 24
minority health, 65, 66
miracle of modern medicine, 68
mistakes, 117–21, 123
Monaco, 176
monasteries, 186
monkeys, calorie-restricted, 89
Monopoli, Sara Thomas, 366–67

Morales, Angela, 174
Morgagni, Giovanni, 27
morphine, 203, 298–99, 382, 384–85, 391
Mount, Balford, 103, 190–91
multicellular organisms, 174
multimorbidity, 28, 120, 156
Munro, Alice, 223
Murdoch, Iris, 51
muscle atrophy, 29
*My Struggle* (Knausgaard), 171

Napoléon, 27
Nascher, Ignatz, 146–48, 156–57, 158,
    188–89, 194, 289
National Academy of Medicine, 24
National Council on Aging, 71
national health care systems, 111
National Institute on Minority Health and
    Health Disparities, 65
National Institutes of Health, 134–35
National Institutes on Aging, 70
National Library of Medicine, 112
Native Americans, 177
natural death, 368–69
natural selection, 175
*The Nature of Prejudice* (Allport), 69–70
needs, Maslow's hierarchy of, 318
Neeta, 182–84, 185
Neugarten, Bernice, 193
neurological disorders, 380, 382
neurologists, 53, 54, 93–94, 239
neurosurgeons, 205, 206
*New England Journal of Medicine*, 238
Newton, Huey P., 129–31, 134
New York City Farm Colony, 289
*New York Times*, 142–43
Nina, 267
"Nine Days of Ruth" (Morales), 174
Ninetieth Psalm, 192
non-compliance, 96, 185
normality, 63–69, 120, 135, 148, 248–49, 267,
    343–44
nurses, 30–33, 42, 110, 151, 154
nursing homes. *See also* assisted living; old-age
    institutions; skilled nursing facilities
    current health care system and, 155
    doctors and, 183–84
    fear of, 171
    history of, 185–88
    low-quality, 182–85

medical education and, 67
prevention of placement in, 111
proportion of older Americans in, 71–72
in twentieth century, 110

obesity, 29, 56, 260
Occam's razor, 95
occupational therapy and therapists, 200,
    283–84
Oedipus, 87
Okinawa, Japan, 89, 263
old, definition of, 17, 76, 81, 268–69
old age. *See also* advanced old age
    diversity in, 73, 321–23
    gradual transition to, 76–77, 79–80, 317
    medicalization of, 248–49
    perspectives on, 81, 201, 249, 254–56, 358–62
    resistance to, 268–69
    stages of, 193, 270
    stories of, 397–400
    on television, 221–22
old-age institutions, 185–87, 201, 204, 293–98.
    *See also* nursing homes
"old lady smell," 359–60
old-old and oldest old people, 36, 193, 243, 321,
    323. *See also* advanced old age
old *vs.* elder, 4–7
old *vs.* old school, 142–43
Olivier, Laurence, 223
Olshansky, Jay, 92
oncologists, 189–90
oncology training, 86
*Ongoingness* (Manguso), 60–61
"On Sixty-Five" (Fox Gordon), 397
*Opuscula Medica* (Ranchin), 27, 146–47
orthopedists, 205, 233–35
Osborne, James, 304
osteoporosis, 96
othering, 59–62, 142, 179
overpopulation, 27

pain, 172, 284–85, 310–11
palliative care
    death outsourced to, 191
    death *vs.* aging and, 367–68, 370, 372
    lower status of, as specialty, 205
    old age disassociated with, 156
    oncology training programs and, 86
    resistance to, 366
    as term, 190

Palo Alto Longevity Prize, 71
paradigms and paradigm shifts, 373, 378–80
paramedics, 34, 36–39, 123, 190, 210
Parkinson's disease, 45–49, 121, 198, 200, 364
pathological aging, 28, 30, 120, 147, 148, 247–49
patient-centered care, 221, 355, 369, 374
Peabody, Francis Weld, 377–78
pediatrics and pediatricians, 44, 63–64, 101, 205, 206, 207, 265
perversion of brutal treatments, 82–86
Phormio (Terence), 249
physical therapy and therapists, 200, 283–84
physician assistants, 234
physicians
    burnout in, 214–21, 229–32, 238–40, 305, 345–47, 377
    gender differences and, 207
    mistakes by, 117–21, 123
    nurses compared to, 42
    physical challenges and, 229–30
    specialties, prestige, and salaries of, 204–8, 235–36
physiological theories of aging, 175
Plato, 24, 256
pneuma, 24, 80
pneumonia, 201–2
pocket talkers, 125
Poison Prevention Packaging Act (1970), 265, 267
police departments, 40
polypharmacy, 168
Poor Laws, 186
Population Health, 207–8, 358
poverty, 28, 79, 334, 336–37
prescribing cascades, 45–49
pressure ulcers/sores, 29, 182, 202, 217
prestige in medicine, 204–8
preventative care, 93–94
prevention of disease, 278–80
primary care medicine, 21–22, 205, 208, 233, 236, 239
prison inmates, 177
privacy and technology, 305–8
privilege and successful aging, 276, 277
prokaryotes, 174
The Prolongation of Life (Metchnikoff), 89
"Prolonging the Prime of Life" (McFarlane), 92
prostate disease, 98–99

psychiatrists and psychiatry, 53, 101–2, 205, 206
psychosocial theories of aging, 175
PubMed, 112
Puritans and Puritanism, 59–60, 227, 277

Quality of Life Technology Center, Carnegie Mellon, 304

racial and ethnic disparities in health care, 65, 66, 129–34, 136
radiation treatment, 189–90, 322–23, 374
radiologists, 206, 207
Rafael, 285
RAISE Act, 24
Ranchin, François, 27, 146–47, 288–89
Rankine, Claudia, 61
rapamycin, 90–91
Ray, 124–25
realism vs. romance, 372
reclamation of elderhood, 268–70
rectal exams, 180–81
redundancy, 177
red wine, 90
Reformation, 186
refugees, Southeast Asian, 42–43
Regimen Sanitatis, 25
rehabilitation, 29, 145–46
rejuvenation, 86–93
relevance, 289–90
religion
    care for aged and, 185–86
    chosen death and, 387
    history of ideas about aging and, 25–26, 81, 88, 274
    longevity and, 263
    sanctity of life and, 203, 246
    success and happiness and, 142, 277
Remnick, David, 75
Renaissance, 242
reproduction and aging, 175
Republic (Plato), 24, 256
research, exclusion of old people from, 95, 96, 97
resilience, 217, 232, 274, 276, 311, 344–48
resilience therapies, 88
resveratrol, 90
retirement age, 76
review of symptoms (ROS), 38
Rhetoric (Aristotle), 274

rheumatologists, 205
Riley, Matilda White, 193
robot caregivers, 301–5
Roman authors, 242
romance *vs.* realism, 372
Roman Empire, 186
Roman writers, 242
Rome, ancient, 24
ROS (review of symptoms), 38
Rosin, Heinrich, 27
Rossellini, Isabella, 362
Roth, Philip, 177
Rowe, Anne, 17–23
Rowe, John W., 274
Rowling, J. K., 312–13
Ruefle, Mary, 255
Rush, Benjamin, 27–28, 368–69

Sacks, Oliver, 253, 291–93
safety, 172–73, 202, 265–68, 296, 305–8
Said, Laila, 208–12
Sakovich, Dimitri, 45–49
*Salvaging Old Age* (Martin), 194
Sandberg, Sheryl, 156
San Francisco General Hospital, 16, 105
Sardinia, Italy, 263
Sarton, May, 398–99
science
    aging, attempts to affect, 90–91, 92
    anti-aging products and, 87
    dementia and, 54–55
    history of medicine and aging and, 26–28, 30
    human health and, 278
    imagination and, 313–14
    limits of, 403
    as medical education focus, 3–4, 43–44, 45
    medical paradigm shift and, 373, 377, 378, 379–80
Scientific Revolution, 26–27
scribes, 233, 234
selective serotonin reuptake inhibitors, 23
senescence, 26, 27, 174, 175, 193, 194, 368
senility (cognitive impairment), 49, 50, 144.
    *See also* dementia
senility (old age), 146, 156–57, 194
senior moments, 260
senolytics, 90
Seventh-day Adventists, 263
sexiness in health care, 226–27
sexuality, 221–28

sexual orientation, 117–19
sexual vitality and vigor, 88–89, 91, 222
Shakespeare, William, 173
shame, 125–29
Shannon, Diane, 231
Shaw, Byers "Bud," 230–31
Sheen, Martin, 221
Shem, Samuel, 44
Shoven, John, 260–61
sickness, childhood, 30–34
Silicon Valley, 290
silver architecture and design, 352–56
silver economy, 290
Silverman, Sarah, 264
silver tsunami, 16, 140, 261
single-celled organisms, 174
sirtuins, 90
skilled nursing facilities, 110, 154, 182–84.
    *See also* nursing homes
sleeping medications, 98–99
smoking, 56
social care combined with medical care, 111
social inequality, 56, 57
social policies, 28
Social Security, 76
Solnit, Rebecca, 116
Sontag, Susan, 142, 143
Springsteen, Bruce, 75–76, 77
stages of life, 192–95, 241–47
standards of care, 56–59, 95
Steinem, Gloria, 179
stem cells, 91
sterilization of poor and disabled, 65
stress, 79, 80, 115–16, 255, 262–63, 277–78
stress resistance, 90
strokes
    blood pressure and, 66, 135
    blood thinners and, 94–95
    confusion and, 34–39
    dementia and, 53
    disabling effects of, 198, 200, 202, 210
    falls compared to, 170–71
    medical advances to prevent, 68
    minimizing risk factors for, 56
    rehabilitation after, 29
structural inequality, 237
structural violence, 237
*The Structure of Scientific Revolutions* (Kuhn), 373
successful aging, 140, 273–78

suffering, caring about, 190–91, 376–77
suicide attempts and suicidal thinking
  geriatric patients and, 195, 198–99, 202
  physicians and, 217, 231, 240
Super Bowl (2016), 189
surgery rotations, 100–101
Susan (Frank's daughter), 195, 198, 199, 200
Suzman, Richard, 193
Sweden, 302
Swift, Jonathan, 27
Switzerland, 386
sympathy, lack of, 240

tachyphylaxis, 115
technology, 301–8, 378, 403
teenage years, 41
teeth, 78
Terence, 249
Thane, Pat, 146, 147
*That Senescence Itself Is an Illness* (Hutter), 27
Third Age, 243–45, 261, 268
*This Chair Rocks* (Applewhite), 361
Thoms, William, 26
Tokoni, 326–35
Tolstoy, Leo, 252–53
Tomlin, Lily, 221
touch, need for, 360–61
toxicology screens, 132–33
transitions, 156
trauma, 105–9
treatments, perversion of brutal, 82–86
treatment *vs.* care, 343
trigeminal neuralgia, 121
Tuskegee syphilis experiments, 65

UCLA geriatrics conference, 144–46, 148
UCSF (University of California, San
  Francisco), 53, 144, 148
ugliness, 290–91
UK Ministry of Health, 189
undertreatment, 72–73
United Kingdom, 24, 28, 29, 72–73, 110, 120,
  318–19, 358. *See also* Britain; England
United States
  ageism in, 70
  aging *vs.* dying in, 367–70
  anti-aging medicine in, 92
  baby boomer blip and, 263
  deinstitutionalization in, 187
  geriatrics in, history of, 110, 111

health care spending in, 237
history of medicine and ideas about aging in,
  24, 27–28, 29–30
history of old-age institutions in, 185
hormone injections in, 89
life expectancy in, 176–77, 260, 262
medical education requirements in, 341
medication safety regulation in, 265
old age definition in, 76
overtreatment in, 73
patient health outcomes in, 45
pediatrics in, 64
primary care in, 205
robot caregivers, reaction to, in, 302–3
weight in, 90
well-being in, 255
youth as metaphor in, 142
Universities of the Third Age, 243
University Hospitals of Cleveland, 281
University of California, Berkeley, 4–7
University of California, San Francisco
  (UCSF), 53, 144, 148
*The Unknown Profession*, 137
unretiring, 288
urinary problems, 98–99. *See also*
  incontinence
urinary tract infections, 330, 382
urologic conditions, treatments for, 322
urologists, 205, 336
usefulness, 290, 310–11

vaccine schedules, 321–22, 323
van Gogh, Vincent, 358
vascular dementia, 210, 338
Vedas, 88
violence by doctors, 112–17
vision loss and impairments, 26, 98–99, 111,
  226, 334–35, 348
vital force, waning, 88–89
Voltaire, 72
Volunteer Corps, 311
Voronoff, Serge, 89

Warren, Marjory, 29, 160, 189, 311
Waterston, Sam, 221
*Ways of Seeing* (Berger), 358
Weinstein, Michael S., 238
well-being, 172–73, 253–56, 261
West Middlesex hospital old age unit, 29, 189,
  311

*The White Album* (Didion), 129–31
"Why I Hope to Die at Seventy-Five"
  (Emanuel), 308–10
*Why Survive?: Being Old in America* (Butler), 70
Williams, Clarence, Sr., 82–86
Winakur, Jerald, 302
*A Woman's Story* (Ernaux), 184–85
*Women and Power* (Beard), 227
women's health, 64–65, 67, 373–74
workhouses, 185, 187, 189
World Health Organization, 113, 205, 286
World War II, 111
worthiness, 287–91
wound infections, 182

Yolanda, and daughters, 150–54
Young, Robin, 189
young adulthood, 42, 77, 270
young-old people. *See also* Third Age
  cancer treatment and aging of, 85
  expressions about aging and, 141
  Neugarten's definition of, 193
  old-old compared to, 321, 323
  packaging testing and, 266
  Third Age and, 243–45, 261, 268
youth, 59–60, 88, 142, 222

Zerbi, Gabriele, 26
Zuckerberg, Mark, 278–80

# A NOTE ON THE AUTHOR

**Louise Aronson, MD,** is the author of *A History of the Present Illness* and a geriatrician, educator, and professor of medicine at the University of California, San Francisco (UCSF), where she directs UCSF Medical Humanities. A graduate of Harvard Medical School and the MFA Program for Writers at Warren Wilson College, Dr. Aronson has received the Gold Professorship in Humanism, the California Home Care Physician of the Year Award, and the American Geriatrics Society Outstanding Mid-Career Clinician Educator of the Year Award, as well as numerous awards for her teaching, educational research, and writing, including being named one of Next Avenue's 2019 Influencers in Aging. The recipient of a MacDowell fellowship and four Pushcart nominations, her articles and stories have appeared in many publications, including the *New York Times*, the *New England Journal of Medicine*, the *Lancet*, and *Bellevue Literary Review*. She lives in San Francisco.